POINT-OF-CARE
ULTRASOUND
IN CRITICAL CARE

POINT-OF-CARE ULTRASOUND IN CRITICAL CARE

Editors:

Luke Flower MBChB, BSc (Hons), MRCP, MAcadMEd

Trainee in Anaesthesia and Honorary Clinical Research Fellow in Intensive Care Medicine, Central London School of Anaesthesia, London, UK

Pradeep Madhivathanan MBBS, FRCA, MRCP, EDIC, FFICM

Consultant in Anaesthesia and Intensive Care Medicine, Royal Papworth Hospital, Cambridge, UK

Scion

First edition © Scion Publishing Ltd, 2022

ISBN 978 1 911510 99 4

A CIP catalogue record for this book is available from the British Library.

Scion Publishing Limited

The Old Hayloft, Vantage Business Park, Bloxham Road, Banbury OX16 9UX, UK

www.scionpublishing.com

Important Note from the Publisher

The information contained within this book was obtained by Scion Publishing Ltd from sources believed by us to be reliable. However, while every effort has been made to ensure its accuracy, no responsibility for loss or injury whatsoever occasioned to any person acting or refraining from action as a result of information contained herein can be accepted by the authors or publishers.

Readers are reminded that medicine is a constantly evolving science and while the authors and publishers have ensured that all dosages, applications and practices are based on current indications, there may be specific practices which differ between communities. You should always follow the guidelines laid down by the manufacturers of specific products and the relevant authorities in the country in which you are practising.

Although every effort has been made to ensure that all owners of copyright material have been acknowledged in this publication, we would be pleased to acknowledge in subsequent reprints or editions any omissions brought to our attention.

Registered names, trademarks, etc. used in this book, even when not marked as such, are not to be considered unprotected by law.

Feedback, errors and omissions

We are always pleased to receive feedback (good and bad) about our books – if you would like to comment, please email info@scionpublishing.com.

We've worked really hard with the editors and authors to ensure that everything in the book is correct. However, errors and ambiguities can still slip through in books as complex as this. If you spot anything you think might be wrong, please email us and we will look into it straight away. If an error has occurred, we will correct it for future printings and post a note about it on our website so that other readers of the book are alerted to this.

Thank you for your help.

Cover design by AM Graphic Design Ltd
Typeset by Evolution Design & Digital Ltd (Kent), UK
Printed in the UK
Last digit is the print number: 10 9 8 7 6 5 4

Contents

*Chapters marked with an asterisk have accompanying video clips; these can be viewed at: www.scionpublishing.com/POCUS – click on the "Resources" tab for access.

Contributors

Jonathan Aron – *Consultant in General and Cardiothoracic Intensive Care Medicine and Anaesthesia, St George's University Hospitals NHS Foundation Trust, London, UK*

Dan Aston – *Consultant in Cardiothoracic Anaesthesia and Critical Care, Royal Papworth Hospital NHS Foundation Trust, Cambridge, UK*

Zdenek Bares – *Clinical Fellow in Critical Care, University College London Hospitals NHS Foundation Trust, UK*

Rosie Baruah – *Consultant in Critical Care and Anaesthesia, Western General Hospital, Edinburgh, UK*

Jim Buckley – *Consultant in Critical Care, Royal Free Hospital NHS Foundation Trust, London, UK*

Alejandra Ceballos – *Clinical Fellow in Cardiothoracic Anaesthesia, Royal Papworth Hospital, Cambridge, UK*

Sam Clark – *Consultant in Anaesthesia and Critical Care, University College London Hospitals NHS Foundation Trust, London, UK*

John Dick – *Consultant in Anaesthesia and Clinical lead for Obstetric Anaesthesia, University College London Hospitals NHS Foundation Trust, London, UK*

Richard Fisher – *Consultant in Intensive Care Medicine, King's College Hospital, London, UK*

Luke Flower – *Clinical Research Fellow in Critical Care and Trainee in Anaesthesia, Central London School of Anaesthesia, London, UK*

Luna Gargani – *Senior Researcher, Italian National Research Council, Pisa, Italy*

Stuart Gillon – *Consultant in Critical Care, Royal Infirmary Edinburgh, Edinburgh, UK*

David Hall – *Defence Military Services, Consultant in Anaesthesia and Critical Care, Royal Infirmary of Edinburgh, UK*

Charlotte Hateley – *Clinical Research Fellow, Imperial College London, London, UK*

Abhishek Jha – *Senior Clinical Fellow in Cardiothoracic Intensive Care, Royal Papworth Hospital, Cambridge, UK*

Tim Keady – *Clinical Fellow in Anaesthesia and Critical Care, Royal Papworth Hospital, Cambridge, UK*

Angus McKnight – *Specialty Registrar in Anaesthesia and Intensive Care Medicine, Royal Infirmary Edinburgh, Edinburgh, UK*

Maryam Khosravi – *Specialist Registrar in Nephrology and Intensive Care Medicine, Barts NHS Trust, London, UK*

Chuen Khwan – *Specialist Registrar in Respiratory Medicine, Royal Free Hospital NHS Foundation Trust, London, UK*

Luigi La Via – *Consultant in Critical Care, University AOU Policlinico–Vittorio Emanuele, University of Catania, Catania, Italy*

Pradeep Madhivathanan – *Consultant in Anaesthesia and Intensive Care Medicine, Royal Papworth Hospital, Cambridge, UK*

Kay Mak – *Research Fellow in Obstetric Anaesthesia, University College London Hospitals NHS Foundation Trust, London, UK*

Ashley Miller – *Consultant in Intensive Care, Shrewsbury and Telford Hospital NHS Trust, Shrewsbury, UK*

Dipak Mistry – *Consultant in Emergency Medicine, University College London Hospitals NHS Foundation Trust, London, UK*

Sarah Morton – *Core Trainee in Anaesthesia, St George's University Hospitals NHS Foundation Trust, London, UK*

Colum O'Hare – *Consultant Interventional Radiologist, Royal Infirmary of Edinburgh, UK*

Olusegun Olusanya – *Consultant in Intensive Care Medicine, Barts Heart Centre, London, UK*

Sunil Patel – *Specialist Registrar in Respiratory and Intensive Care Medicine, London, UK; Clinical Research Fellow in Anaesthesia, Pain Medicine and Intensive Care, Imperial College London, UK*

Gianluca Paternoster – *Consultant in Critical Care, San Carlo Hospital, Potenza, Italy*

Marcus Peck – *Consultant in Anaesthesia and Intensive Care Medicine, Frimley Park Hospital, Surrey, UK*

Zudin Puthucheary – *Clinical Senior Lecturer, Queen Mary University of London, Consultant in Intensive Care Medicine, Royal London Hospital, London, UK*

Julian Andres Rios Rios – *Clinical Fellow in Cardiothoracic Anaesthesia, Royal Papworth Hospital, Cambridge, UK*

Ashraf Roshdy – *Consultant in Intensive Care Medicine, North Middlesex University Hospital, London, UK; Lecturer of Critical Care Medicine, Faculty of Medicine, Alexandria University, Egypt*

Filippo Sanfilippo – *Consultant in Critical Care, AOU Policlinico–Vittorio Emanuele, University of Catania, Catania, Italy*

Arun Sivananthan – *Clinical Research Fellow, Imperial College Healthcare NHS Trust, London, UK*

Elliot Smith – *Clinical Scientist and Lead Echocardiographer, St George's Hospital NHS Foundation Trust, London, UK*

Hatem Soliman-Aboumaire – *Consultant in Cardiothoracic Intensive Care, Harefield Hospital, London; King's College, London, UK*

Manni Waraich – *Consultant in Neurocritical Care, National Hospital for Neurology and Neurosurgery, University College London Hospitals NHS Foundation Trust, UK*

Jonny Wilkinson – *Consultant in Anaesthesia and Critical Care, Northampton General Hospital NHS Trust, Northampton, UK*

Adrian Wong – *Consultant in Anaesthesia and Intensive Care Medicine, King's College Hospital, London, UK*

Pablo Rojas Zamora – *Core Trainee in Anaesthesia, Royal Papworth Hospital NHS Foundation Trust, Cambridge, UK*

Foreword

In writing the foreword to this exciting new text, I'm reminded of my own medical career and how it has evolved in parallel with the growing clinical utility of medical ultrasound imaging. Thinking back to my medical school days, it would have been impossible even then to imagine that a woman would not undergo serial ultrasound scanning for both diagnostic and monitoring purposes during her pregnancy. Perhaps back then equally unimaginable would have been the idea that one day doctors would be conducting ward rounds with a portable ultrasound scanner attached to their person. How times change, and it has now come to pass that ultrasound use in a wide range of emergency/ward-based settings has emerged as an important diagnostic and monitoring modality.

I was an early adopter of such technology and was excited by the opportunities afforded by powerful new imaging tools, serviced on ever smaller and more versatile platforms. Today, a new generation of medical professionals have led the way to an era which is no longer about unhelpful professional boundaries dictating who can and who cannot engage with ultrasound technology. Instead, what has emerged is a more forward-thinking approach, which rightly asks, what are the medical problems which need to be solved, who is trained to use ultrasound and in what capacity, and what does training and competence look like?

Even before this enlightened age it appeared, to me at least, that ultrasound users all wanted the same thing: safe and responsible ultrasound use, often in a population of patients in whom, at times, clinical medicine had left their clinicians stumbling in the dark. It's not surprising therefore that some years on we are fast approaching a tipping point, one where it appears deficient not to have assessed at least some of our most unstable patients with ultrasound, or not to have benefited from the added assurance of clear images of vital anatomical structures during elective and emergency interventions.

However, if we are to truly capitalise on this unfolding revolution, we must not be afraid to tell it how it is. Whether talking about sound wave velocity or anatomical acoustic windows, each should be approached from an understanding of first principles made simple, but not simpler. Students must have a willingness to put time aside to wrestle with practical haptic mastery of sound wave imaging and its interpretation. Not that long ago the voices of those intent on harnessing powerful ultrasound technology were drowned out by those most content with the status quo. Today, with those unhelpful days behind us, textbooks such as this, written by clinician–sonographers, will find a welcome home with the many professionals eager to improve the outcome and experiences of their patients in widely differing clinical settings.

Professor David Walker
University College London
Consultant in Anaesthesia, Perioperative and Critical Care Medicine
June 2022

Preface

Point-of-care ultrasound, commonly referred to as POCUS, has revolutionized clinical practice, something we the editors have experienced first-hand. Our own POCUS knowledge has been accrued through innumerable hours of hunting for experienced mentors, scouring journals and teaching colleagues. Whilst a rewarding process, this is also an inefficient and inaccessible one for many. Throughout our journey we found ourselves longing for a central reference text to guide us. It was this that inspired us to bring together some of the greatest POCUS minds on the planet to create this book and, after much contemplation, we finally put pen to paper.

Our initial timeline was somewhat disrupted by a pandemic rivalling any in modern history, one that further highlighted the vital role POCUS plays in clinical practice. Despite the hurdles, through perseverance and the exceptional support of our contributing authors, we were able to create this book. We are extremely proud of the world-renowned ultrasound experts we have been able to bring together, to cover everything from cerebral perfusion to thrombosis of the lower limb – a literal head to toe of POCUS.

Whilst primarily aimed at critical care clinicians, the skills taught in this book can be utilized anywhere from the roadside through to the emergency department, medical and surgical wards, during the perioperative period, and on the intensive care unit.

We sincerely hope you find this book as enjoyable and educational to read as we have found creating it.

Luke Flower and Pradeep Madhivathanan

Library of video clips

We have put together a series of video clips to accompany chapters 7, 8, 9, 10, 11, 16 and 22 (with more to follow) and these can be viewed at: www.scionpublishing.com/POCUS – click on the "Resources" tab for access.

Acknowledgments

We would firstly like to thank our brilliant panel of contributing authors for their hard work and dedication, without whom this book would not have been possible. We would also like to thank Dr Carlos Corredor, Dr Jonny Wilkinson, and Dr Olusegun Olusanya for generously allowing us the use of their extensive image libraries.

A special thank you needs to go to Dr Jonathan Ray and all the team at Scion Publishing, for their continuous support and flexibility through what has been a challenging time for all.

Finally, a huge thank you to our families, who have supported us through the highs and lows of this project and have been a source of inspiration throughout our careers. We would like to dedicate this book to them: Rachel, Richard, Jake and Maxim; and Dr S Madhivathanan and Mrs Josephine Jessy.

Abbreviations

A2Ch	apical two-chamber view	EDEC	European Diploma in Echocardiography
A4Ch	apical four-chamber view	EDV	end-diastolic velocity
A5Ch	apical five-chamber view	EF	ejection fraction
AAA	abdominal aortic aneurysm	eFAST	Extended Focused Assessment with Sonography for Trauma
ACA	anterior cerebral artery	ELS	echocardiography in life support
AKI	acute kidney injury	ETT	endotracheal tube
AMVL	anterior mitral valve leaflet	EVLW	extravascular lung water
AR	aortic regurgitation	FAC	fractional area change
ARDS	acute respiratory distress syndrome	FAFF	focused assessment of free fluid
aSAH	aneurysmal subarachnoid haemorrhage	FAST	focused assessment with sonography for trauma
ASD	atrial septal defect	FCU	focused cardiac ultrasound
AV	aortic valve	FEEL	focused echocardiography in emergency life support
BSA	body surface area	FICE	focused intensive care echocardiography
BSE	British Society of Echocardiography	FR	fluid responsiveness
CABG	coronary artery bypass grafting	FRC	functional residual capacity
CBD	common bile duct	FUSIC	focused ultrasound for intensive care
CBF	cerebral blood flow	GLS	global longitudinal strain
CFD	colour flow Doppler	GSV	great saphenous vein
CFV	common femoral vein	IAS	interatrial septum
CHS	cerebral hyperperfusion syndrome	ICA	internal cerebral artery
CKD	chronic kidney disease	ICC	intra/inter-class correlation coefficient
CNB	central neuraxial block	ICM	intercostal muscles
CO	cardiac output	ICP	intracranial pressure
COPD	chronic obstructive pulmonary disease	ICS	Intensive Care Society
CPP	cerebral perfusion pressure	ICU	intensive care unit
CPR	cardiopulmonary resuscitation	ICUAW	intensive care unit acquired weakness
CSA	cross-sectional area	IJV	internal jugular vein
CSE	combined spinal epidural	IVC	inferior vena cava
CSF	cerebral spinal fluid	IVS	interventricular septum
CT	computed tomography	LA	left atrium
CVC	central venous catheter	LAA	left atrial appendage
CVP	central venous pressure	LAD	left anterior descending
CWD	continuous wave Doppler	LAP	left atrial pressure
Cx	circumflex	LAX	long-axis
CXR	chest X-ray	LCC	left coronary cusp
DDU	Diploma of Diagnostic Ultrasound	LCx	left circumflex artery
DEX	diaphragmatic excursion	LMS	left main stem
DPAP	diastolic pulmonary artery pressure	LRV	left renal vein
DTF	diaphragm thickening fraction	LUS	lung ultrasound
DTG	deep trans-gastric	LV	left ventricle
DVT	deep vein thrombosis		
ECG	electrocardiogram		
ED	Emergency Department		

LVEDP/V	left ventricular end-diastolic pressure/volume	RRI	renal resistive index
LVEF	left ventricular ejection fraction	RV	right ventricle
LVOT	left ventricular outflow tract	RVEDV/P	right ventricular end-diastolic pressure/volume
MAPSE	mitral annular plane systolic excursion	RVEF	right ventricular ejection fraction
MCA	middle cerebral artery	RVFAC	right ventricular fractional area change
ME	mid-oesophageal	RVOT	right ventricular outflow tract
ME2Ch	mid-oesophageal two-chamber	RVSP	right ventricular systolic pressure
ME4Ch	mid-oesophageal four-chamber	RWMA	regional wall motion abnormality
ME5Ch	mid-oesophageal five-chamber	SAAG	serum–ascites albumin gradient
MELAX	mid-oesophageal long-axis	SAM	systolic anterior motion
MPAP	mean pulmonary artery pressure	SAX	short-axis
MR	mitral regurgitation	SBP	spontaneous bacterial peritonitis
MV	mitral valve	SC4Ch	sub-costal four-chamber
NBE CCE	National Board of Echocardiography Critical Care Echocardiography	SCM	spontaneous cardiac movement
		SFV	superficial femoral vein
NCC	non-coronary cusp	SMA	superior mesenteric artery
ONSD	optic nerve sheath diameter	STE	speckle tracking echocardiography
PA	pulmonary angiography	SV	stroke volume
PASP	pulmonary artery systolic pressure	SVC	superior vena cava
PAT	pulmonary acceleration time	SVR	systemic vascular resistance
PDA	posterior descending artery	SVV	stroke volume variation
PDT	percutaneous dilatational tracheostomy	TAM	time average mean flow velocity
		TAPSE	tricuspid annular plane systolic excursion
PE	pulmonary embolism	TCCD	transcranial colour-coded duplex
PEA	pulseless electrical activity	TCD	transcranial Doppler
PEEP	positive end-expiratory pressure	TDI	tissue Doppler imaging
PICC	peripherally inserted central catheter	TG	trans-gastric
		TG2Ch	trans-gastric two-chamber view
PLAX	parasternal long-axis view	TGC	time gain compensation
PMVL	posterior mitral valve leaflet	TGLAX	trans-gastric long-axis
POCUS	point-of-care ultrasound	TOE	transoesophageal echocardiography
PR	pulmonary regurgitation		
PSAX	parasternal short-axis view	TR	tricuspid regurgitation
PSV	peak systolic velocity	TTE	transthoracic echocardiography
PV	pulmonary valve	TV	tricuspid valve
PVR	pulmonary vascular resistance	VExUS	venous excess ultrasound
PWD	pulsed wave Doppler	VIDD	ventilator-induced diaphragm dysfunction
PZT	piezoelectric material (lead zirconate titanate)		
		VSD	ventricular septal defect
RA	right atrium	VTE	venous thromboembolism
RaCeVA	rapid central vein assessment	VTI	velocity–time integral
RCA	right coronary artery	VV-ECMO	veno-venous extracorporeal membrane oxygenation
RCC	right coronary cusp		
RF	rectus femoris		

CHAPTER 1

THE EVOLUTION OF CRITICAL CARE ULTRASOUND

Luke Flower & Pradeep Madhivathanan

Recent years have seen a dramatic rise in the use of point-of-care ultrasound (POCUS) in critical care, perioperative, acute, and emergency medicine. In the correct hands POCUS has an almost unrivalled ability to provide a rapid, non-invasive and comprehensive assessment of the critically unwell patient. Its use has increased to the point whereby many specialties, including critical care, now require at least basic POCUS competencies as part of their curriculum.

1.1 A brief history of POCUS

Recognition of the acoustic properties of sound waves can be traced as far back as ancient Greece. The ability to harness these properties for human use was catalysed following the sinking of the Titanic and for the use of sonar navigation in World War I.

The potential diagnostic benefits of ultrasound were first recognized in the 1940s, initially by the Austrian physician Karl Theodore Dussik for identifying cancerous tissue. Echocardiography became established in the 1950s, with the Japanese physician Shigeo Satomura first credited with its use in assessing the motion of cardiac valves.

As technology advanced, so did ultrasound, with more advanced scanning modes and probes allowing its use to expand. The first real-time ultrasound scanner, the Vidoson, was developed in 1965 and had the ability to show 15 images per second. From here, its potential use for rapid diagnosis of life-threatening conditions was noticed. This led to the development of the focused assessment with sonography for trauma (FAST) protocol in the 1970s, with its inclusion in the advanced trauma life support algorithm seen in the late 1990s. This period saw a rapid uptake in the use of ultrasound to assess several organ systems, with lung ultrasound (previously thought to be an impossible exercise) developed from the mid-1980s by Daniel Lichtenstein.

As technology has advanced, and probes have become less expensive and smaller in size (including the development of hand-held probes), POCUS use has continued to grow. A huge number of training and accreditation pathways have been developed across multiple specialties, including critical care. In the UK, arguably the most recognized of these is the Focused Ultrasound for Intensive Care (FUSIC) accreditation, with modules available covering everything from neurological POCUS through to deep vein thrombosis scanning. Other worldwide accreditations include the Diploma of Diagnostic Ultrasound (DDU) available in Australasia, the European Diploma in Echocardiography (EDEC), and the National Board of Echocardiography Critical Care Echocardiography accreditation (NBE CCE) to name but a few.

1.2 When to use POCUS?

POCUS provides clinicians with a unique ability to rapidly assess multiple organ systems in the critically ill patient, in a relatively non-invasive fashion, at the bedside. It thus has huge potential in correctly trained hands, with its use now widely recommended as a first-line diagnostic tool when assessing the shocked patient.

Some have described the ultrasound probe as the stethoscope of the next generation, and indeed we are seeing an increase in POCUS education in medical schools. It is, however, vital that we acknowledge the limitation of POCUS, the potential dangers of misdiagnosis, and the importance of strict clinical governance and ongoing skill maintenance.

1.3 Summary

So, whilst stethoscopes may not quite be ready to be cast aside as mere 'wheeze detectors', it is paramount that the critical care community acknowledges the advances we have seen in medical imaging. To not embrace POCUS is to ignore some of this progress and the advantages it can provide our patients.

CHAPTER 2

BASIC ULTRASOUND PHYSICS

Abhishek Jha & Pablo Rojas Zamora

Ultrasound is a high frequency sound wave that allows non-invasive imaging of tissues in real time. Ultrasound waves are considered longitudinal mechanical waves with a frequency higher than the upper limit of unaided human hearing (20,000kHz). Characteristically, diagnostic ultrasound frequencies range from 1 to 20MHz and are chosen according to the tissue of interest [1].

There are two basic parameters of a wave that help characterize its properties – wavelength and frequency:

- **Wavelength** is the distance travelled by sound in 1 second. It is inversely proportional to frequency.

- **Frequency** is the number of cycles per second and is expressed in hertz. An inverse relationship means there is always a trade-off between depth of imaging and resolution: a higher frequency produces a sharper image but the depth of field is shallow; whereas a lower frequency allows imaging of deeper structures but with poorer resolution. Commonly used frequencies include:
  - abdomen: 3–5MHz
  - echocardiography: 1.5–7.5MHz
  - superficial and musculoskeletal structures: 10–15MHz.

Ultrasound waves are generated from a transducer when an alternating electrical current is passed through a piezoelectric material, normally lead zirconate titanate (PZT). These materials can transform the electrical voltage into mechanical waves (i.e. ultrasound waves) through an alteration of its thickness [1,2]. In turn, they are also able to convert mechanical waves received into electric signals.

To create an image, ultrasound waves are usually emitted in short pulses and travel through the tissues, but when they encounter an interface between two substances with different acoustic impedance the waves are reflected. Some of these reflected waves are received by the piezoelectric crystals in the transducer (when they are not emitting a pulse), allowing an image to be formed.

2.1 Sound wave properties

Sound waves are a succession of pressure changes (compressions (high pressure) and rarefactions (low pressure)) transmitted through a medium (i.e. tissue) from one particle to the next, due to elastic forces between them. These pressure changes form a sinusoid wave which can be defined by time and magnitude parameters (*Fig. 2.1*).

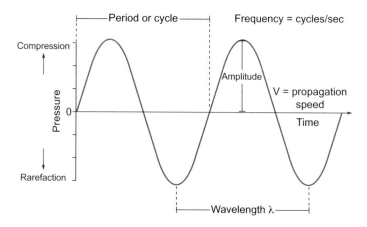

Figure 2.1. Sound wave properties.

2.1.1 Time parameters

- **Frequency (f):** refers to the number of cycles that occur in 1 second. It is only influenced by the sound source. It is measured in hertz (Hz).

- **Period (T):** the time for a sound wave to complete a single cycle. It is measured in microseconds and has an inverse relationship with the frequency of the wave.

- **Wavelength (λ):** the distance over which one cycle occurs; equal to the distance from the beginning to the end of one cycle. It has an inverse relationship with the frequency and its multiplication results in the propagation speed of a wave in a medium. It is expressed in metres.

- **Propagation speed (v):** the speed (m/sec) at which the sound travels through a medium. It is influenced by the characteristics of the medium through which it propagates, especially stiffness and density. It is approximately 1540m/s in soft tissue and can be up to 4100m/sec in denser tissues.

The relationship between frequency, wavelength and propagation speed can be described by the following formula:

$$v = f \cdot \lambda$$

2.1.2 Magnitude parameters

- **Amplitude (A):** the wave's height. It is measured in metres from the wave's average value to its peak.

- **Intensity (I):** the total power in the cross-section of a sound beam. It has important influences on the bioeffects of ultrasound. It is higher at the centre of the beam and is decreased in the periphery.

- **Power (P):** the energy produced per unit of time. In a practical setting, the higher the power, the higher the vibration of the crystal, resulting in a brighter image.

2.2 Interactions of ultrasound

As ultrasound waves meet human tissue, they undergo a process called attenuation, diminishing their amplitude as they travel deeper. Higher frequencies and deeper tissues tend to attenuate sound waves the most. Attenuation mainly happens due to four types of interactions: reflection, refraction, absorption, and scattering [3].

2.2.1 Reflection

When a sound wave is incident on a tissue interface with different acoustic properties, some of the original wave is reflected and the remainder is transmitted through to the next medium. Reflection describes the process through which the sound beam is sent back to the medium from which it came. This reflected beam is called an echo.

The amount of ultrasound wave reflected is directly proportional to the difference in acoustic impedance (resistance to the passage of ultrasound) between the two mediums. The bigger the difference, the stronger the reflection and, therefore, the higher the attenuation.

For example, the acoustic impedance difference between air and soft tissue is high, because air has an extremely low relative acoustic impedance, and this creates a strong reflection. This is the reason why an acoustic coupling medium (i.e. conducting gel) must be placed between the transducer and the skin.

Reflection intensity is also dependent on the angle at which the ultrasound waves enter the second medium. The ultrasound probe should be perpendicular to the target to get a clear image, otherwise the ultrasound will be deflected, and the echo will be weakened [3,4].

2.2.2 Refraction

This is the change of direction that the transmitted sound wave undergoes when it travels through an interface. The angle of refraction is dependent on its velocity in the medium distal to the tissue interface. Its angle of incidence depends on the propagation speed in the second medium. If it is slower than in the first medium, the angle of refraction is smaller [3,4].

2.2.3 Absorption

This is the main cause of attenuation. It is the transformation of acoustic energy into heat and is mainly influenced by wave frequency and tissue composition and structure. The particles in the medium start to vibrate as the ultrasound wave penetrates the tissue. At low wave frequencies, particles adapt to the vibrations of the wave and there is low absorption; however, at high frequencies particles cannot move at the same speed and so some energy is retained by the medium [3,4].

2.2.4 Scattering

This is the process whereby the ultrasound beam disperses after hitting an interface that is smaller than the wavelength of the ultrasound itself. It also happens when the beam encounters a rough surface. This process is responsible for viewing different echogenic structures within a specific tissue. The amount of scattering is directly proportional to the frequency of the incident wave.

It is possible to compensate for attenuation by amplifying the received echo signal, although this will also amplify unwanted background noise. The degree of amplification is called gain. Time gain compensation (TGC) is the machine's capacity to adjust gain to allow for absorption and thus ensure a uniformly dense image. For example, on detecting the first returning waves the gain is initially low because these pulse echoes have returned from superficial tissues with little attenuation, but as time progresses the gain is increased to compensate for lower amplitude pulses returning from deeper tissues.

2.3 Resolution

In the context of ultrasound, resolution may be described as three main types: spatial, temporal, and contrast resolution.

2.3.1 Spatial resolution

This is the capacity of the ultrasound machine to distinguish between two adjacent objects. A low spatial resolution implies that the ultrasound machine is more precise at differentiating objects that are close together. It may be further classified into axial resolution and lateral resolution:

- **Axial resolution** is the minimum distance that can be differentiated between two objects parallel (longitudinal) to the beam. Shorter pulses and therefore higher frequencies enhance accuracy.

- **Lateral resolution** is the minimum distance that can be detected between two structures perpendicular to the beam. A narrower ultrasound beam increases the lateral resolution. Of note, ultrasound transducers tend to be more accurate in the axial than the lateral plane.

2.3.2 Temporal resolution

This is the capacity of the ultrasound machine to observe movement; defined as the time from the beginning of one frame to the next. This is increased by a high frame rate which may be achieved by reducing the depth of penetration, reducing the number of focal points, and using narrower frames.

2.3.3 Contrast resolution

This refers to the ability to identify differences in echogenicity between adjacent tissues. Contrast resolution is particularly relevant when considering two tissues of similar echogenicity such as the spleen and kidney. It may be altered at various stages in the image processing via compression, image memory, and the use of contrast agents.

2.4 Types of probes

Modern ultrasound machines found on critical care units usually have three different transducers available, differing from each other in their emitting wave frequency and shape. The choice of probe will depend on the depth and nature of the structure being viewed:

- **Linear transducers** are normally used for superficial structures, such as nerves or blood vessels. They typically have frequency ranges from 6 to 15MHz.

- **Curvilinear transducers** are used for deeper tissues. The frequency ranges are commonly below 6MHz.

- **Phased array transducers** are usually used for cardiac imaging, because they have a small acoustic footprint. They typically use frequencies between 1.5 and 7.5MHz.

2.5 Ultrasound image modes

2.5.1 A-mode

This is the oldest ultrasound mode. It consists of a one-dimension graphic display of vertical peaks versus time that represent the amplitude of the returning wave every time it encounters an interface. The distance between each amplitude peak is representative of the depth of the encounter. The transducer in this mode emits a single pulse.

2.5.2 B-mode

This is a two-dimensional mode where an anatomical image is created through the transformation of peaks from A-mode scans into dots of varying grey-scale brightness. The brightness represents the echo strength and the two-dimensional image the real distances in the tissue.

2.5.3 M-mode

This is a one-dimension mode that shows tissue movement over time at one specific point. Moving structures are represented as curved lines and static structures as straight lines. It is commonly used in echocardiography, lung ultrasound and in assessment of the inferior vena cava.

2.5.4 Doppler mode

This mode is based on the Doppler effect, which describes the phenomenon whereby a stationary source of sound may detect changes in the frequency of the reflected sound wave secondary to movement of the object they reflect from. The difference in frequency (Δf) is called Doppler shift and increases as the speed of the moving object increases. Two shifts can be observed when analyzing a blood vessel: a positive shift when red blood cells move towards the transducer and the Doppler frequency is higher than the transmitted ultrasound wave, and a negative shift when the red blood cells move away, resulting in a Doppler frequency lower than the transmitted ultrasound wave.

The Doppler shift is subject to the velocity of the object, the angle between the object's direction and the observer, the velocity of sound and the emitted frequency, and is described by the Doppler equation (below) [4,5]. Based on this equation, if the angle is 90°, no movement is detected because cos 90° is 0.

$$F_d = \frac{2 \cdot F_t \cdot v \cdot \cos\theta}{c}$$

where F_d is the Doppler shift, F_t is the frequency of the transmitted ultrasound, v is the velocity of sound in tissue, and θ is the angle between the incident beam and the direction of flow.

This equation demonstrates that frequency is inversely proportional to velocity. Therefore, when using Doppler mode, it is better to have lower frequencies because high flow velocities can be measured. In practice, this mode is normally used to detect blood vessels or blood flow (*Fig. 2.2*).

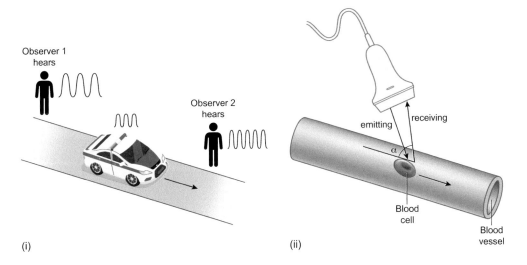

Figure 2.2. An illustration of the Doppler effect. (i) This demonstrates an everyday example of the Doppler effect. The sound of a police siren is lower in pitch if it is moving away from an observer (observer 1) than if the vehicle is moving towards an observer (observer 2). (ii) The Doppler effect as used to assess movement of a red blood cell with ultrasound.

2.5.5 Colour flow Doppler

In colour flow Doppler, the echoes are represented by varying colours that relate to the direction of the flow. If the flow is moving towards the sound source, the received sound wave will have a higher frequency and will be depicted in red. If flow is moving away from the sound source, the frequency will be lower and will be depicted in blue. The intensity of the flow will be represented by the varying brightness of the colours.

2.5.6 Power Doppler

Power Doppler displays the amplitude of a signal and provides greater detail of flow than standard colour flow Doppler. However, it does not provide information about the direction and the speed of the flow [4,5].

2.5.7 Pulsed wave Doppler

In this mode the user defines an area of interest within the image and only Doppler shifts within this zone are recorded. It is achieved through the transmission of pulsed impulses by PZT, which then also detect the reflected wave. This allows for the recording of 'site specific' information. It is, however, subject to aliasing at higher flow velocities (1.5–1.7m/sec) and thus is best avoided in these circumstances [4,5].

2.5.8 Continuous wave Doppler

This mode allows the detection of velocities along the whole length of the ultrasound beam path. It is achieved via the use of separate emitting and detecting piezoelectric materials. In contrast to pulsed wave Doppler, it can reliably record flow at high velocities but cannot specify where they originate from [4,5].

2.6 Artefacts

Artefacts are erroneous ultrasound images; in other words, they do not represent real tissues, shapes, or organs. These errors are due to non-anatomical reflections that tweak the assumptions the ultrasound machine makes about the beam. Nonetheless, valuable information can be taken from these artefacts [4,5]. They are discussed in more detail in *Chapter 3*.

2.6.1 Reverberation

This artefact occurs when an ultrasound wave encounters two strong acoustic interfaces, and the wave bounces between them before returning to the transducer. This creates an image of various equally spaced echoes along a ray line.

2.6.2 Mirror artefact

This artefact occurs when the ultrasound beam is strongly reflected from a smooth reflector into a second tissue, creating a duplicate deeper than the original structure.

2.6.3 Edge shadowing

This happens when a curved interface refracts the ultrasound wave and, consequently, a hypoechoic area appears along the edge of the curved structure.

2.6.4 Acoustic enhancement

This effect takes place when the ultrasound beam penetrates down through a tissue with a lower attenuation rate than the adjacent tissues. This produces reflectors with an abnormally high brightness. It may appear in ducts and cysts.

2.6.5 Acoustic shadowing

This is seen when the ultrasound beam encounters a strong attenuating medium, and therefore a hypoechoic area is formed below it as nearly all the sound is reflected. This is seen in gallstones.

2.7 Summary

An understanding of the basic principles underpinning the use of ultrasound is vital. It allows users to optimize their images, accurately interpret findings and explain any artefacts seen.

2.8 References

1. Buscarini E, Lutz H, Mirk P (2013) *Manual of Diagnostic Ultrasound*, volume 2. Geneva: World Health Organization.

2. Shriki J (2014) Ultrasound physics. *Critical Care Clinics*, 30(1): 1.

3. Ziskin MC (1993) Fundamental physics of ultrasound and its propagation in tissue. *RadioGraphics*, 13(3): 705.

4. Aldrich JE (2007) Basic physics of ultrasound imaging. *Critical Care Medicine*, 35(Suppl): S131.

5. Magee P (2020) Essential notes on the physics of Doppler ultrasound. *BJA Educ.* 20(4): 112.

CHAPTER 3

IMAGE OPTIMIZATION AND ARTEFACTS

Elliot Smith

Whether performing a focused or a comprehensive sonographic assessment, an understanding of image optimization and commonly encountered artefacts is essential. Optimized images enable better visualization of anatomy and associated pathology, which may enable better diagnosis, treatment and patient outcomes. Conversely, poorly optimized images and/or the misinterpretation of an artefact could result in misdiagnosis, unnecessary further investigations and associated risks and increased healthcare costs. This chapter discusses the basic principles of image optimization, ultrasound machine controls, and some of the most frequently faced image artefacts. Whilst we will primarily focus on echocardiography, many of the concepts discussed are applicable to other forms of ultrasound.

3.1 Image optimization and machine controls

To optimize ultrasound images, it is important to understand machine controls. The variety of controls and settings available will be dependent upon a few factors:

1. **Machine vendor** – different vendors may have varying names or button positions for the same control.

2. **Model of machine** – larger machines tend to have more advanced software, settings and imaging probes compared to portable machines.

3. **Age of machine** – newer machine versions often come equipped with 'auto-optimization' technologies which are designed to simplify the optimization process.

It is therefore important when first learning POCUS to get hands-on experience with all vendors and machines available in your department. Considering the often urgent nature of POCUS, time wasted on finding the correct control could have potentially negative consequences for the patient. If you are unsure of where a certain control or setting is, then ask a senior colleague or sonographer.

3.1.1 Resolution

Consider optimizing ultrasound images to be improving image resolution. There are two main types of resolution when it comes to echocardiography:

1. **Spatial resolution** – the ability to differentiate between two separate objects close in space, separated into two sub-types:

   - axial resolution – points along the ultrasound beam (vertically)

   - lateral resolution – points adjacent to each other (horizontally)

2. **Temporal resolution** – the ability to detect motion over time.

When optimizing ultrasound images, always keep in mind these types of resolution and how the following controls can affect them.

3.1.2 Receiver gain

Commonly described as 2D gain or overall gain, this control adjusts the amplitude of all returning signals to the ultrasound probe. When performing echocardiography, it should be adjusted so that the blood pool appears black and the myocardial tissues grey. Increase the gain to improve visualization of poor reflectors and decrease the gain to improve visualization of strong reflectors.

However, be aware that over-gained images are common in the hands of inexperienced sonographers. Over-gaining decreases spatial resolution and can make structures appear thicker than they are, which could lead to misdiagnosis, e.g. incorrect diagnosis of a calcified aortic valve.

3.1.3 Time gain compensation (TGC)

Like overall gain, the TGC control can adjust the amplitude of returning signals, but rather than for the overall picture, it can be adjusted at varying depths. This is useful to counteract the effect of attenuation, where ultrasound energy is lost when it interacts with tissues as it propagates through the body. Attenuation increases exponentially with imaging depth, resulting in lower amplitude signals returning from deeper structures. Hence the TGC sliders can be manipulated to ensure gains are higher in the far-field where attenuation is the greatest (see *Fig. 3.1*). Note that modern portable machines often have touchscreen TGC controls, rather than physical sliders.

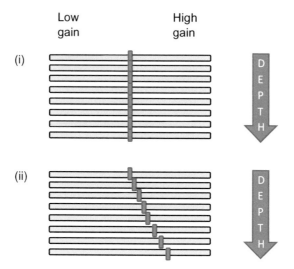

Figure 3.1. TGC controls typically consist of a series of sliders placed in horizontal bars that are vertically aligned. The bars represent different imaging depth levels, with the top representing the near-field and bottom representing the far-field. The further a slider is pushed to the left, the lower the gain will be at that corresponding imaging depth. Conversely the further the slider is pushed to the right, the higher the gain at that depth.

(i) TGC sliders are level at all imaging depths resulting in equal gain throughout the ultrasound image. Based on standard probe settings, structures in the far-field may appear under-gained due to attenuation.

(ii) TGC sliders adjusted to compensate for the effect of attenuation – gains are increased in the far-field.

3.1.4 Focus

As the ultrasound beam is generated by the transducer, the pulses of ultrasound are directed slightly inward (near-field) before they diverge outwards at greater depths (far-field). The point at which the beam diverges is where the ultrasound pulses are most concentrated, and hence have the best spatial resolution. This area is called the focal zone and its position can often be adjusted by the sonographer to optimize resolution at certain depths (see *Fig. 3.2*). The focal zone should be positioned at the area of interest (e.g. at the left ventricular apex for assessment of thrombus in apical views). *Note: some modern ultrasound machines have auto-focusing software and therefore may not have a focus control.*

3.1.5 Sector width and depth

Both these controls affect temporal resolution, also known as frame rate. High frame rates are required to assess for abnormalities on rapidly moving structures such as the heart valves (see *Fig. 3.3*). When creating a 2D image, the transducer sweeps a series of parallel scan lines across the screen [1]. The wider the sector width, the more scan lines the machine must generate before starting a new sweep, resulting in a lower rate. Likewise, the deeper

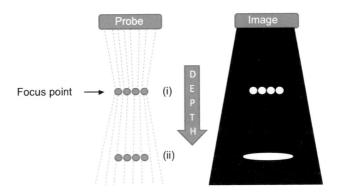

Figure 3.2. The greater lateral resolution at the level of the focal zone enables four distinct structures to be visualized on the image (i). However, if the same four structures were situated in the far-field where the beam is unfocused then the spatial resolution will be worse, and they may appear as less distinct structures (ii).

the machine samples, the longer it must wait for pulses to return before generating a new pulse. Hence to optimize temporal resolution, both sector width and depth should be kept to a minimum (see *Fig. 3.3*).

3.1.6 Frequency

Imaging at higher frequencies enables greater resolution due to shorter wavelengths. However, high frequency probes have poorer imaging at greater depths (penetration) compared to lower frequency probes. Adult echocardiography probes are designed to image at a lower set range of frequencies (typically ~2–5MHz) than paediatric probes (~5–10MHz), because adults generally have more tissue through which the ultrasound must propagate to generate the image. If scanning a large patient, consider decreasing the probe frequency to achieve better penetration. Conversely, if scanning a small patient, try increasing this control or selecting a higher frequency probe.

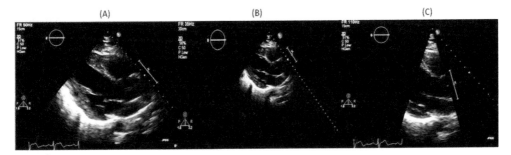

Figure 3.3. Three parasternal long axis images demonstrating the effect of sector width and depth on temporal resolution (Hz). (A) Well optimized depth (15cm) with maximal sector width (90°) results in reasonable temporal resolution – 50Hz. (B) By doubling the imaging depth to 30cm the temporal resolution has reduced to 35Hz. (C) Both the sector width and depth have been optimized resulting in excellent temporal resolution of 110Hz for the visualization of the aortic and mitral valves.

3.1.7 Probe manipulation

Correct manipulation of the ultrasound probe is also essential for image optimization. Even when all the above controls are optimized, image resolution will always be highest at the centre of the beam at the focal zone. Therefore, the structures of interest should always remain in the centre of the image. This can be achieved through a series of probe movements, dependent on the imaging window:

- moving up and down a rib space

- moving the probe medially or laterally

- rotating the probe clockwise and anticlockwise

- tilting the probe – superiorly (tail downwards, probe face upwards) or inferiorly (tail upwards, probe face downwards)

- rocking the probe – leftwards or rightwards (see *Fig. 3.4*).

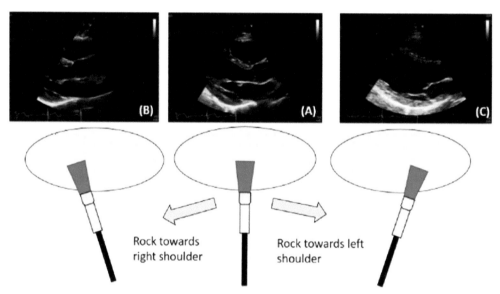

Figure 3.4. Three parasternal long axis pictures demonstrate the effect of 'rocking' the probe on moving different structures into the area of highest resolution. (A) With the probe placed flat against the chest a standard parasternal long-axis view can be seen. (B) By rocking the probe face towards the patient's right shoulder, more of the left atrium, proximal aorta and right ventricular outflow tract can be seen. (C) Rocking the probe towards the left shoulder enables more of the mid to apical left ventricular walls to be visualized.

3.2 Ultrasound artefacts

Artefacts can be defined as structures seen on an ultrasound image that are *not* actually present in the body, or structures that *are* present but which appear absent on the ultrasound image [1]. Causes can include machine settings, patient anatomy and prosthetic materials. There are several different types of artefacts encountered in echocardiography and a few are discussed below.

3.2.1 Acoustic shadowing

This occurs when the ultrasound beam encounters a very strong reflector. Most of the beam is reflected back to the transducer, resulting in a lack of echoes (shadow) beyond that structure. This artefact is typically caused by heavily calcified valves, prosthetic valves or pacemaker/implantable cardioverter defibrillator leads (*Fig. 3.5*). Acoustic shadowing may also limit the assessment of valvular function with both colour and spectral Doppler [2].

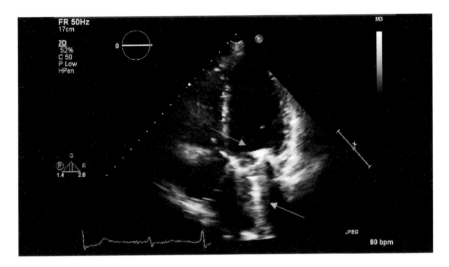

Figure 3.5. Apical four-chamber view demonstrating acoustic shadowing (orange arrow) caused by a metallic mitral valve (green arrow).

3.2.2 Reverberation artefact

This occurs when the ultrasound beam encounters two strong, usually large flat parallel reflectors close to each other (e.g. the walls of the proximal aorta in the parasternal long axis view). If a reflected ultrasound pulse encounters another strong reflector on its return to the transducer, some of the ultrasound will return to the transducer, whilst a smaller amount will reflect back away from the transducer. This process repeats itself, but with a progressively smaller amount of ultrasound reflected to the transducer each time. On the ultrasound image this manifests as regularly spaced linear echoes that gradually diminish in intensity, separated by the exact distance between the two reflectors [3].

3.2.3 Mirror image artefact

A similar process to reverberation artefacts, mirror images occur when the ultrasound beam reflects off a strong flat reflector at an angle and then encounters a structure. It then travels back to the strong flat reflector and returns to the transducer. The machine interprets this as two identical structures, one true structure above the reflector, and one false structure equally spaced below the reflector (*Fig. 3.6*).

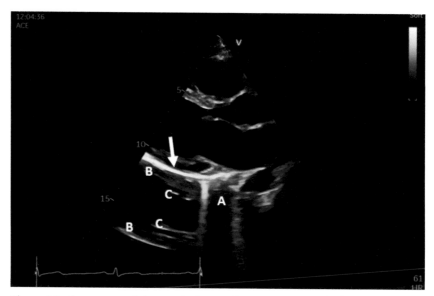

Figure 3.6. A parasternal long axis image demonstrating a thickened echogenic pericardium (arrow) that is causing two separate artefacts.
Acoustic shadowing is demonstrated at (A) – the pericardium reflects back all the ultrasound causing no echoes below this point. A mirror image artefact can be seen of the LV walls (B) and mitral valve leaflets (C) below the bright pericardium. This could be falsely diagnosed as a left pleural effusion.

3.2.4 Artefact or real?

Determining an artefact from real anatomy can be challenging. The following tips may prove useful when trying to distinguish between the two.

- **Optimize images** – use the controls mentioned earlier; many artefacts are caused by over-gained images and strong reflectors.

- **Can the structure be seen in multiple image planes?** If it can only be seen from a single window and not the rest of the POCUS views, it is likely an artefact. If visualized in several imaging planes it is more likely to be genuine.

- **Identify causes of artefacts** such as strong reflectors, and try an imaging window which avoids visualization of these.

- **Does the motion of the structure match that of other cardiac structures?** The movement of artefacts typically matches the motion of whatever is causing it. For example, a reverberation artefact mimicking an aortic dissection flap will match the motion of the bright aortic walls in the PLAX view. Whereas genuine structures, such as a dissection flap, tend to have independent motion to the structures around them.

- **Does the appearance of the structure mirror that of other cardiac structures?** Mirror image artefacts have the same appearance and motion as a genuine cardiac structure that is adjacent to a flat strong reflector. The distance between the artefact and reflector will also match the distance between the reflector and the genuine structure.

- **Ask a senior colleague/request a formal echocardiogram** – experienced and accredited sonographers are well-versed in distinguishing fact from artefact.

3.3 Summary

Whether performing a focused or comprehensive study, the ability to optimize images and recognize artefacts is essential. Adjusting basic controls such as gain, focus, sector width and depth can improve image resolution and therefore the visualization of anatomy. Knowledge of common artefacts and how to differentiate them from true anatomy can help reduce misdiagnoses and referrals for further imaging.

3.4 References

1. Houghton AR (2009) *Making Sense of Echocardiography.* Hodder Arnold.

2. Bertrand PB, Levine RA, Isselbacher EM, Vandervoort PM (2016) Fact or artifact in two-dimensional echocardiography: avoiding misdiagnosis and missed diagnosis. *J Am Soc Echocardiogr,* 29(5): 381.

3. Le HT, Hangiandreou N, Timmerman R, *et al.* (2016) Imaging artifacts in echocardiography. *Anesthes Analg,* 122: 633.

CHAPTER 4

FOCUSED VERSUS ADVANCED ECHOCARDIOGRAPHY

04

Angus McKnight & Stuart Gillon

Although formal echocardiography, performed by a suitably qualified clinician or cardiac physiologist, has an important role in acute care settings, there is an increasing role for focused cardiac ultrasound (FCU) performed at the bedside. This chapter discusses the differences between these techniques and highlights some of the indications for each.

4.1 Definition of FCU

FCU is described by the American Society of Echocardiography as an examination of the cardiovascular system by a physician as an adjunct to a physical examination [1]. This examination, in a similar way to a traditional physical examination, seeks to identify specific signs that point towards a potential diagnosis. Other terminology used to describe this technique includes point-of-care ultrasound (POCUS).

FCU is typically performed at the bedside and can be conducted in less time than a formal examination. FCU may be performed on lower specification ultrasound equipment, such as hand-held scanners, and thus the advanced features (such as spectral Doppler) required for formal echocardiography may be missing. FCU typically relies on a visual assessment of cardiac function (qualitative measures) rather than a quantitative assessment, although some protocols may include basic measurements. The study is typically limited to simple, binary questions such as the presence or absence of a particular abnormality. There is minimal grading of any abnormalities seen. As FCU is quick to perform, it may be repeated regularly and can be used to assess the effect of a therapeutic intervention (e.g. the effect of a fluid bolus or a vasopressor infusion).

A number of organizations have published guidelines as to which views should be obtained during a FCU scan. These include the Intensive Care

Society (ICS) which has developed the FUSIC (Focused Ultrasound in Intensive Care) Heart accreditation, the Resuscitation Council (UK) which has developed a FEEL (Focused Echocardiography in Emergency Life Support) accreditation, and the British Society of Echocardiography which has developed the slightly more advanced Level 1 accreditation (see *Table 4.1*) [2,3].

Table 4.1. A comparison of FCU accreditation schemes in the UK

Accreditation scheme	Responsible organization	Course length	Structures assessed	Logbook requirement	Completion process
Focused Echo-cardiography in Emergency Life Support (FEEL)	Resuscitation Council UK	1 day	Visual assessment of LV and RV size and function, IVC and pericardium	50 cases (25 under direct supervision)	Sign off by local mentor
British Society of Echocardio-graphy Level 1	British Society of Echocardio-graphy	Not required	Visual and basic quantitative assessment of LV, RV and IVC; visual and colour Doppler valvular assessment; visual aortic root, atrial and pericardial assessment	75 cases with specified case mix	Practical assessment at external centre
Focused Ultra-sound in Critical Care (FUSIC Heart)	Intensive Care Society	1–2 days	Visual assessment of LV and RV size and function, IVC and pericardium	50 cases (10 under direct supervision)	Triggered assessment by local supervisor

IVC – inferior vena cava; LV – left ventricle; RV – right ventricle.

Despite subtle differences in protocol, the aim of all FCU guidelines is to identify key pathology which may be of significance in the acutely unwell patient. As illustrated by the ICS FUSIC Heart model report, this process takes the form of several binary questions:

- Is the LV function significantly impaired?

- Is the LV dilated?

- Is the RV dilated or severely impaired?

- Is there pericardial fluid?

- Is there evidence of hypovolaemia?

- Is there pleural fluid?

These questions can be answered using four standard views: the parasternal long-axis, parasternal short-axis, apical four-chamber and subcostal windows.

4.2 Difference between FCU and comprehensive echocardiography

In contrast to FCU, a full echocardiogram is a comprehensive examination of the heart using ultrasound. This technique is suitable for patients with chronic, stable disease as well as in the acute setting. The equipment used for echocardiography should be designed specifically for this purpose. A high-performance phased array transducer should be available, as well as a free-standing Doppler probe. Comprehensive controls should allow the operator to optimize the obtained images and steer the ultrasound beam towards areas of interest. The operator may be a physician or a sonographer and may perform the scan as a stand-alone study without otherwise being involved in the clinical care of the patient.

A formal echocardiogram, to the standard of the British Society of Echocardiography Level 2 minimum dataset, can consist of more than 60 individual images and includes, in addition to 2D views, images taken using a variety of ultrasound techniques including M-mode, pulsed wave and continuous wave Doppler and tissue Doppler imaging [4,5]. Additional images may be taken if an abnormality is identified. The American Society of Echocardiography has produced a similar minimum dataset covering a suggested sequence of views taken in a comprehensive echocardiogram [6].

Following image acquisition, facility should be available for offline analysis of the images and reporting. A comprehensive echocardiogram, covering the minimum dataset, may take in the region of one hour to perform and fully report.

The term 'limited echocardiogram' refers to an echocardiographic study performed to the same standard as a full or comprehensive echocardiogram, but with fewer images acquired, in order to focus on a particular area of the heart. The American Intersocietal Accreditation Commission suggests that a limited examination should only be performed after a recent comprehensive examination and when changes outside of a specific area of interest are unlikely [7].

4.2.1 Indications for FCU

There are a wide variety of indications for FCU:

- Acutely unwell patient where the diagnosis is uncertain, e.g. patients who are hypotensive, shocked or have symptoms of chest pain or dyspnoea.

- Rapid assessment of the heart during cardiac arrest.

- Assessment of effect of an intervention such as fluid resuscitation or initiation of inotropic therapy in an unwell patient.

- Suspicion of a cardiovascular pathology causing acute illness, e.g. suspected pulmonary embolism, cardiac tamponade, left or right ventricular dysfunction.

FCU is most valuable in the assessment of the acutely unwell patient where rapid diagnostic information is needed.

4.2.2 Information available from FCU

As is evident from the list of binary questions in *Section 4.1*, FCU can answer a wide variety of questions about cardiac function which are of interest to a clinician. This technique has a particular role in the assessment of a deteriorating or shocked patient and can help in trying to ascertain the cause of critical illness (see *Table 4.2*).

An important area of assessment is the left ventricle. Studies have been conducted to compare the assessment of left ventricular systolic function by FCU and formal echocardiography. Johnson *et al.* [8] conducted a prospective observational study involving FCU scans performed by a cohort of physicians who had undergone a short period of bedside training. This study included a wide variety of patients, some of whom had technically challenging examinations secondary to chronic obstructive pulmonary disease or obesity. The estimate of left ventricular function made by these physicians correlated closely with comprehensive echocardiographic findings and the ejection fraction as interpreted by a cardiologist.

A focused ultrasound scan of the left ventricle can identify patients with impaired left ventricular systolic function and give an indication of the severity. Therapy to improve left ventricular function can be instigated and the ultrasound repeated to monitor the response. This may therefore identify a patient with pump failure and help differentiate this from other causes of shock.

FCU is useful in the assessment of intravascular fluid status, which can be difficult to determine using traditional physical examination in critically ill patients. A hyperdynamic circulatory state seen in a shocked patient may indicate that they are intravascularly depleted. A collapsible inferior vena cava can suggest a reduced central venous pressure (see *Chapter 24* for more detail on this subject). This may aid the clinician in choosing between further intravascular filling or a vasopressor infusion. This real-time assessment is extremely valuable in unstable patients.

FCU of the right ventricle can be helpful in a variety of pathologies affecting the right heart, lungs and pulmonary vasculature. The finding of a dilated right heart can occur in a patient with pulmonary embolism. Although FCU is not sufficiently sensitive or specific on its own to diagnose pulmonary embolism, it can indicate that further investigations towards this potential diagnosis are required.

Impaired right ventricular systolic function is found following an inferior myocardial infarction. Patients with respiratory compromise may have a

Table 4.2. A comparison of information available from FCU and formal echocardiography

		FCU	Formal echocardiography
Left ventricle	Systolic function	Qualitative assessment only; typically only focuses on severe dysfunction and more subtle abnormalities may be missed	Quantitative assessment including ejection fraction; will identify subtle changes
	Diastolic function	Generally not assessed, although some protocols evaluate left atrial size and motion of intra-atrial septum	Assessed by quantitative means and classified into grades of diastolic dysfunction
	Size	Visual impression or single plane measurement	Three-dimensional volume measurement using methods such as Simpson's biplane method of disks
	Regional wall motion abnormalities	Qualitative visual impression only	Categorized, e.g. using a standard 17 segment model
Right ventricle	Size	Qualitative assessment only	Two-dimensional measurement such as area in systole and diastole
	Systolic function	Qualitative assessment only or single measurement of function (e.g. TAPSE)	Assessment of both longitudinal and radial function
Valves		Commonly not assessed, although some protocols include a visual and colour Doppler evaluation	Valve structure and function assessed by colour, pulsed wave and continuous wave Doppler; valve pathology accurately classified
Peri-cardium		Visual impression of pericardial pathology, e.g. a pericardial effusion	Measurement of pericardial effusion size in multiple echo views; identification of restrictive or constrictive pathology

dilated right heart secondary to raised pulmonary pressures. Abnormalities of the right ventricle found using ultrasound can therefore be considered together with the clinical picture to aid diagnosis or indicate what further investigations might be useful (for more details on right ventricular assessment see *Chapter 8*).

FCU is also useful to identify pericardial or pleural fluid. The presence of significant pericardial fluid in a shocked patient suggests the possibility of cardiac tamponade. Unilateral or bilateral pleural effusions may be a significant finding, for example, in thoracic trauma when this may represent a haemothorax. All images taken during a study should be interpreted in the context of the clinical picture, with attention paid to the haemodynamics of the patient at the time of the study.

4.2.3 Pitfalls of FCU

The pitfalls of focused ultrasound examination must be borne in mind. Because detailed assessment of valvular function is often not performed, caution must be used in interpreting a focused ultrasound in a patient with suspected valvular heart disease. A patient with impaired left ventricular systolic function seen on a focused study may have aortic stenosis as an underlying cause which is not detected on this scan. Similarly, a hyperdynamic ventricle might be due to incompetent valves. If there is a suspicion of a valvular lesion, then a formal echocardiogram is likely to be required. Subtle lesions, such as regional wall motion abnormalities, or ventricular dyssynchrony, may also be missed on a focused ultrasound.

It is also possible that findings may be due to chronic disease rather than an acute change. For example, a patient with right ventricular dilation seen on FCU might have underlying chronic lung disease, rather than a new acute event such as a pulmonary embolism.

The clinician performing a focused ultrasound must be aware of these limitations and have the ability to integrate the echocardiographic findings with the full clinical picture. The choice of investigation depends on the question to be answered and the urgency and availability of the investigation. Clinicians must have an awareness of when to refer for a full study.

4.2.4 Information available from a comprehensive echocardiogram

A comprehensive echocardiogram is the investigation of choice for chronic structural heart disease, because it involves an assessment of all areas of the heart and the grading of any abnormalities found. A patient who is acutely unwell may have underlying chronic structural heart disease as a contributing factor to their illness. Indications for a comprehensive echocardiogram include, but are not limited to, assessment of valvular lesions, detailed assessment of left and right ventricular function and assessment of the pericardium, aorta and great vessels (see *Table 4.2*) [9]. Patients with intracardiac shunts or congenital heart disease can then have these lesions characterized. A transthoracic echocardiogram (TTE) can be used to investigate suspected intracardiac masses or thrombus and suspected infective endocarditis.

Alongside capturing images detailing all areas of the heart, a comprehensive echocardiogram uses quantitative and visual measures to characterize any identified lesions. For example, in the assessment of the left ventricle there are a variety of methods to measure size and function, and cardiac chamber volumes can be calculated. It is possible to measure a quantitative ejection fraction which can be used to guide therapy or for prognosis (for more details on left ventricular assessment see *Chapter 7*).

In the assessment of valvular lesions, a comprehensive echocardiogram involves the measurement of flow velocity across valves using Doppler.

Multiple measurements can be taken in different views and both stenotic and regurgitant valvular lesions can be graded mild, moderate or severe. The categorization of lesions is standardized and reproducible, and information available from echocardiography can be used to determine the timing of any intervention that may be required (for more details on valvular assessment see *Chapter 9*).

TTE is not without its limitations, and a transoesophageal echocardiogram (TOE) may be required where the images obtained from a transthoracic study are not of sufficient quality to answer the clinical question.

4.3 Governance and training

In most institutions in the UK, clinicians performing full echocardiographic studies undergo a significant period of formal training. Additionally, they are required to undertake formal examinations towards a certificate of accreditation. The British Society of Echocardiography Level 2 transthoracic certificate of accreditation requires the completion of a theory and practical examination and a logbook consisting of 250 cases. Clinicians are required to keep their practice up-to-date and revalidate after a period of time (often every 5 years). Images taken as part of echocardiographic studies are saved and form part of the permanent medical record. There are systems in place for these images to be reviewed at multidisciplinary meetings.

Training schemes, such as the ICS's FUSIC programme, exist to promote training and standards in focused ultrasound. Accreditation in focused ultrasound may consist of a short 1 or 2 day training course, followed by a period of supervised practice and a bedside assessment by an experienced clinician. It is equally important that institutions have systems in place to store and review these studies and that it is possible to access a clinician who can perform a formal echocardiogram when this is indicated [10].

The concept of a short training course has been described elsewhere in Europe. Breitkreutz *et al.* [11] described the implementation of a blended learning course, which consisted of web-based electronic learning materials followed by a 1 day course. The authors demonstrated that this was an effective method of teaching basic skills which could then be further developed during a period of mentored practice.

4.4 Impact on clinical decision making

The impact of FCU on clinical decision making has been studied. Hall *et al.* [12] looked at a case series of scans performed in an ICU, and found that FCU provided new diagnostic information in 68% of scans performed and changed management in 47% of cases. Similar assessments on the impact of formal TTE and TOE in a mixed intensive care population demonstrated an impact on management in 51% of patients [13]. Types of intervention instituted in intensive care based on scan findings included commencing or changing intravenous fluids, initiation of diuretics and the commencement of inotropes [14].

A prospective study has been conducted looking at the use of FCU in the prehospital setting in Germany. Over 200 patients who were either in cardiac arrest or in a shocked state were included. Emergency physicians performing FCU recorded their findings and any change in management as a result. The authors found that management was altered by the ultrasound findings in 78% of cases.

Despite the promising results of these studies, there have not yet been any randomized controlled trials published comparing the use of FCU to usual care. A systematic review conducted by Heiberg *et al.* [15] recognized that there is emerging evidence for this technique, but further work is needed to link the use of FCU to patient outcomes.

4.5 Summary

FCU is a useful tool in a clinician's armoury that provides timely diagnostic information rapidly at the bedside. Emerging evidence is showing this to be a valuable adjunct to physical examination in decision making in acutely unwell patients.

4.6 References

1. Spencer KT, Kimura BJ, Korcarz CE, Pellikka PA, Rahko PS, Siegel RJ (2013) Focused cardiac ultrasound: recommendations from the American Society of Echocardiography. *J Am Soc Echocardiogr Off Publ Am Soc Echocardiogr*, 26:567.

2. FUSIC Heart Accreditation Pack. Intensive Care Society [Internet]. Available from www.ics.ac.uk/.

3. Resuscitation Council UK. FEEL Course Programme [Internet]. Available from www.resus.org.uk/sites/default/files/2020-05/FEEL_Programme.pdf [cited 2021 Jan 20]

4. Popescu BA, Stefanidis A, Nihoyannopoulos P, *et al.* (2014) Updated standards and processes for accreditation of echocardiographic laboratories from The European Association of Cardiovascular Imaging. *Eur Heart J - Cardiovasc Imaging*, 15:717.

5. Wharton G, Steeds R, Allen J, *et al.* (2015) A minimum dataset for a standard adult transthoracic echocardiogram: a guideline protocol from the British Society of Echocardiography. *Echo Res Pract*, 2:G9.

6. Mitchell C, Rahko PS, Blauwet LA, *et al.* (2019) Guidelines for performing a comprehensive transthoracic echocardiographic examination in adults: recommendations from the American Society of Echocardiography. *J Am Soc Echocardiogr*, 32:1.

7. IAC Standards and Guidelines for Adult Echocardiography Accreditation (2017) https://intersocietal.org/programs/echocardiography/standards/

8. Johnson BK, Tierney DM, Rosborough TK, Harris KM, Newell MC (2016) Internal medicine point-of-care ultrasound assessment of left ventricular function correlates with formal echocardiography. *J Clin Ultrasound*, 44:92.

9. Cheitlin MD, Alpert JS, Armstrong WF, *et al.* (1997) ACC/AHA Guidelines for the Clinical Application of Echocardiography. *Circulation*, 95:1686.

10. Neskovic AN, Edvardsen T, Galderisi M, *et al.* (2014) Focus cardiac ultrasound: the European Association of Cardiovascular Imaging viewpoint. *Eur Heart J - Cardiovasc Imaging*, 15:956.

11. Breitkreutz R, Uddin S, Steiger H, *et al.* (2009) Focused echocardiography entry level: new concept of a 1-day training course. *Minerva Anestesiol*, 75:285.

12. Hall DP, Jordan H, Alam S, Gillies MA (2017) The impact of focused echocardiography using the Focused Intensive Care Echo protocol on the management of critically ill patients, and comparison with full echocardiographic studies by BSE-accredited sonographers. *J Intensive Care Soc*, 18:206.

13. Orme RML, Oram MP, McKinstry CE (2009) Impact of echocardiography on patient management in the intensive care unit: an audit of district general hospital practice. *Br J Anaes*, 102:340.

14. Breitkreutz R, Price S, Steiger HV, *et al.* (2010) Focused echocardiographic evaluation in life support and peri-resuscitation of emergency patients: a prospective trial. *Resuscitation*, 81:1527.

15. Heiberg J, El-Ansary D, Canty DJ, Royse AG, Royse CF (2016) Focused echocardiography: a systematic review of diagnostic and clinical decision-making in anaesthesia and critical care. *Anaesthesia*, 71:1091.

CHAPTER 5:

FUNDAMENTALS OF TRANSTHORACIC ECHOCARDIOGRAPHY

Richard Fisher

During the first two decades of the 21st century, POCUS has proliferated in critical care to such an extent that trainees in Intensive Care Medicine are now expected to be able to interpret echocardiographic studies in critically ill patients and integrate these findings into a patient assessment [1].

To aid healthcare professionals, numerous focused echocardiography protocols have been developed. It is not practical to discuss all the protocols that have been developed here, and so this chapter will concentrate on two protocols developed by professional bodies within the UK, namely the Intensive Care Society's FUSIC (Focused UltraSound in Intensive Care) Heart protocol and the British Society of Echocardiography's Level 1 (BSE L1) protocol [2,3]. There is an emphasis on how images should be acquired and the role of these protocols in critical care. More detailed guidance on analysis of specific anatomical structures is provided in subsequent chapters.

5.1 Indications for focused echocardiography

The European Society of Intensive Care Medicine recommends that echocardiography be considered 'the first-line evaluation modality' of shocked patients in whom the nature of shock is uncertain. Transthoracic echocardiography (TTE) explicitly is non-invasive, can be performed rapidly in almost any environment where a patient may be cared for and can be repeated as often as is required as the patient's situation evolves.

Focused echocardiography is best suited to be used as a 'rule-in' test for life-threatening pathologies that require immediate intervention. However, focused echocardiography protocols do not evaluate the heart with the same detail as a comprehensive study and therefore subtle abnormalities may be missed and these protocols are not designed to be used to label patients as having normal anatomy and function. Both FUSIC Heart and BSE L1 provide structured reporting templates to guide sonographers. Common to both protocols are gross assessments of ventricular size and systolic function, and evaluation of the pericardial and pleural spaces for fluid. In addition, the BSE L1 protocol adds colour Doppler to 2D imaging to allow identification of significant valvular stenosis (based primarily on the 2D appearance of the valve) or regurgitation.

By understanding the strengths as well as the limitations of focused echocardiography it is easy to consider clinical scenarios where it may have some utility: shock or hypotension of uncertain aetiology; in trauma for detection of cardiac tamponade; in septic shock for detection of myocardial dysfunction; in patients undergoing mechanical ventilation to assess for cor pulmonale; in cardiac arrest to identify reversible causes [4].

5.2 Preparing to scan

The steps required prior to performing a study will vary depending upon the situation. Whilst the following general considerations require time and effort up-front, they should ultimately pay that time and effort back in spades.

Always enter the patient demographic details and save clips, ideally on a central server. This will allow serial studies to be compared to each other and changes to be tracked over time, and it is essential for departmental governance.

5.2.1 Patient positioning

When possible, position the patient in the left lateral decubitus position for parasternal and apical windows to bring the heart up against the anterior chest wall. Place supports such as pillows or rolled blankets behind the patient's back to stabilize them in the optimal position. Comfort of both the patient and the sonographer is essential. An uncomfortable conscious patient will move around, making image acquisition more challenging, whilst your own discomfort will be a distraction from performing the best study you can. Clear the patient's chest adequately including moving electrocardiogram (ECG) leads and removing clothing that interferes with your ability to access the chest (whilst ensuring that you maintain patient comfort and dignity).

If your ultrasound system permits, then use ECG leads to allow the phase of the cardiac cycle to be easily identifiable in clips and still images. Two caveats to this advice include:

- avoiding using ECG leads when it would pose an infection control risk (for example, in a patient with a high consequence infectious disease)

- during cardiac arrest when activity around the bed frequently leads to artefacts detected by the ECG leads which results in inappropriately short clips being recorded.

5.3 Focused echocardiography protocols

Whilst there is no inherently 'correct' sequence of echocardiographic views, following the same sequence with every scan will reduce the risk of missing out key views or measurements. Both FUSIC Heart and BSE L1 follow the same structure, starting with the parasternal window, before moving to the apical window and then the sub-costal window. As a general rule, when time is critical one should spend the most time on those views that provide the most information about the clinical question. It is unusual to encounter a patient in whom all the windows are universally excellent. So, if the patient has a poor parasternal window but other windows are good, one should concentrate on extracting as much diagnostic information as possible from those windows which provide it, and then return to the parasternal window if time allows.

TTE is performed with a phased array probe which has a rectangular footprint behind which the grid of piezoelectric crystals is housed. On one side of the probe is an orientation marker which marries up with the orientation marker on the right-hand side of the image as displayed.

5.4 Basic probe movements

For each of the views below, the description of the probe position refers to the starting position which will then need to be adjusted to achieve a correctly aligned image. We will limit descriptions of probe movements to one of four terms when describing how the probe should be manipulated.

- **Sliding** is the only probe movement whereby the point of contact between the probe and the patient changes. The probe can be slid superiorly or inferiorly, laterally or medially. When a structure in the near-field casts acoustic shadowing over structures in the far-field (for example, when trying to image through a rib) then sliding will likely be the most useful manipulation to get around this obstacle.

- **Rotation** occurs through the centre of the probe and can either be clockwise or anticlockwise, and is the manipulation required to move between long- and short-axis views.

- **Rocking** is movement in parallel to the orientation marker. When the probe is rocked the viewed structures remain the same but appear to swing left and right within the displayed imaging sector.

- **Tilting** is movement perpendicular to the orientation marker. Tilting the body of the probe will cause you to move the imaging sector back and forth, demonstrating structures in front and behind the imaging sector.

Figure 5.1 demonstrates the four key probe manipulations.

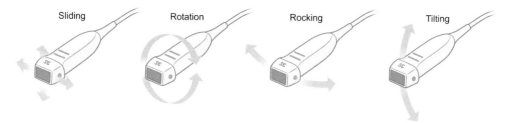

Figure 5.1. Descriptions of probe manipulations.

5.5 Performing the scan

5.5.1 Parasternal long-axis (PLAX)

The probe should be placed to the left of the sternum, usually in either the second, third or fourth intercostal space, and with the orientation marker pointing towards the patient's right shoulder. An example of the PLAX view is seen in *Figure 5.2a*. To correctly align the view, first experiment with moving the probe up and down between the different available intercostal spaces; the aim is to achieve a view whereby the inferolateral wall of the left ventricle (LV) is parallel with the ultrasound beams. This is not always achievable in patients with elevated lung functional residual capacity (FRC) (for example, those with obstructive lung disease or undergoing mechanical ventilation with positive end-expiratory pressure). In such cases the diaphragm can be displaced inferiorly, meaning the heart sits lower in the chest and the inferolateral LV wall is shifted such that it lies less horizontally.

Next the probe should be rotated to ensure that the inferolateral and anteroseptal LV walls are parallel with each other along the viewed section. If you are struggling to achieve a view, the most likely explanation is that the left lung is sitting between your probe and the heart. The lung tends to encroach on the heart from above and laterally, therefore try sliding the probe as medially as possible (right up to the sternum, without trying to image through the sternum) and then slowly slide the probe inferiorly until the heart becomes visible. A well aligned view will not include the left ventricular apex, demonstrating only the basal and mid LV segments.

It is useful to have a sequence for image interpretation in each of the views, in much the same way you may already have learnt a sequence for interpreting chest radiographs. For the PLAX view I recommend starting in the far-field and then working through to the near-field.

The pericardium
First identify the descending thoracic aorta in short-axis. This is an essential landmark for helping to characterize effusions as either pericardial or pleural. Fluid that tracks far to the aorta will be in the left pleural space (this fluid will not track beyond the aorta because this is where the pleural space ends). Fluid that tracks between the aorta and the left atrium (LA) is within the pericardial space.

The left atrium

Next turn to the LA. Three structures sitting one in front of the other along the right-hand side of the image are the right ventricular outflow tract (RVOT), aortic root and LA. In healthy individuals these three structures all appear to have broadly similar diameters when seen in the PLAX view. It is unusual to see any of these structures get smaller due to disease, therefore if one (or two) of these structures seem to be larger than the others consider that they may be dilated. Whilst it is unlikely that dilatation of the LA is itself the reason why your patient is sick, it may be evidence of another process such as mitral valve disease, elevated LV filling pressures or atrial fibrillation.

The mitral valve

Next consider the mitral valve (MV). Here our imaging sector is cutting through the anterior mitral valve leaflet (AMVL) in the near-field and posterior mitral valve leaflet (PMVL) in the far-field. The AMVL is larger than the PMVL by area and appears much larger when viewed in this plane. Consider the thickness of the leaflets, inspect for attached masses and assess the motion in both systole (when the leaflets should meet on the ventricular side of the imaginary line drawn between the MV hinge points, without prolapsing or flailing back into the LA) and diastole (when the leaflets should open to allow blood to pass from the LA to the LV). During early diastole, the AMVL should open such that it reaches within 5mm of the interventricular septum (IVS). Failure of the AMVL to get close to the IVS may be due to restricted opening due to structural MV disease, eccentric aortic regurgitation (AR) angled across the ventricular face of the AMVL, or may represent decreased cardiac output with low left ventricular ejection fraction (LVEF).

The left ventricle

Follow the blood leaving the LA and now consider the LV. The PLAX view allows for perpendicular alignment of the LV walls with the ultrasound beams, which is ideal for assessing thickness as well as thickening throughout the cardiac cycle. Four (of 17) LV segments are visible here, the basal (third of LV nearest the MV) and mid inferolateral and anteroseptal segments. Inspect for wall thickening which may be a sign of chronically elevated LV afterload (for example, in chronic systemic hypertension or aortic stenosis), hypertrophic cardiomyopathy or infiltrative cardiomyopathy. Assess LV walls for movement and thickening in systole. Normal walls should increase their thickness by ~50% during systole (when compared to end-diastole). Segments whose thickening is reduced are termed hypokinetic, whilst walls which do not thicken (or barely thicken) are termed akinetic. Be aware that akinetic segments may move if they are adjacent to moving segments, therefore it is essential to look for both movement and thickening.

The LV cavity diameter at end-diastole should be visually assessed and, if following the BSE L1 minimum dataset, should be measured. Freeze the moving image and scroll to end-diastole using a combination of both the synced ECG and 2D image (the aortic valve must be closed and the

MV should just be closing). Measure the perpendicular distance between the basal anteroseptal and inferolateral segments. Different international associations quote slightly different reference ranges, but in the UK the BSE's upper reference limit for men is 56mm and for women is 51mm [5]. Assess the change in the LV cavity diameter as the heart moves from end-diastole to peak-systole (this can be visually assessed or measured to calculate fractional shortening). Remember that this is a 1D assessment of a 3D structure and if there are regional variations in LV performance this may be misleading, for example, in takotsubo stress cardiomyopathy where the basal segments are spared (or are hyperkinetic) whilst the more apical segments are most affected.

The aortic valve and aorta

Next turn your attention to the aortic valve (AV) and aortic root. Assuming that the patient has a tri-leaflet AV then the right coronary cusp (RCC) leaflet will be visible in the near-field, whilst either the left coronary cusp (LCC) leaflet or non-coronary cusp (NCC) leaflet will be visible in the far-field. As with the MV, the assessment of the AV includes describing leaflet thickness, associated masses and leaflet movement when opening (systole) and closing (diastole). Focused echocardiography does not include spectral Doppler, therefore focused echocardiography protocols do not allow for quantification of valvular stenosis. However, a thickened or calcified valve with limited visible opening should raise the suspicion of stenosis and prompt referral for a comprehensive study. Inspect the root for evidence of dilatation (visually assess by comparing with the diameters of the LA and RVOT) and presence of a dissection flap.

The right ventricle

Finally, in the near-field we have a small section of the right ventricle (RV), namely the RVOT. As with the LV, consider wall thickness, cavity diameter and wall thickening and motion. Whilst the RV free wall is usually measured in the sub-costal window (where the upper limit of the reference range is 5mm), it may be appreciably thickened when first viewed here, and this finding should raise the suspicion of hypertrophy secondary to chronic elevation of pulmonary artery pressure. The cavity size is assessed by comparing it with the aortic root and LA, as well as looking for posterior displacement of the IVS. RV systolic function can be considered in terms of longitudinal and radial contractility, and it is radial contractility which should be assessed here.

Use of colour flow Doppler

After inspection of the 2D images, sonographers following the BSE L1 protocol should apply colour flow Doppler. First, place a colour box covering the aortic root, AV, LVOT and basal portion of the LV (*Fig. 5.2b*). The key pathologies to be identified here are turbulence within the LVOT (occurring in systole), which may represent sub-valvular stenosis or dynamic LVOT obstruction, and aortic regurgitation (occurring in diastole) which will present as a high velocity jet, arising at the AV and directed into the LV.

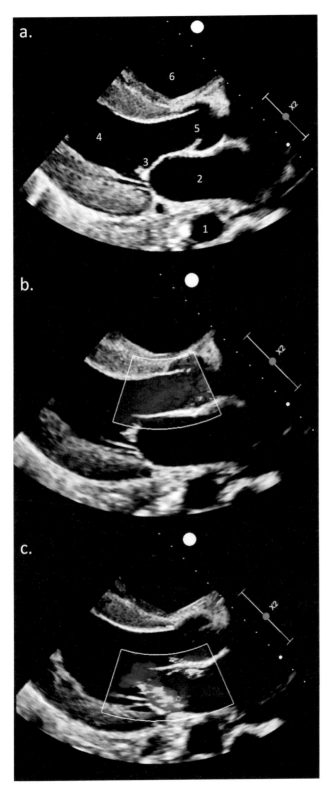

Figure 5.2. (a) Parasternal long-axis (PLAX) view: 1 – descending aorta; 2 – left atrium (LA); 3 – mitral valve (MV); 4 – left ventricle; 5 – aortic valve (AV); 6 – right ventricular outflow tract. (b) PLAX view with colour flow mapping over the AV and left ventricular outflow tract during ventricular systole. (c) PLAX view with colour flow mapping over the MV and LA during ventricular systole, demonstrating mitral regurgitation.

The colour box should then be moved over the MV and LA (*Fig. 5.2c*), primarily to assess for the presence of mitral regurgitation. Here, as with any colour Doppler interrogation of cardiac valves, the probe should be tilted slowly over several cardiac cycles, such that you pan from the most inferior border of the valve to the most superior border. It is not uncommon for regurgitant jets to arise away from the centre of the valve and failing to pan through the entirety of the valve may lead to regurgitant jets being underestimated or missed entirely. When regurgitant jets are identified, describe both the volume of blood that is moving backwards (consider the proportion of the preceding chamber which fills with regurgitant flow) as well as the direction of the jet (which may be central or eccentric and will provide clues as to the aetiology of the regurgitation).

5.5.2 Parasternal short-axis (PSAX)

The simplest way to achieve the PSAX view is to start by obtaining a well optimized PLAX view, then rotating the probe ~90° clockwise. To achieve a true short-axis view it is likely that the probe will need to be rotated such that the orientation marker is pointing somewhere between the mid-clavicular line and the left shoulder (the exact position will vary patient to patient). As the probe is rotating, whichever structure lies in the centre of the image in the PLAX view will remain in the centre of the image in the PSAX view. In the FUSIC Heart protocol one PSAX view is obtained, a slice through the mid sections of the LV, whilst the BSE L1 protocol adds slices at the level of AV (sometimes referred to as the level of the great vessels), the level of the MV (sometimes referred to as the basal level) and, most laterally, at the LV apex. In this section we will describe each of these four views moving from most medial to most lateral.

The aortic valve

The PSAX AV view (*Fig. 5.3a*) shows the AV in the centre of the image, surrounded by the LA (in the far-field), the RA (in the bottom left of the image), tricuspid valve (TV – to the left of the AV), RVOT (in the near-field) and pulmonary valve (PV – anterior and to the right of the AV). The LV is not seen because it lies lateral to the AV. For the purposes of focused echocardiography this view is most useful in inspecting the morphology of the AV. When viewed from this position the coaptation lines of the closed tri-leaflet valve form the shape of the letter 'Y'. The valve leaflets are named after the coronary arteries which arise from the corresponding aortic sinus. The most anterior leaflet is the RCC, posterior and to the right is the LCC (above which arises the left main stem (LMS)), whilst posterior and to the left is the NCC, so named because it has no associated coronary artery. The valve should be inspected for number of leaflets (the prevalence of bicuspid AV is estimated at 0.5–2%), thickening and calcification, excursion during systole and attached masses.

Basal left ventricular / mitral valve view

Tilting the probe such that the imaging sector sweeps laterally brings you to the PSAX MV view (*Fig. 5.3b*). Here it is possible to see the en-face view of the MV, with its large AMVL occupying approximately two-thirds of the valve area, whilst deep to this is the PMVL which, despite being smaller, occupies the majority of the annular circumference. Again, consider leaflet thickness, motion and attached masses. Surrounding the MV are the basal segments of the LV.

For the purposes of aiding the description of findings, the LV is divided into 17 segments (six at the base, six at the mid-level, four at the apex and a single apical cap), with the six basal segments being on view here. Starting from the attachment of the RV and LV in the near-field and moving clockwise around the LV, these six segments are termed: anterior, anterolateral, inferolateral, inferior, inferoseptal and anteroseptal. As for all views where LV walls are visible, consider the motion and the degree of thickening in systole.

Mid-papillary muscle view

Tilting further still takes you below the MV and through the sub-valvular apparatus, initially the chordae and then the papillary muscles. Continue to tilt the probe until the two papillary muscles form part of the LV wall, to reach the mid-level (*Fig. 5.3c*). Here the circular LV is again arbitrarily divided into six segments named identically to the basal segments. Arising from the inferior wall of the LV is the posteromedial papillary muscle, whilst the anterolateral papillary muscle unsurprisingly arises from the anterolateral wall.

This view is useful for identifying regional wall motion abnormalities (RWMAs). The three main coronary arteries all have territories on display here, and whilst there is a degree of variation between normal patients, the anteroseptal and anterior segments are typically supplied by the left anterior descending (LAD) artery, the anterolateral and inferolateral segments tend to be supplied by the left circumflex (LCx) artery and the inferior and inferoseptal segments are usually supplied by the right coronary artery (RCA). Interrogate each segment in turn, comparing contractility between adjacent and opposing segments. The presence of regional discrepancies is often a clue suggesting underlying coronary artery disease.

Pay particular attention to the position of the IVS. In healthy individuals the RV pressure is typically lower than LV pressure throughout the cardiac cycle, especially during ventricular systole. Conditions that lead to increased RV volume, both chronic and acute, will lead to progressive displacement of the IVS from right to left, leading to flattening of the IVS and a 'D-shaped' LV during diastole. When RV systolic pressure is also increased then this flattening can be seen during systole.

Figure 5.3. (a) Parasternal short-axis (PSAX) view at the level of the aortic valve (AV): 1 – AV; 2 – left atrium; 3 – right atrium; 4 – right ventricular outflow tract; 5 – pulmonary valve; 6 – pulmonary artery. (b) PSAX view at the level of the mitral valve: 7 – anterior mitral valve leaflet; 8 – posterior mitral valve leaflet; 9 – right ventricle (RV). (c) PSAX view at the mid-level: 9 – RV; 10 – left ventricle.

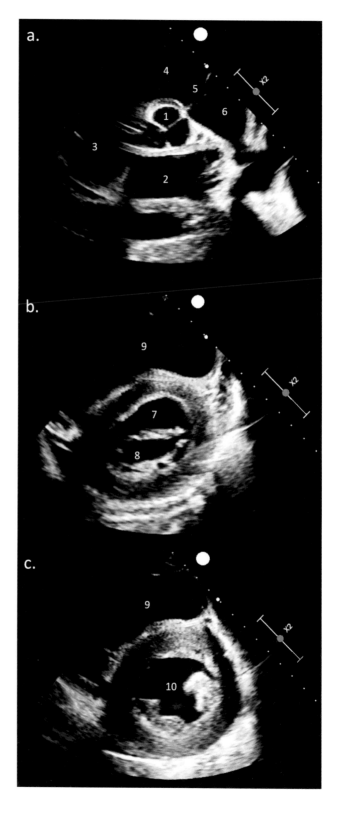

The apex

Finally, tilt the probe such that the image moves beyond the papillary muscles to find the LV apex. Here we find four LV segments, clockwise from the near field: anterior, lateral, inferior, and septal. As previously, inspect for thickening and motion of the LV walls.

5.5.3 Apical four-chamber (A4Ch)

The probe should be placed over the apex of the heart with the orientation marker turned to the patient's left (3 o'clock position). The probe should then be tilted slightly such that the imaging sector sweeps superiorly and anteriorly. This will produce a view of the heart with all four intracardiac chambers on display, with the ventricles in the near-field and the atria in the far-field (*Fig. 5.4a*).

The left ventricle

The LV apex should sit directly below the probe, whilst the IVS should run parallel to the ultrasound beams, running straight down the length of the image. Care should be taken to avoid foreshortening, i.e. placing the probe on the chest wall either superior or inferior to the apex, such that the true apex is not included within the view, resulting in ventricles with a short and squashed appearance. In healthy individuals the LV cavity should appear to have the shape of a bullet, whilst the RV appears triangular. Foreshortening should be suspected when there is unexpected rounding of the apex, especially if the apex appears disproportionately thick with excessive thickening during systole (this appearance is caused by cutting obliquely through the LV wall).

First inspect the LV. As always, consider wall thickness, thickening and motion. The A4Ch view is (along with the apical two-chamber view (A2Ch)) one of the two views used in comprehensive echocardiography in the Simpson's biplane method of estimation of LVEF. Whilst this measurement is not performed during focused echocardiography, the view is useful for a global assessment of LV contractility, and with practice and experience the novice sonographer will improve in being able to visually estimate LV systolic function. The LV walls on view here are the inferoseptal and anterolateral. The basal segment of the inferoseptal wall is usually supplied by the RCA, whilst the anterolateral wall may be supplied by either the LAD or LCx artery.

The right ventricle

None of the views obtained during 2D echocardiography adequately reflect the geometry of the RV, which wraps around the LV. However, one advantage of the A4Ch view is that it allows direct comparison of LV and RV in terms of size and function. In healthy individuals the RV should appear significantly smaller than the LV (assuming the LV is of normal size), and in the standard A4Ch view the area of the RV should not exceed two-thirds of the area of the LV [6]. If the RV appears larger than the LV it suggests significant RV dilatation.

To assess RV contractility, consider both the longitudinal function (how much the tricuspid annulus is drawn towards the apex during systole) and radial function (how much the RV free wall moves in towards the IVS), and combine these two assessments to produce an overall impression of RV systolic function. A simple measure of longitudinal shortening is tricuspid annular plane systolic excursion (TAPSE). To perform this measurement, zoom in on the lateral annulus of the TV, place the cursor through the annulus just beyond the TV hinge point and record an M-mode clip (*Fig. 5.4b*). The TV annulus position should be traced from immediately prior to ventricular systole to peak systole, and the *y*-axis component of that movement measured (if you perform a labelled measurement most ultrasound machines will ignore the *x*-axis component of the measurement and automatically quote only the *y*-axis component). A TAPSE measurement <17mm is considered highly suggestive of RV systolic dysfunction [7].

RV fractional area change (RVFAC) offers a measure of RV systolic function that correlates well with RV ejection fraction (RVEF) as measured on MRI [8]. The RV area can be measured by tracing from the TV hinge point on the free wall, up to the apex, then back down the IVS to the TV septal hinge point in both end-diastole (RVEDA) and end-systole (RVESA), and using the formula:

$$RVFAC = (RVEDA - RVESA) / RVEDA$$

RVFAC <30% in males and <35% in females is considered abnormal [7].

The mitral and tricuspid valves

Inspect the MV and TV and, just as previously, consider the thickness and motion of the valve leaflets. Look for restricted motion in either diastole (inadequate opening) or systole (inadequate closing) as well as excessive motion in systole (with leaflets prolapsing behind the imaginary line drawn between the valve hinge points).

The atria

Inspect the atria for relative and absolute size. In healthy individuals the interatrial septum (IAS) usually sits between the two atria, moving gently from side to side throughout the cardiac cycle. If either atrium unilaterally develops elevated pressure then this will cause fixed bowing of the IAS away from the atrium with elevated pressure. Whilst it is of course possible to have lesions on both sides of the heart, as a general rule, if the IAS is fixed bowing towards the right this suggests a predominantly left-heart issue, whilst fixed bowing towards the left may well be a sign of significant right heart disease.

Colour flow Doppler

If performing a scan according to the BSE L1 data set, colour boxes should now be placed over the MV and LA and then the TV and RA to assess for incompetence (*Figs 5.4c and d*).

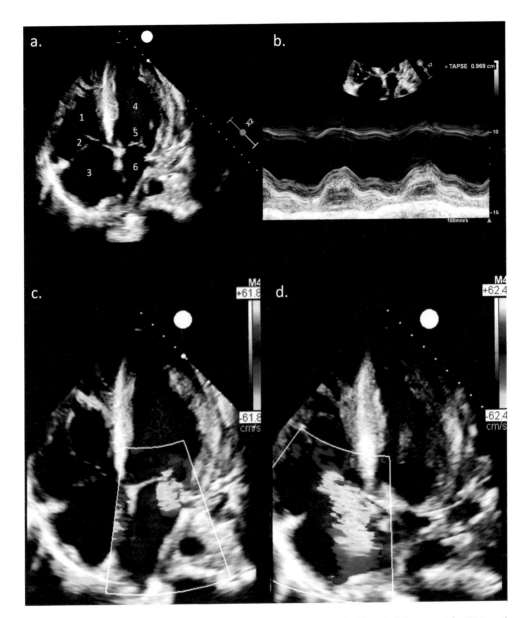

Figure 5.4. (a) Apical four-chamber (A4Ch) view in a patient with dilated right ventricle (RV) and atrium (RA): 1 – RV; 2 – tricuspid valve (TV); 3 – RA; 4 – left ventricle (LV); 5 – mitral valve (MV); 6 – left atrium (LA). (b) M-mode graph used to measure the TAPSE. (c) A4Ch view with colour flow mapping over the MV and LA during ventricular systole, demonstrating mitral regurgitation. (d) A4Ch view with colour flow mapping over the TV and RA during ventricular systole, demonstrating tricuspid regurgitation.

5.5.4 Apical five-chamber (A5Ch)

This view is not included in the FUSIC Heart protocol but does form part of the BSE L1 minimum dataset. Starting from the A4Ch view the probe is tilted such that the imaging sector sweeps further anteriorly bringing the LVOT and AV into view (remember from the PLAX view that the AV sits

anterior to the MV), which may result in loss of some or all of the MV and/
or TV (*Fig. 5.5a*). The principal reason for performing this view in focused
echocardiography is to place a colour box over the LVOT, AV and aortic root
(*Fig. 5.5b*). Here you should examine for turbulent flow within the LVOT
occurring during systole (suggesting LVOT obstruction) and for jets of AR,
originating at the AoV and travelling back into the LV.

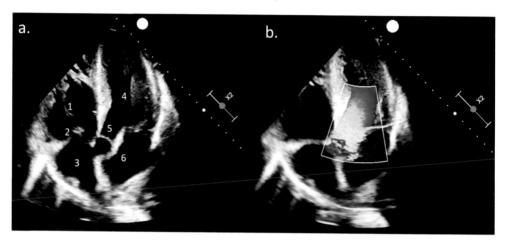

Figure 5.5. (a) Apical five-chamber (A5Ch) view in a patient with a dilated right ventricle (RV) and atrium (RA): 1 – RV; 2 – tricuspid valve; 3 – RA; 4 – left ventricle; 5 – left ventricular outflow tract (LVOT); 6 – left atrium. (b) A5Ch view with colour flow mapping over the aortic valve and LVOT during ventricular systole.

5.5.5 Sub-costal four-chamber (SC4Ch)

The patient is now laid in the supine position. If the patient is awake,
asking them to flex their knees may allow abdominal wall muscles to relax
and improve both your view and their comfort. The probe should be placed
inferior to the xiphisternum, angled up into the anterior chest, with the
orientation towards the patient's left (3 o'clock position). This will produce an
off-axis four-chamber view of the heart, with atria to the left of the image and
ventricles to the right of the image (*Fig. 5.6a*). This view is often challenging
in obese patients or those with elevated intra-abdominal pressure, but can
be surprisingly useful in patients with elevated FRC where hyper-expanded
lungs cause inferior displacement of the diaphragm and subsequently the
heart.

The structures on view here are the same as in the A4Ch view, and a similar
step-wise assessment should be made. This view is useful for detecting
inferior pericardial fluid collections. It is also of particular use during cardiac
arrest, where it can be employed whilst causing minimal disruption to chest
compressions.

5.5.6 The inferior vena cava

Following assessment of cardiac structures, the probe should be rotated 90° anticlockwise (such that the orientation marker is pointing towards the patient's chin, the 12 o'clock position) and the probe lifted such that the imaging sector is pointing towards both the lower thorax (which will appear on the right of the image) and the upper abdomen (which will appear on the left). The probe should then be tilted to identify the IVC in its long-axis running into the RA (*Fig. 5.6b*). When first starting out in focused echocardiography it can be challenging to distinguish between the IVC and the descending aorta (which runs parallel). In general, the descending aorta is slightly to the left of the IVC, slightly deeper and runs posterior to the LV rather than into the RA.

Measurements of the IVC diameter and change in diameter over the course of the respiratory cycle are sometimes used as part of an approach to establish likely response to the administration of intravenous fluids (discussed in *Chapter 24*). These measurements should be taken approximately 2cm inferior to the RA/IVC junction, just below the point at which the confluence of the hepatic veins enters the IVC. Measurement errors here are easy to make, and you should ensure that the measurement is made perpendicular to the IVC walls, and that changes in vessel calibre are not overestimated as the vein moves in and out of the scan plane with respiration.

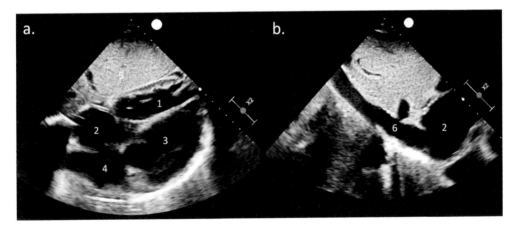

Figure 5.6. (a) Sub-costal four-chamber (SC4Ch) view: 1 – right ventricle; 2 – right atrium (RA); 3 – left ventricle; 4 – left atrium; 5 – liver. (b) Sub-costal IVC view: 2 – RA; 6 – inferior vena cava.

5.5.7 Reporting and communication

Following completion of your study it is important that you record your findings and inform the referring team (assuming that you are not the responsible healthcare provider). Both the ICS and BSE provide reporting templates which allow for binary answers to fundamental questions regarding your findings (for example, 'LV significantly impaired?'; see *Section 4.1*). You should decide at a trust/departmental level which reporting tool you will adopt and use a standardized approach. Regardless of whether you use one of these reporting tools or something bespoke to your own department, there should be a clearly marked area for conclusions. These conclusions should be written in such a way that emphasis is given to immediately life-threatening pathologies (for example, pericardial effusion potentially causing tamponade), so that it should be impossible to read the report without grasping the gravity of the finding.

5.6 Summary

Focused echocardiography is increasingly being utilized throughout critical care. It provides clinicians with the ability to rapidly assess a patient's cardiac function at the bedside and identify several significant pathologies. Its focused nature means more subtle abnormalities may be missed and it is therefore vital that clinicians are aware of their limitations and understand when a more advanced assessment is indicated.

5.7 References

1. Competency-Based Training In Intensive Care Medicine In Europe Syllabus. European Society of Intensive Care Medicine, 2006.

2. FUSIC Accreditation pack – for more information see www.ics.ac.uk/Society/ Learning/Focused_Ultrasound/FUSIC/Society/Learning/FUSIC_Accreditation. aspx

3. British Society of Echocardiography Level 1 pack – for more information see www.bsecho.org/Public/Accreditation/Personal-accreditation/Level-1/Public/ Accreditation/Accreditation-subpages/Personal-accreditation-subpages/Level-1-accreditation.aspx

4. Vieillard-Baron A, Millington SJ, Sanfilippo F, *et al.* (2019) A decade of progress in critical care echocardiography: a narrative review. *Intensive Care Med*, 45:770.

5. Harkness A, Ring L, Augustine DX, *et al.* (2020) Normal reference intervals for cardiac dimensions and function for use in echocardiographic practice: a guideline from the British Society of Echocardiography. *Echo Res Pract*, 7:G1. [published correction appears in *Echo Res Pract*, 2020;7:X1]

6. Rudski LG, Lai WW, Afilalo J, *et al.* (2010) Guidelines for the echocardiographic assessment of the right heart in adults: a report from the American Society of Echocardiography endorsed by the European Association of Echocardiography, a registered branch of the European Society of Cardiology, and the Canadian Society of Echocardiography. *J Am Soc Echocardiogr*, 23:685.

7. Zaidi A, Knight DS, Augustine DX, *et al.* (2020) Echocardiographic assessment of the right heart in adults: a practical guideline from the British Society of Echocardiography. *Echo Res Pract*, 7:G19.

8. Spruijt OA, Di Pasqua MC, Bogaard HJ, *et al.* (2017) Serial assessment of right ventricular systolic function in patients with precapillary pulmonary hypertension using simple echocardiographic parameters: a comparison with cardiac magnetic resonance imaging. *J Cardiol*, 69:182.

CHAPTER 6

FUNDAMENTALS OF TRANSOESOPHAGEAL ECHOCARDIOGRAPHY

Dan Aston

Imaging of the heart and great vessels using ultrasound passed through the oesophageal wall was first developed in the 1970s. Early probes were mounted in a fixed orientation at the tip of rigid endoscopes and could only transmit a single frequency. They were able to examine blood flow in the aorta and structures in the heart using only continuous-wave Doppler and M-mode, but images as we know them today were not possible.

Transoesophageal echocardiography (TOE) technology progressed rapidly. Two-dimensional imaging soon became available and modified flexible gastroscopes started to be used, allowing far greater mobility of the scope and the acquisition of a much wider range of images. Over time, scopes became smaller, probes became more sophisticated and, by the 1980s, TOE had become a well-established diagnostic tool for use both perioperatively and in cardiology practice.

Today, TOE probes are available in several sizes, are highly flexible in different planes, can utilize ultrasound at different frequencies, use pulsed flow and colour flow Doppler, and have omniplane transducers that allow rotation of the scanning angle and the ability to obtain high resolution 2D and 3D images. They are widely used in cardiothoracic surgery, cardiology practice and intensive care.

6.1 Indications, risks and contraindications

Updated recommendations for the use of TOE in three groups of patients (those undergoing cardiac surgery, those undergoing non-cardiac surgery and those on critical care units) were issued by both the European Association of Echocardiography [1] and the American Society of Anesthesiologists (ASA) and Society of Cardiovascular Anesthesiologists (SCA) [2] in 2010. The two sets of recommendations are similar.

For patients without contraindications, who are having thoracic aortic surgery, cardiac surgery involving valvular procedures (including for endocarditis), complex pericardial drainage, or the placement of intracardiac devices, the use of TOE is recommended. The ASA/SCA guidelines also recommend that TOE should be considered in patients having coronary artery bypass grafting (CABG) surgery. TOE may also be required for the pre-operative assessment or diagnosis of infective endocarditis and aortic dissection, or the evaluation of prosthetic valves, and it is used to exclude the presence of thrombus in the left atrial appendage before cardioversion under certain circumstances.

In non-cardiac surgery, TOE is recommended where severe haemodynamic, pulmonary or neurological compromise might result from the nature of the surgery or known cardiovascular pathology. Examples include lung or liver transplantation, major vascular surgery (including that for trauma), neurosurgery where there is a risk of venous thromboembolism, or in patients who have severe coronary or valvular heart disease or those with heart failure. TOE is recommended in critical care settings where there is severe or life-threatening haemodynamic disturbance in patients who are known to have, or are suspected to have, cardiac disease and where assessment using transthoracic echocardiography (TTE) or other imaging modalities is inadequate or not possible in a timely manner. TOE may also be used during investigation for sources of emboli, such as a thrombus in the left atrial appendage.

Complications due to TOE are generally rare. They range from relatively minor problems, such as oral and dental damage and a sore throat, to major injuries including gastrointestinal bleeding, tearing or perforation of the oesophagus or stomach, and even death in rare circumstances. Major complications are generally more common in patients who are under general anaesthesia than for those having the procedure under conscious sedation. For gastro-oesophageal perforation, a variety of studies of different sizes have reported an incidence of between one and nine perforations per 10,000 TOE studies (0.01–0.09%) [3]. A large multi-centre prospective audit conducted over 1 year in the UK and Ireland in 2017 collected data on over 22,000 TOE examinations and found 17 patients who suffered major complications such as palatal injury or gastro-oesophageal perforation – an incidence of 1:1300 (just under 0.08%) [4]. Seven deaths were directly attributed to these complications, which equates to an overall incidence of 1:3000. Moreover, the mortality rate among patients who were unfortunate enough to suffer a major complication was 41%. In comparison, the mortality and perforation rates found in a study of more than 100,000 upper gastrointestinal endoscopies was 0.01% and 0.03%, respectively [1, 5].

With the exception of patient refusal, absolute contraindications to TOE are controversial, and the ASA/SCA taskforce declared that there was insufficient literature to assess which might exist. There was also no consensus among the taskforce regarding what they might be, apart from a history of oesophagectomy or oesophagogastrectomy. The European Association of Echocardiography also does not give a list of contraindications to TOE, but warns that if resistance to insertion of the probe is encountered, the procedure should be abandoned and upper gastrointestinal endoscopy performed before TOE is attempted again. A suggested list of contraindications to TOE is shown in *Table 6.1*[6].

Table 6.1. Suggested absolute and relative contraindications to TOE

Suggested absolute contraindications	Suggested relative contraindications
Known oesophageal pathology: • Stricture • Trauma • Tumour • Mallory–Weiss tear • Diverticulum	Atlanto–axial joint pathology or severe cervical arthritis that restricts cervical mobility
	Prior radiation therapy to the thorax
	Symptomatic hiatus hernia
	History of GI surgery
	Recent upper GI bleeding or oesophageal varices
	Oesophagitis or peptic ulcer disease
Oesophagectomy or oesophagogastrectomy	Thoraco-abdominal aneurysm
Active upper GI bleeding	Barrett's oesophagus
Perforated viscus	History of dysphagia
Recent upper GI surgery	Coagulopathy or thrombocytopenia

Adapted from Table 4 in *J Am Soc Echocardiogr*, 2010;23:1115, with permission from Elsevier. GI – gastrointestinal.

6.2 Transoesophageal versus transthoracic echocardiography

TOE and TTE are complementary, and both are useful in the complete and comprehensive assessment of the heart. Many structures can be visualized or measured equally well using either technique, but there are some differences and some advantages of one over the other under certain circumstances.

The most obvious difference is the position and design of the probes. While TTE is a relatively benign procedure that can be performed with awake patients while causing little or no discomfort and carrying no specific risks, TOE is much more unpleasant and may require sedation or occasionally general anaesthesia. Indeed, the absence of sedation while performing TOE can lead to stress causing hypertension and increased myocardial oxygen demand – both undesirable when cardiovascular instability and pathology are likely.

Since TTE is performed with the probe on the front of the thorax and TOE with the probe behind the heart, it is unsurprising that images of anterior structures (such as the cardiac apex) tend to be of superior quality using TTE while those lying more posteriorly (such as the left atrial appendage, interatrial septum and thoracic aorta) are better seen with TOE. The latter may also provide better images in circumstances such as after cardiac surgery when there are dressings and drains preventing the acquisition of good echocardiographic windows anteriorly. Similarly, in some patients with a high BMI, TOE images may prove to be superior to TTE.

For measurements of cardiac chamber sizes and Doppler interrogation of valves, TTE is considered the more reliable technique, while TOE is needed to thoroughly evaluate the mitral valve and look for signs of endocarditis. TOE provides high resolution images of most of the thoracic aorta but images of the proximal arch and distal ascending aorta are better visualized using TTE, albeit at a lower resolution [7].

6.3 TOE imaging planes and probe movements

In the main, echocardiography provides 2D representations of 3D anatomy. Therefore, to properly assess a structure, it must be viewed from several different angles and the TOE probe and transducer are designed to allow a wide range of imaging views.

The probe can be advanced into the oesophagus to view deeper and more inferior structures or withdrawn to view superior structures. It can be rotated clockwise (to the patient's right) or anticlockwise (to the patient's left). The tip of the probe can be ante- or retroflexed using the large wheel on the probe handle and can be flexed to the left or right using the smaller wheel. These wheels can be fixed in place to hold the probe tip at a particular angle using the flexion control lock, although this should not be used while the probe is being advanced or withdrawn due to the risk of pulling a flexed probe through the relatively narrow oesophagus. Similarly, unless the probe is in the stomach large flexion movements should be avoided to reduce the risk of oesophageal damage.

While transducers on most ultrasound probes in clinical practice produce an ultrasound beam as a sector that is at a fixed orientation and parallel with the long axis of the probe, the sector produced by the omniplane transducer on the TOE probe can be rotated using buttons on the probe handle or a switch on the machine. The angle of the beam is displayed on the ultrasound image. An angle of 0° means that the beam is orientated transversely and is perpendicular to the long axis of the probe and to the oesophagus. If the angle is rotated to 90°, the beam is orientated longitudinally and is parallel with the probe and oesophagus. At 180°, the ultrasound beam is in the same plane as at 0°, but the image is inverted left-to-right.

6.4 Imaging modes and Doppler

Ultrasound can be used to examine the anatomy of interest in several different ways, as outlined in the following sections.

6.4.1 A-mode

A-mode, or amplitude mode, is an old-fashioned way of using ultrasound that is now obsolete. Pulses of ultrasound are emitted from a single piezoelectric crystal to form a narrow beam. As the ultrasound passes into the body and hits different structures, some of the energy is reflected back to the transducer. The output in A-mode is displayed as a line graph showing a series of spikes, with the amplitude (strength) of the reflected signal on the y-axis and the time taken for the reflected signal to return to the transducer on the x-axis. Since the velocity of ultrasound in soft tissue is known, the x-axis more usually shows the distance travelled by the ultrasound pulse, and therefore the depth of the structure from which it was reflected.

6.4.2 B-mode / two-dimensional mode

In B-mode, or brightness mode, the output is displayed as a horizontal line of dots. The x-axis still represents the depth of the signal, but the amplitude is displayed by the brightness of the dot. A very strong signal is shown as bright white whereas a weak signal is shown as a dim shade of grey.

Transducers capable of producing 2D images consist of more than one piezoelectric crystal arranged in a line. Each crystal produces ultrasound pulses that together form a broader beam than that produced by a single crystal alone. The output can then be displayed in the same way as B-mode, but with many lines of dots stitched together, each corresponding to a different crystal. When the lines of dots are viewed together, they form a 2D image.

As ultrasound pulses are transmitted and received, each line is updated, and the image can move. The speed at which the lines update depends on how often the ultrasound pulses are sent out (known as the pulse repetition frequency). The speed at which the whole image is updated is known as the frame rate, and this dictates the temporal resolution. The typical frame rate for 2D ultrasound is 30–60 frames per second and this provides a high enough temporal resolution to see the majority of cardiac movement.

6.4.3 M-mode

If accurate measurement of very short periods of time is required, M-mode provides a higher temporal resolution than 2D imaging. This is achieved using a single scan line again (as in B-mode) but plotting depth (represented by the line of dots) against time. Because only one scan line needs to be updated per 'frame', instead of the many that make up a whole 2D image, the update rate can be much faster (up to 2000 times per second).

6.4.4 Doppler

The Doppler principle states that the frequency of an energy wave rises as the source of the wave moves towards the receiver and falls as it moves away [8]. The magnitude of the change in frequency is proportional to the velocity of the source relative to the receiver. If a sound wave is transmitted at a known frequency and the reflected wave has a different ('shifted') frequency, then the velocity of the reflector can be calculated. To detect a Doppler shift, the energy wave must ideally be parallel with the direction of travel of the reflector. The greater the angle between the wave and the direction of travel, the more the measured Doppler shift will underestimate the velocity.

In TOE this principle can be used to calculate the velocity of blood flow through the heart and great vessels. This technique can be used in several ways, as follows.

- In continuous wave Doppler (CWD) one crystal continuously transmits ultrasound at a constant frequency down a single scan line, and another crystal continuously receives reflected signals. The Doppler shifts are then used to calculate the velocity of structures along the scan line and this is plotted as velocity against time. CWD can measure very high velocities but is unable to pinpoint their source other than somewhere along the scan line.

- In pulsed wave Doppler (PWD), a single crystal transmits a pulse and then waits for the reflected signal before transmitting the next pulse. Using this method, the exact distance of the reflector along the scan line can be measured and its location pinpointed. However, PWD cannot be used to measure velocities above approximately 150–200cm/sec due to the development of aliasing artefact when the measured velocity becomes too fast relative to the ultrasound pulse repetition frequency. PWD is also plotted as velocity against time. Neither CWD nor PWD produce an 'image' because they utilize single scan lines.

- Colour flow Doppler (CFD) is a form of PWD where the Doppler shift is coded as a colour and superimposed onto a 2D ultrasound image. An area of the 2D image is selected for CFD. Any movement in the area with a positive Doppler shift (i.e. travelling towards the transducer) is coloured red while anything with a negative shift is coloured blue. Like PWD, CFD is also subject to aliasing.

- In most measurements made using Doppler, it is the movement and velocity of the blood that is of interest, but in tissue Doppler imaging (TDI), it is the movement of tissue structures in the heart that is being studied. This motion is of a much slower velocity than that of blood and the signals are of higher intensity. TDI is similar to PWD in that it can be used to look at specific parts of the heart (e.g. the lateral and medial aspects of the mitral annulus as part of the assessment of diastolic function).

6.4.5 Three-dimensional mode

3D images of static structures can be obtained following the acquisition of a series of 2D images which are then stitched together using 'offline' software. Similarly, if the ECG is used to take pictures at the same point in the cardiac cycle, then static 3D images of objects that are moving can be obtained. However, this technique relies on sinus rhythm and no ectopic beats being present to work well. Alternatively, live, real-time 3D imaging is possible using advanced transducers which transmit ultrasound pulses from a phased array. CFD can also be superimposed onto 3D images, although the frame rate can be slow.

3D echocardiography is used in tandem with 2D images. It can be particularly useful in the assessment of the mitral valve to diagnose the exact mechanism of regurgitation, and during closure of atrial septal defects.

6.5 Standard views

To ensure that all the relevant structures are assessed properly and consistently, it is important that there is a standardized method of performing a TOE examination. In 1999, the American Society of Echocardiography and the SCA produced a set of guidelines for performing a comprehensive TOE examination [9]. They recommend imaging using 20 standard views (see *Figures 6.1–6.3* for all of these core views and *Table 6.2* for a list of left ventricle wall segments). A further eight views were added in updated guidelines in 2013 [10].

Table 6.2. Left ventricle wall segments

Number	Segment	Showing
1	Basal anterior	LAD
2	Basal anteroseptal	LAD
3	Basal interseptal	RCA
4	Basal inferior	RCA
5	Basal inferolateral	RCA/Cx
6	Basal anterolateral	LAD/Cx
7	Mid-anterior	LAD
8	Mid-anteroseptal	LAD
9	Mid-inferoseptal	LAD/RCA
10	Mid-inferior	RCA
11	Mid-inferolateral	RCA/Cx
12	Mid-anterolateral	LAD/Cx
13	Apical anterior	LAD
14	Apical septal	LAD
15	Apical inferior	RCA/LAD
16	Apical lateral	LAD/Cx
17	Apical cap	LAD

The views are broadly divided into the position of the probe in the oesophagus or stomach; upper or mid-oesophageal and trans-gastric or deep trans-gastric. A combination of views and imaging modes is needed to examine different structures. A description of a small number of the structures that can be examined using TOE follows.

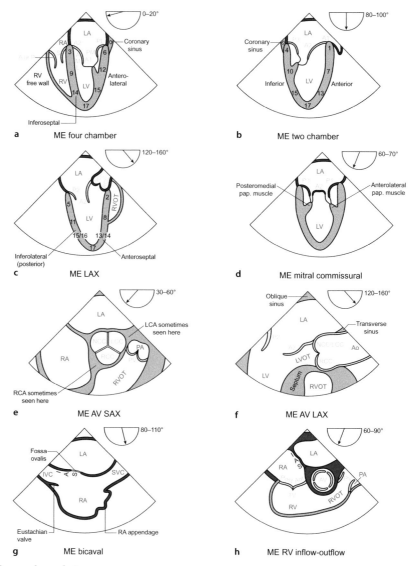

Figure 6.1. Mid-oesophageal views.

(a) Mid-oesophageal four-chamber. (b) Mid-oesophageal mitral commissural. (c) Mid-oesophageal two chamber. (d) Mid-oesophageal long-axis. (e) Mid-oesophageal short-axis aortic valve. (f) Mid-oesophageal long-axis aortic valve. (g) Mid-oesophageal bicaval. (h) Mid-oesophageal right ventricular inflow–outflow.

Ao – aorta; Asc Ao – Ascending aorta; IVC – inferior vena cava; LA – left atrium; LAA – left atrial appendage; LV – left ventricle; LVOT – left ventricular outflow tract; PA – pulmonary artery; RA – right atrium; RPA – right pulmonary artery; RV – right ventricle; RVOT – right ventricular outflow tract; SVC – superior vena cava.

Based on images first published in *J Am Soc Echocardiogr*, 2011:23:1115, with permission from Elsevier.

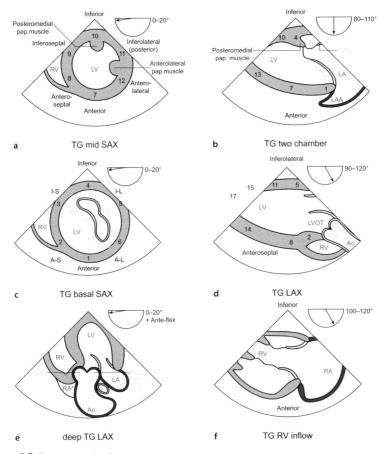

Figure 6.2. Trans-gastric views.

(a) Trans-gastric mid short-axis. (b) Trans-gastric basal short-axis. (c) Deep trans-gastric long-axis. (d) Trans-gastric long-axis. (e) Trans-gastric two-chamber. (f) Trans-gastric mitral valve inflow.

Ao – aorta; Asc Ao – Ascending aorta; IVC – inferior vena cava; LA – left atrium; LAA – left atrial appendage; LV – left ventricle; LVOT – left ventricular outflow tract; PA – pulmonary artery; RA – right atrium; RPA – right pulmonary artery; RV – right ventricle; RVOT – right ventricular outflow tract; SVC – superior vena cava.

Based on images first published in *J Am Soc Echocardiogr*, 2011:23:1115, with permission from Elsevier.

6.5.1 Mitral valve

The mid-oesophageal (ME) four-chamber (0°), commissural (60°), two-chamber (90°), and long-axis (LAX, 120°) views, along with the trans-gastric (TG) basal short-axis (SAX, 0°) and two-chamber (90°) views provide a comprehensive study of the MV.

Starting with the mid-oesophageal four-chamber (ME4Ch) view, the anterior MV leaflet (AMVL) is seen on the left of the image while the posterior leaflet (PMVL) is seen on the right. As the angle is increased past the commissural view, this arrangement is reversed so that in the mid-oesophageal two-chamber (ME2Ch) and mid-oesophageal long-axis (MELAX) views, the AMVL is on the right and the PMVL is on the left.

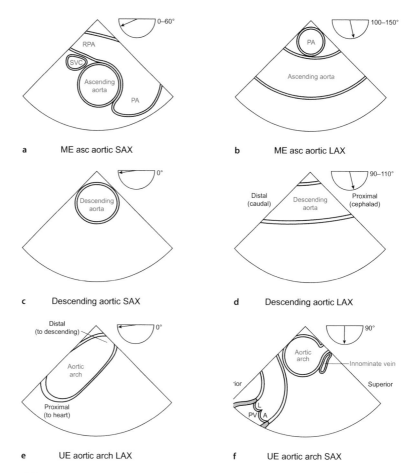

Figure 6.3. Views of the aorta.
(a) Mid-oesophageal ascending aorta short-axis. (b) Mid-oesophageal ascending aorta long-axis.
(c) Descending aorta short-axis. (d) Descending aorta long-axis. (e) Upper oesophageal aortic arch
short-axis. (f) Upper oesophageal aortic arch long-axis.
Ao – aorta; Asc Ao – Ascending aorta; IVC – inferior vena cava; LA – left atrium; LAA – left atrial
appendage; LV – left ventricle; LVOT – left ventricular outflow tract; PA – pulmonary artery; RA –
right atrium; RPA – right pulmonary artery; RV – right ventricle; RVOT – right ventricular outflow
tract; SVC – superior vena cava.
Based on images first published in *J Am Soc Echocardiogr*, 2011:23:1115, with permission from Elsevier.

At the level of the ME4Ch view, the scan sector bisects the valve so that the
middle thirds of the leaflets (A2 and P2) are visible. Withdrawing the probe
by 2–3cm to show the mid-oesophageal five-chamber (ME5Ch) view brings
the lateral thirds of the leaflets (A1 and P1) into view, while advancing the
probe by 2–3cm from the ME4Ch view allows examination of the medial
thirds of the leaflets (A3 and P3).

The TG basal SAX view shows an *en face* ('fish mouth') view of the MV,
allowing further evaluation of the annulus or leaflet pathology, while the TG
two-chamber (TG2Ch) view reveals good views of the papillary muscles and
chordae tendineae.

Doppler measurements through the MV are easy in the ME views because the direction of blood flow through the valve is parallel with the ultrasound beam. Doppler measurements through the MV are not possible in the TG2Ch view as the direction of blood flow is perpendicular to the ultrasound beam.

6.5.2 Aortic valve

The ME AV SAX view is found by withdrawing the probe by 3–5cm from the ME4Ch view and increasing the scan angle to 30°. This view shows a good cross-sectional image of the three aortic valve cusps and CFD can be used to visualize regurgitation if it is present. In the MELAX view, the AV is seen to the right of the MV, with either the non-coronary cusp (NCC) or left coronary cusp (LCC) above and the right coronary cusp (RCC) below. Measurements of the diameters of the left ventricular outflow tract (LVOT), aortic annulus, and aortic root structures can also be made in this view.

Using the deep trans-gastric (DTG) view at 0° or the TGLAX view at 90–100°, the LVOT and aortic valve are seen at the bottom left or right of the image, respectively. Both views allow alignment of a scan line with the direction of blood flow through the LVOT, which is not possible in the ME views. CWD can therefore be used to measure velocities through the LVOT and AV using these views.

6.5.3 Left ventricle

The left ventricle (LV) can be seen best in the ME4Ch, ME2Ch, MELAX, TG basal and mid SAX, and TG2Ch views. For echocardiographic purposes, the LV is divided into four parts: basal, mid, apical and apex. The basal and mid sections are each divided into six segments: anterior, anteroseptal, anterolateral, inferior, inferoseptal and inferolateral. The apical section is divided into four segments: anterior, septal, inferior and lateral. The apex is a single segment in its own right, making a total of 17 segments.

Each segment should be seen to thicken during systole and fully relax during diastole. Ischaemia of the LV wall produces characteristic abnormalities of movement in different segments, depending on which coronary artery has inadequate flow.

6.5.4 Right ventricle and tricuspid valve

There are four main views used for examining the right ventricle (RV). These are the ME4Ch, ME RV inflow–outflow (60°), TG RV inflow (110°) and TG mid SAX (0°) views.

The RV should have thin walls and the cavity should appear small in comparison with the more muscular LV. The septal wall bulges into the RV cavity, leaving the latter with a crescent shape in short-axis. The wall becomes less trabeculated from the inflow to the outflow portions, and the crista supraventricularis (a muscular ridge that contains the proximal right coronary artery) is found between the two. A moderator band that contains the right bundle branch of the cardiac conducting tissue is often seen stretching from the septum to the anterior RV free wall.

The tricuspid valve in the ME4Ch view has the septal leaflet on the right of the image and either the anterior or posterior leaflet on the left. Advancing or withdrawing the probe a short distance may help fully visualize the valve. In the ME RV inflow–outflow view, the anterior leaflet of the valve is seen on the right while the posterior leaflet is seen on the left.

The pulmonary valve can also be seen on the ME RV inflow–outflow view, but the image is usually unclear since it is an anterior structure and a considerable distance from the TOE probe. It is better visualized using TTE.

6.5.5 Atria, interatrial septum and vena cavae

The left atrium (LA) can be seen in all the ME views, being the chamber closest to the probe and it has been called 'the window into the heart' for this reason. The atria and interatrial septum are best seen in the ME4Ch and ME bicaval (90°) views and, as the name suggests, the vena cavae are also visible in the latter with the SVC on the right of the image and the IVC on the left.

Several structures may be visible in the right atrium (RA) which are normal but which can sometimes be mistaken for pathological processes such as thrombi or vegetations. The crista terminalis is a ridge of muscle seen at the junction of the RA and SVC. The eustachian valve is a remnant of part of the foetal circulation that directed blood from the IVC across the foramen ovale and into the LA. It is sometimes seen at the junction of the IVC and the RA. The Thebesian valve is sometimes seen at the opening of the coronary sinus as it drains into the RA, and the sinus itself can be mistaken for other structures if it is enlarged, as is seen when there are anatomical variants such as a persistent left-sided SVC or anomalous pulmonary venous drainage. The Chiari network is a fine, filamentous mesh or lattice-like structure that is seen to randomly move around in the RA. It is attached to the eustachian or Thebesian valve and is a remnant of a valve of the embryonic sinus venosus.

Similarly, in the LA, a band of tissue separating the left atrial appendage (LAA) from the left upper pulmonary vein is sometimes mistaken for a thrombus and is known as the coumarin ridge.

The ME bicaval view allows reasonable alignment for CFD interrogation of the interatrial septum to help identify or study atrial septal defects (ASDs). However, the presence of an ASD cannot be ruled out using this technique alone.

6.5.6 Aorta

With the exception of the distal ascending aorta and the proximal aortic arch, which are hidden from view behind the trachea and left main bronchus, the whole thoracic aorta can be visualized using TOE. Images of the proximal ascending aorta may not be completely clear since it is an anterior structure and therefore lies a reasonable distance from the probe.

The aortic root and first part of the ascending aorta are seen in the MELAX view along with the AV, and these structures are also seen in the ME AV SAX view with the pulmonary arteries. The probe must be withdrawn from here and the aorta followed as it elongates into the arch in the upper oesophageal arch long-axis (UE arch LAX) view. It can then be followed as it descends behind the heart and passes posteriorly to the oesophagus, meaning the probe must be rotated by 180° so that the transducer faces the patient's back. The aorta can then be viewed in long- or short-axis by changing the scan angle between 0° and 90°, respectively, and Doppler measurements can be made. Pathology that can be identified in the aorta on TOE includes atheroma and dissection.

6.6 Measurements possible with TOE

There are many measurements that can be made using TOE to assess cardiac anatomy and function [11]. Below are just a small number of examples.

6.6.1 Left ventricular function

LV systolic function can be assessed in several ways. Fractional shortening gives an estimation of systolic function. In the TG mid SAX view, the diameter of the LV at end-systole is compared with that at end-diastole. A change in diameter of 27–45% is considered normal. The absolute diameters are also used to indicate the size of the LV cavity, with a normal end-diastolic diameter being gender dependent (often quoted in the region of 3.3–5.5cm) and over 7.5cm indicating severe dilation. A similar method is fractional area change (FAC), where the 2D area of the LV cavity is measured instead of the diameter, and the change expressed as a percentage.

Probably the most accepted approach used to assess LV systolic function is Simpson's biplane method. In this method, the ME4Ch and ME2Ch views are used because they are perpendicular to each other. In each view, the LV is split up into a series of 20 discs stacked on top of each other. The shape of each disc is assumed to be an ellipse with the two diameters taken from the perpendicular views. The sum of the volumes of all the discs is used to estimate the overall volume of the LV. The change in volume between end-systole and end-diastole is expressed as a percentage of the end-diastolic volume and is known as the ejection fraction (EF); normal EF is considered to be 55–75%.

The LV filling pressure is used to assess LV diastolic function. This is estimated using a combination of the transmitral inflow and pulmonary venous pulse wave Doppler waveforms and TDI of the mitral annulus. The LA volume index and peak velocity of a tricuspid regurgitation jet are also used [12].

6.6.2 Right ventricular function

A normal RV is used for propelling blood through the low-resistance pulmonary circulation. It is thin walled and low pressure in comparison with the LV. An increase in venous return is accommodated without a significant rise in RV pressure due to its high compliance, but the chamber is sensitive to changes in afterload and a sudden rise in pulmonary vascular resistance can lead to RV failure. In comparison, the function of the LV is relatively independent of afterload.

RV function can be assessed using the ME4Ch and TG mid SAX views. The size of the RV chamber, especially in comparison with the LV, is helpful in its evaluation. Fractional shortening and FAC can be used in the same way as for the LV. The end-diastolic area of the RV can be up to 60% of the LV area before it is judged to be dilated [13].

As the RV contracts during systole, its longitudinal axis shortens. The distance that the base of the RV moves towards the apex can be measured and correlates well with overall RV function. The distance from the lateral aspect of the tricuspid valve annulus to the RV apex in systole is subtracted from the same distance in diastole to give the tricuspid annular plane systolic excursion (TAPSE) and should be approximately 2–2.5cm with normal RV function.

6.6.3 Aortic valve

In the DTG or TG LAX views, a single scan line can be placed in parallel with blood flow as it leaves the LV through the LVOT and AV. Using CWD, the velocity of the blood through these structures can be measured. If the AV is stenotic, the blood must accelerate as it passes through the narrowing to maintain the same flow as through the wide LVOT. Therefore, comparison of the velocity of the blood through the LVOT with that through the AV can be used to help grade the severity of the stenosis. An LVOT:AV velocity ratio of less than 0.25 is indicative of severe aortic stenosis.

6.7 Haemodynamic calculations using TOE-derived parameters

There is a large array of calculations that can be performed using TOE in the assessment of cardiac structure and function. Many of these are carried out by the machine without any input from the operator. However, it is important to understand how the machine arrives at its conclusions. Here are examples of some principles that are commonly used in echocardiographic calculations.

6.7.1 The Bernoulli equation

The Bernoulli equation describes the relationship between the velocity of a fluid through a system to its pressure:

$$P_1 - P_2 = \frac{4\rho(V_2^2 - V_1^2)}{2}$$

where P = pressure ρ = density and V = velocity. By adding a conversion factor and assuming that the density of blood $(\rho) = 1$, this can be simplified to:

$$P_1 - P_2 = 4(V_2^2 - V_1^2)$$

Flow across an orifice only occurs if there is a pressure difference across it. As fluid passes through the orifice down its pressure gradient, the velocity of the fluid increases. The increase in velocity is inversely proportional to the orifice area. If the starting pressure (P_1) and the starting velocity (V_1) are taken to be very small, the equation can be further simplified to:

$$\Delta P = 4V^2$$

Using this equation, a peak velocity of 4m/sec measured across a stenotic AV equates to a peak pressure gradient of 64mmHg (as the pressure and velocity through the LVOT are both low), which is consistent with severe aortic stenosis.

In another example, if the peak velocity of a tricuspid regurgitation jet is measured to be 2.5m/sec and the right atrial pressure is 8mmHg, then the pressure gradient between the right ventricular systolic pressure (RVSP) and the right atrium pressure (RVSP – RAP) is equal to $(4 \times 2.5^2) = 25$mmHg. Therefore, the RVSP is equal to $25 + 8 = 33$mmHg. If the pulmonary valve is normal, then pulmonary artery systolic pressure is approximately equal to RVSP.

6.7.2 Velocity–time integrals (VTI)

The area under a graph of velocity (cm/sec) against time (sec) gives the distance (cm) travelled. If the graph is square, then the distance is simply velocity × time. However, velocity does not change instantaneously, and a period of acceleration and deceleration occurs. To take this into account, velocity is integrated with time to give distance. This is known as the VTI.

If this is applied to blood flow, then the distance the blood travels multiplied by the cross-sectional area of the vessel through which it is travelling gives the volume flowing. The VTI can be obtained by passing a CWD scan line through the LVOT and measuring the velocity during a single cardiac cycle. Therefore, if the measured LVOT VTI is 16cm and the diameter of the LVOT is measured as 2.2cm, then stroke volume is equal to:

$$SV = VTI_{LVOT} \cdot \pi \cdot r^2$$

Stroke volume is therefore 60.8ml and cardiac output is calculated by multiplying this by heart rate. The cardiac index can then be calculated by dividing by body surface area.

6.7.3 The continuity equation

Provided that nothing is added or removed, flow into a system must equal the flow out of it. For example, at steady state, cardiac output and venous return must be equal. Stroke volume through the MV must equal stroke volume through the AV or, in the presence of a VSD, stroke volume through the MV must equal stroke volume through the AV plus the volume lost via the VSD.

This can be used to calculate the area of a stenotic AV. If VTIs are measured using the TGLAX view through the LVOT and AV, and the diameter of the LVOT is measured in the MELAX view, then the AV cross-sectional area (CSA) can be calculated. This is because flow through the LVOT must equal flow through the aortic valve. Therefore:

$$CSA_{LVOT} \cdot VTI_{LVOT} = CSA_{AV} \cdot VTI_{AV}$$

So, if the LVOT diameter is 1.8cm, the VTI_{LVOT} is 20cm and the VTI_{AV} is 75cm, then the AV area is:

$$\pi \cdot \left(\frac{1.8}{2}\right)^2 \cdot 20 = CSA_{AV} \cdot 75$$

Therefore, the AV area is 0.68cm², and corresponds to severe aortic stenosis.

An incompetent AV can also be assessed using this equation. As mentioned above, the stroke volume through the MV must be equal to the stroke volume through the AV. If there is aortic regurgitation, then trans-mitral stroke volume must equal aortic ejected volume minus the regurgitant volume. Therefore:

$$Regurgitant\ volume = (CSA_{LVOT} \cdot VTI_{LVOT}) - (CSA_{MV} \cdot VTI_{MV})$$

Similarly, the regurgitant fraction is the proportion of blood ejected from the AV in systole which then regurgitates back through it in diastole:

$$Regurgitant\ fraction = \frac{Regurgitant\ volume}{Stroke\ volume}$$

6.8 TOE training

As TOE becomes more widely used, it is important that standards are adopted to ensure that patients gain the maximum benefit of the technology. One aspect of this is the guidelines and recommendations that are issued by learned societies regarding how comprehensive examinations should be performed. However, another aspect of maintaining standards is ensuring a minimum level of training occurs.

There are currently three main routes to accrediting in comprehensive TOE: the US National Board of Echocardiography, the European Association of Echocardiography / European Association of Cardiothoracic Anaesthesiologists, and the British Society of Echocardiography all offer formal certification and accreditation pathways. Most involve a combination of written examination and a logbook of experience.

A novel accreditation pathway in basic TOE was recently introduced by the ICS in collaboration with the Association of Anaesthetists of Great Britain and Ireland. This pathway, called Focused Transoesophageal Echocardiography, is best suited for intensive care specialists who wish to advance their echocardiography skills beyond TTE [14].

6.9 Summary

TOE is widely used in cardiac surgery and increasingly in critical care. It possesses several advantages over TTE, including an often-superior image quality. However, its associated limitations and comparatively increased risk profile should be acknowledged. A thorough understanding of underlying principles and structured training is key to allowing clinicians to use TOE to its full potential and for patients to benefit from this.

6.10 References

1. Flachskampf FA, Badano L, Daniel WG, *et al.* (2010) *Recommendations for transoesophageal echocardiography: update 2010. Eur J Echocardiogr*, 11:557.

2. American Society of Anaesthesiologists and Society of Cardiovascular Anesthesiologists Task Force on Transesophageal Echocardiography (2010) Practice guidelines for perioperative transesophageal echocardiography. *Anesthesiology*, 112:1084.

3. Hauser ND, Swanevelder J (2018) Transoesophageal echocardiography (TOE): contra-indications, complications and safety of perioperative TOE. *Echo Res Pract*, 5:R101.

4. Ramalingam G, Choi S-W, Agarwal S, *et al.* (2020) Complications related to peri-operative transoesophageal echocardiography – a one-year prospective national audit by the Association of Cardiothoracic Anaesthesia and Critical Care. *Anaesthesia*, 75: 21.

5. Jenssen C, Faiss S, Nurnberg D (2008) Complications of endoscopic ultrasound and endoscopic ultrasound-guided interventions – results of a survey among German centers. *Z Gastroenterol*, 46:1177.

6. Hilberath JN, Oates DA, Shernan SK, *et al.* (2010) Safety of transesophageal echocardiography. *J Am Soc Echocardiogr*, 23:1115.

7. Shillcutt SK, Bick JS (2013) Echo didactics: a comparison of basic transthoracic and transesophageal echocardiography views in the perioperative setting. *Anesth Analg*, 116:1231.

8. Edelman SK (2012) *Understanding Ultrasound Physics: fundamentals and exam review*, 4th ed. ESP Ultrasound, Houston.

9. Shanewise JS, Cheung AT, Aronson S, *et al.* (1999) ASE/SCA guidelines for performing a comprehensive intraoperative multiplane transesophageal echocardiography examination. *J Am Soc Echocardiogr*, 12:884.

10. Hahn RT, Abraham T, Adams MS, *et al.* (2013) Guidelines for performing a comprehensive transesophageal echocardiographic examination. *J Am Soc Echocardiogr,* 26:921.

11. Sidebotham D, Merry AF, Legget ME, Edwards ML (2011) *Practical Perioperative Transesophageal Echocardiography with Critical Care Echocardiography,* 2nd ed. Elsevier Saunders.

12. Nagueh SF, Smiseth OA, Appleton CP, *et al.* (2016) Recommendations for the evaluation of left ventricular diastolic function by echocardiography. *Eur Heart J Cardiovasc Imaging,* 17:1321.

13. Feneck RO, Kneeshaw J, Ranucci M (2010) *Core Topics in Transesophageal Echocardiography,* 1st ed. Cambridge University Press.

14. fTOE Accreditation pathway: www.ics.ac.uk/Society/Learning/focused_TOE.aspx

CHAPTER 7

ASSESSMENT OF THE LEFT HEART

Filippo Sanfilippo, Luigi La Via & Gianluca Paternoster

The most common approach used to quantify the size and function of heart chambers is echocardiography. Its main advantages are its ability to noninvasively and reliably estimate cardiac chamber size, its unique ability to provide real-time images with repeated measurements and follow-up, and the availability and portability of echocardiography machines. The guidelines for assessment of chambers' size and function suggest that echocardiography measurements should be averaged over several cardiac cycles to account for inter-beat variability. For patients in normal sinus rhythm this should be averaged over three beats whilst for those in atrial fibrillation this should be over five beats.

When performing an echocardiographic exam, measurements of size and function are usually classified as normal or abnormal. When an abnormality is detected, operators should try to estimate/calculate its degree, commonly classified as mild, moderate or severe.

7.1 Left ventricle: anatomy, blood supply and size

7.1.1 Left ventricular anatomy

The left ventricle (LV) is one of the four heart chambers. It has a conical shape with an antero-inferiorly projecting apex and is longer and has thicker walls than the right ventricle (RV). It is separated from the RV by the interventricular septum, which is concave in shape (the LV bulges into the RV). The ventricular wall is thickest at the LV base and thins by just 1–2mm at the apex. Oxygenated blood flows from the left atrium (LA) through the mitral valve (MV) into the LV cavity during diastole and it is pumped through the LV outflow tract (LVOT) and the aortic valve (AV) into the aorta. The LVOT is the region of the LV lying between the anterior cusp of the MV and the interventricular septum. Within the LV cavity, there are two papillary muscles (anterolateral and posteromedial) attached to the MV via chordae.

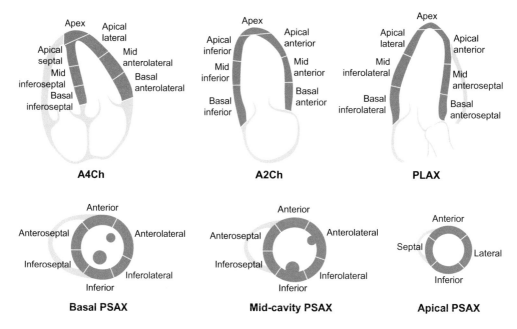

Figure 7.1. An illustration highlighting the 17 left ventricular segments.

A cardiac segmentation model is now widely used for the description of disease-affected myocardial territories and wall function. There are 17 segments that have a reasonably consistent vascular supply from one of the three main coronary arteries, the right (RCA), the left anterior descending (LAD) and the circumflex (Cx), although anatomic variations are described.

In its long-axis, the LV is divided into equal thirds named basal, mid and apical, accounting for 16 segments, while the tip of the apex forms a separate segment (the final 17th segment) (*Fig. 7.1*).

The basal and mid LV thirds are divided into six segments each, while the apical region is separated in four segments. Dividing these LV thirds in short-axis allows rings to be described, which by convention are numbered counterclockwise starting from the anterior segment.

7.1.2 Left ventricular blood supply

The arterial blood supply of the LV is provided by the RCA and by the left main stem (LMS) which splits into the LAD and Cx a few centimetres after its origin. Coronary arterial dominance is defined by the vessel giving origin to the posterior descending artery (PDA), which provides blood supply to the inferior third of the interventricular septum. In most cases (80–85%) hearts are right dominant (PDA supplied by the RCA), whilst the remaining are either left dominant (PDA from Cx or LAD) or co-dominant. Regardless of dominance, most of the LV myocardium and of the interventricular septum receives blood supply from the LAD. Of note, the LAD supplies most of the papillary muscles' territory, and therefore LAD ischaemia may lead to papillary muscle rupture with resultant massive MV regurgitation.

The LV's venous drainage may be directed towards the coronary sinus (great and middle cardiac veins and posterior vein) or to a minor extent directly into the LV cavity (via tiny myocardial Thebesian veins).

7.1.3 Left ventricular size

The normal shape of the LV is symmetrical with two equal short axes (circular in shape) and a long axis running from the base (MV annulus) to the apex. Diagnoses of LV dilation or hypertrophy often provides the first clue of the underlying pathology.

Assessment of LV size includes the calculation of linear internal dimensions and volumes, which are reported both at end-diastole and end-systole. These can then be used to derive parameters of global LV function. Importantly, chamber measurement should be reported indexed to body surface area (BSA) to allow comparison among individuals with different body sizes [1].

Linear and volumetric measurements

Linear internal measurements of the LV walls are performed in the parasternal long-axis view, with values obtained perpendicular to the LV long-axis just

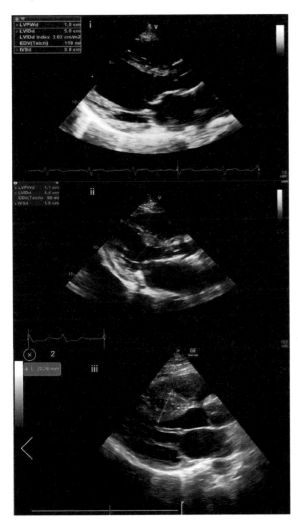

Figure 7.2. Left ventricular wall thickness measurements. (i) Normal LV wall thickness (IVSd 0.8cm, LVPWd 1.0cm). (ii) Hypertrophic LV (IVSd 1.5cm, LVPWd 1.1cm). (iii) Severe left ventricular hypertrophy in a patient with hypertrophic cardiomyopathy.

EDV – end-diastolic volume; IVSd – interventricular septum thickness at end-diastole; LVIDd – left ventricular internal diameter end-diastole; LVPWd – left ventricular posterior wall at end-diastole.

below the level of the MV. Linear measurements are also recommended for LV wall thickness, allowing identification of any hypertrophy present. Calipers are positioned at the interface between myocardial wall and cavity and the interface between wall and pericardium (*Fig. 7.2*). Normal LV wall thickness ranges from 0.6 to 1.0cm (men) or from 0.6 to 0.9cm (women) [1].

When calculating the size of the LV chamber, it is better to use volumetric measurements. These are usually made by tracing the interface between compacted myocardium and the LV cavity. Indeed, LV volume calculations derived from linear measurements are not always accurate. Tracing to obtain volumetric measurements is performed in the apical four- and/or two-chamber views, closing the contour at the MV level with a straight line. LV length is the distance between the middle of such line and the most distant point of the tracing contour. Volume calculations are mostly performed with the biplane method of disc summation (the modified Simpson's rule). An alternative method when apical endocardial definition precludes accurate tracing is the area–length (A–L) method, which assumes a bullet shape of the LV. Current guidelines recommend assessing LV size by means of volumes using the biplane method of disc summation technique (*Figs 7.3 and 7.4*). Normal values for LV chamber size are also referred to in the context of gender and the healthy population (i.e. in the absence of hypertension, diabetes, hypercholesterolaemia, a body mass index >30 kg/m², elevated creatinine levels) [1,2].

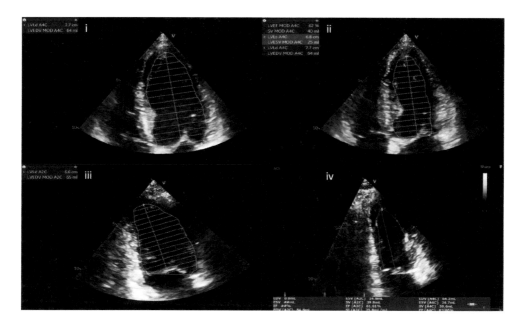

Figure 7.3. Simpson's biplane of normal left ventricular systolic function (ejection fraction of 62%). (i) Left ventricular end-diastolic volume (LVEDV) in apical four-chamber (A4C). (ii) Left ventricular end-systolic volume (LVESV) in A4C. (iii) Left ventricular end-diastolic volume in apical two-chamber (A2C). (iv) Left ventricular end-systolic volume in A2C. EF – ejection fraction; SV – stroke volume.

7.2 The cardiac cycle and assessment of LV systolic function

7.2.1 The cardiac cycle made easy

Understanding the pressure–volume relationship of the LV is essential when estimating LV performance. LV contraction starts when rising cytosol calcium levels stimulate the overlap of actin and myosin filaments resulting in sarcomere shortening. When myocytes are activated, the LV begins to contract with a resultant rise in intraventricular pressure. During the so-called isovolumetric contraction (the period between MV closure and AV opening), the LV pressure continues to rise and, when it exceeds intra-aortic pressure, the AV opens, and the stroke volume is generated. During the ejection phase, the LV pressure peaks and then starts to decrease with AV closure when LV pressure drops below the aortic pressure. At this time, calcium is taken up by the sarcoplasmic reticulum and myofilaments begin the relaxation phase. Initially, because both the MV and AV are closed, the LV volume remains constant (isovolumetric relaxation), but as a consequence of a further drop in LV pressure, the MV opens and LV filling occurs due to a positive LA to LV gradient. In patients with sinus rhythm, this first period (known as early diastolic filling) is followed by a second one occurring after LA contraction (that restores a positive LA to LV gradient). Readers are invited to look at LV pressure–volume loops describing the above-mentioned phases.

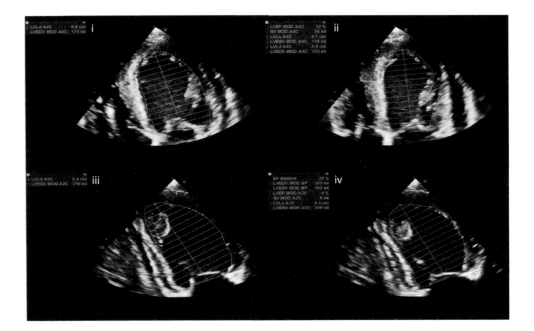

Figure 7.4. Simpson's biplane of severe left ventricular systolic failure (ejection fraction of 20%) with left ventricular thrombus. (i) Left ventricular end-diastolic volume (LVEDV) in apical four-chamber (A4C). (ii) Left ventricular end-systolic volume (LVESV) in A4C. (iii) Left ventricular end-diastolic volume in apical two-chamber (A2C). (iv) Left ventricular end-systolic volume in A2C. EF – ejection fraction.

7.2.2 Assessing global left ventricular systolic function

The assessment of LV systolic function is often performed qualitatively and relies heavily on the ability of the echocardiographer. It must be preliminarily noted that LV systolic performance is a function of intrinsic myocardial contractility and of the LV loading conditions. All parameters commonly used to evaluate LV systolic performance are load dependent, both in terms of preload (wall stress at end-diastole) and afterload (load against which the ventricle ejects). Thus, the load dependence of parameters used to evaluate LV systolic function means that under the same degree of intrinsic LV contractility their indexes will vary.

The echocardiographic assessment of global LV function is usually obtained as the difference between the end-diastolic and end-systolic values of an echocardiographic parameter, divided by its end-diastolic value. End-diastole is defined as either the first frame after MV closure or the frame with the largest LV dimension/volume measurement. Similarly, end-systole is best defined as either the first frame after AV closure or the frame with the smallest cardiac dimension. EF is the most commonly used parameter, and it is calculated with the following formula:

$$EF\ (\%) = ((EDV-ESV)/EDV) \times 100$$

where EDV and ESV stand for end-diastolic and end-systolic volume, respectively. The normal range and the abnormal values cut-offs are only slightly different between genders. Other possible measurements to estimate global LV systolic function rely on the evaluation of diameters (fractional shortening, see *Fig. 7.5*) or areas (fractional area change) measured at end-diastole and end-systole. However, deriving global LV function from linear measurements is problematic when there are regional LV wall motion abnormalities (e.g. due to coronary disease or conduction abnormalities).

Importantly, the evaluation of LV systolic function can also be performed by visual approximation (so called 'eyeballing'), especially in the context of point-of-care echocardiography for diagnosis and treatment. This approach has been proven to be reliable, especially when performed by a skilled operator, and provides a rapid and accurate assessment. For instance, in the case of critical care echocardiography, an error of 5% of LVEF is unlikely to significantly change the therapeutic approach.

Newer echocardiographic techniques, such as tissue Doppler imaging (TDI) and speckle tracking echocardiography (STE), allow other methods of LV assessment to be used.

TDI assessment is a modified pulsed-wave Doppler analysis with high amplitude and low velocity, the opposite settings to those used in assessment of blood flow (high velocity and low amplitude). Regarding the evaluation of LV systolic function, the TDI *s'* wave can be measured at the basal MV annulus level, both in the septal and lateral myocardial region. The annular velocity in systole has some correlation with LVEF. Normal values are usually

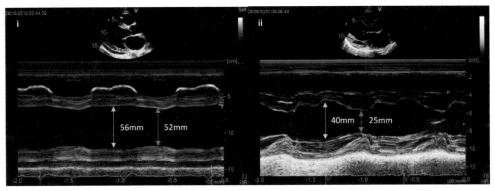

Figure 7.5. Fractional shortening in (i) an LV with severely impaired systolic function (fractional shortening 7%) and (ii) an LV with normal systolic function (fractional shortening 37.5%).

around 8cm/sec (septal region) and 10cm/sec (lateral region). The main advantage of TDI is its ease of use, even in those with challenging cardiac windows (it does not require visualization of the full LV chamber). However, TDI is angle dependent and measures function only in the specific segment where the sample volume is placed. Moreover, whilst cardiology machines are usually equipped with TDI software, only a few intensive care machines have TDI software available [1,2].

Regarding STE, the global longitudinal strain (GLS) is the most adopted parameter because it describes overall LV performance (not only systolic function) in terms of change in the length of the LV in a certain direction related to the baseline length [3].

$$GLS\ (\%) = \frac{(myocardial\ length\ systole - myocardial\ length\ diastole)}{myocardial\ length\ in\ diastole}$$

Therefore, as the LV shortens during contraction, the GLS values are negative by definition and the more negative the GLS, the better the LV performance. GLS is a sensitive early predictor of LV dysfunction and correlates with prognosis in several chronic and acute conditions. This is particularly important because GLS often shows LV impairment before a drop in LVEF is seen. GLS measures the shortening of the myocardium as a correlate to contractility, in contrast to the EF which measures volumes. Disadvantages of GLS include its angle dependency and the availability of software on echocardiography machines. For further information on TDI, strain and strain rate readers are referred elsewhere [3].

Other parameters describing LV systolic function are:

- **MAPSE (mitral annular plane systolic excursion):** an M-mode derived marker of longitudinal LV systolic function. The M-mode is placed in an A4Ch view on the lateral MV annulus, measuring its excursion. A MAPSE above 1cm is considered normal. If the lateral wall of the LV is visualized, MAPSE is easy and feasible.

- **dp/dt:** a parameter describing myocardial isovolumetric contraction measuring the velocity of pressure rise within the LV during systole. The faster the rise, the better the LV is at building up pressure. This rise is captured by the MV regurgitation profile with CWD. Velocity is measured at two different time points (1m/sec and 3m/sec) which represents the time it takes to develop a pressure rise of 32mmHg. This requires a good MV regurgitation profile, and it may be reduced in the presence of dyssynchrony. Normal values are above 1000mmHg/sec; a value below 500mmHg/sec is indicative of severe LV systolic dysfunction.

- **The Tei index, or myocardial performance index (MPI):** a parameter for global LV (and RV) performance. It consists of three variables derived from pulsed wave Doppler. The formula is:

$$MPI = (IVCT + IVRT) / ET$$

where IVCT = isovolumetric contraction time, IVRT = isovolumetric relaxation time and ET = ejection time. The normal value is approximately 0.39. In the presence of LV systolic dysfunction, IVCT increases and ET decreases, with a consequential increase in the Tei index. An MPI over 0.5 would certainly be considered abnormal.

7.2.3 Assessing regional LV systolic function

Regional systolic function evaluation is crucial because acute and chronic ischaemic episodes have repercussions on LV wall thickness and on the contraction of myocardial segments. Regional wall motion abnormalities (RWMAs) describe kinetic alterations in LV wall motion during systole with a possible effect on overall cardiac function. RWMAs are usually categorized not only by their severity but also by their regional pattern to identify a coronary territory responsible for the abnormality. Systolic function of a cardiac segment is usually classified as normokinetic (normal wall thickening and systolic inward movement), hypokinetic (mild or severe and characterized by reduced thickening and inward movement), akinetic (absent wall thickening and systolic movement), or dyskinetic (absent wall thickening and systolic outward movements) (see *Table 7.1*). Any RWMA should be interpreted in the context of the patient's signs and symptoms, their clinical history, ECG and laboratory findings.

Table 7.1. Summary of methods for assessing left ventricular systolic function

LV global function		LV regional function	
Evaluation	**LVEF**	**LV wall thickening**	**Systolic movement**
Hyperkinetic		Normal	Inward
Normal	≥55%	Mild hypokinesia	Inward
Borderline low	50–54%	Severe hypokinesia	Inward
Impaired	36–49%	Akinesia	None
Severely impaired	≤35%	Dyskinesia	Outward

7.3 Left ventricular diastolic assessment: new guidelines and issues in intensive care

From a physiological standpoint, the LV of subjects with normal diastolic function fills smoothly in the presence of low LA pressures and thus with a relatively small LA–LV gradient (the order of a few mmHg). The corresponding echocardiographic appearance of the trans-MV blood flow is represented by a dominant early (E) filling wave over the atrial (A, or late) filling wave. The presence of a normal LA pressure is an important prerequisite for normal LV diastolic function; indeed, the increase of LA pressure (as a pathological response to the increased LV stiffness and reduced compliance) usually restores the LA–LV gradient and the relationship between E and A filling waves. This is one of the reasons behind the complexity of LV diastolic function assessment.

The most recent American Society of Echocardiography and European Association of Cardiovascular Imaging (ASE/EACVI) joint recommendations have made substantial changes to the diagnosis and grading of LV diastolic dysfunction. One of the achievements of these guidelines is the simplification of the approach with a reduction in the number of parameters used [4,5]. For the diagnosis of LV diastolic dysfunction, the recent guidelines recommend an assessment based mainly on four variables (*Fig. 7.6*):

- tricuspid regurgitation (TR) jet velocity
- LA volume
- *e'* wave
- *E/e'* ratio.

The *e'* and *E/e'* ratio are two TDI-derived parameters that measure longitudinal fibre lengthening during early diastole at the MV level. As with the TDI *s'* wave used for the evaluation of LV systolic function, the *e'* maximal velocity can be measured at the septal and lateral MV annulus level and reflects the LV relaxation rate. A septal velocity below 7cm/sec and/or lateral velocity below 10cm/sec would be considered abnormal [4–6].

The *E/e'* ratio also accounts for the blood flow velocity through the MV. This variable has aroused great interest due to its correlation with LV filling pressures. An *E/e'* ratio above 13–15 (depending on whether the *e'* lateral or septal is used) is associated with pulmonary arterial occlusion pressures of >18mmHg [5–8].

Transthoracic echocardiography (TTE) is the recommended approach for measuring LA size. Although the LA is in the far-field, TTE is preferred over transoesophageal echocardiography (TOE) because with TOE the entire LA does not fit in the echo image sector. LA size should be measured when the chamber is at its greatest size. The most widely used linear dimension is the LA antero-posterior measurement in the parasternal long-axis view but it may not be accurate. Measurement of LA volume is recommended over linear dimensions because LA volume has shown strong prognostic value in several cardiac diseases. Measurement of LA volume should be made with the disc summation algorithm, like that used for LV volume. The A–L method is an alternative approach, but it is less accurate.

Care should be taken to avoid foreshortening of the LA, keeping in mind that the axes of the LA and LV frequently lie in different planes. The probe should be tilted throughout the image to identify the LA at its greatest size. The pulmonary veins and the LA appendage should be excluded when tracing the area of the LA. The cut-off for abnormal LA size is 34ml/m².

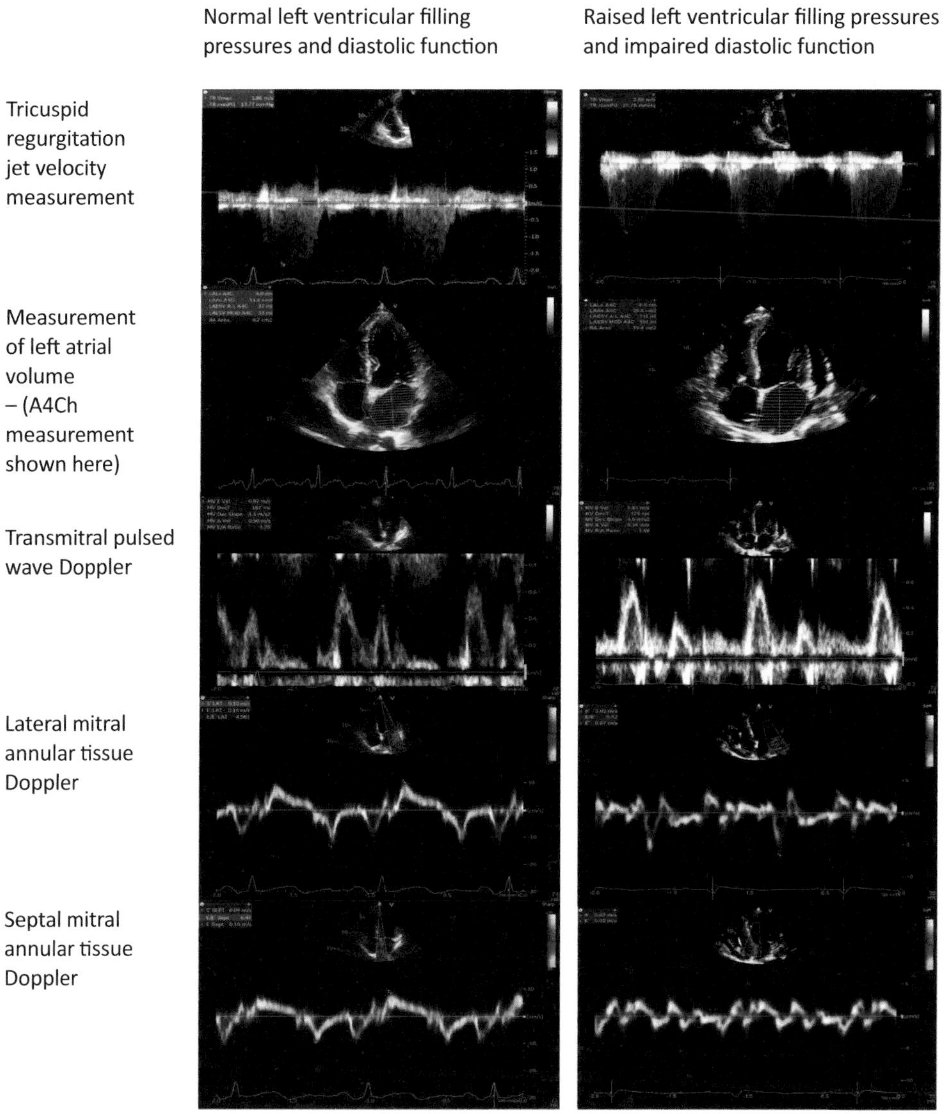

Figure 7.6. Examples of assessments of left ventricular diastolic function. It is important to acknowledge that assessment of diastolic function is not a dichotomous technique, but the culmination of multiple findings. A4Ch – apical four-chamber view.

The TR jet velocity is measured with CWD through the TV with the peak velocity recorded. The TR jet velocity is commonly used to estimate the pulmonary artery systolic pressure using the simplified Bernoulli equation:

$$\Delta P=4v^2$$

where ΔP = pressure difference and v = velocity.

This allows for the translation of a velocity into a pressure gradient. The abnormal cut-off for TR jet velocity is 2.8cm/sec, which represents a ΔP between the RV and right atrium of 31–32mmHg, in turn suggesting pulmonary hypertension [4–6].

In patients with normal LV systolic function, diagnosis of LV diastolic dysfunction is made when abnormalities are detected in more than half of the above four parameters that are measurable (for example, a patient may not have a TR jet).

Another significant acknowledgment made in the new LV diastolic assessment guidelines is that patients with abnormal LV systolic function, by definition, also have impaired myocardial relaxation. Thus, echocardiographic examination should focus on the assessment of LV filling pressures and diastolic dysfunction grade.

Once the echocardiographer has diagnosed LV diastolic dysfunction, the next step is grading of the dysfunction. Grading requires further information from the trans-MV blood flow pattern (E/A ratio and E wave velocity) [4,5]. The following three filling patterns of LV diastolic dysfunction are described by the guidelines:

- E/A <0.8 with E wave velocity below 50cm/sec suggests LV diastolic dysfunction **grade 1**.

- E wave velocity greater than 50cm/sec or E/A ratio is 0.8–2.0, the echocardiographer should evaluate E/e' ratio, LA size and TR jet velocity. If at least two are abnormal, then LV diastolic dysfunction **grade 2** is made (otherwise it will be classified as grade 1).

- E/A >2.0 suggests LV diastolic dysfunction **grade 3**.

Importantly, all the variables described above for the diagnosis and grading of LV diastolic function are obtained from a single view (the A4Ch).

The prevalence of LV diastolic dysfunction in the community is around four times higher than LV systolic dysfunction. Importantly, around half of patients presenting to the Emergency Department with signs of pulmonary oedema have normal LV systolic function and no significant MV abnormalities, suggesting LV diastolic dysfunction as a significant contributor. Similarly, half of hospitalizations for heart failure are made on the basis of preserved LVEF. The importance of LV diastolic dysfunction is becoming increasingly recognized in the perioperative setting and in critically ill patients, but the assessment of LV diastolic dysfunction is challenging and the guidelines' authors themselves state *"...the guidelines are not necessarily applicable to children or in the perioperative setting"*. This should be no surprise because during the perioperative period (and even more so in the context of critical illness) patients undergo mechanical ventilation (with significant influence on RV function and on pulmonary vascular resistances, thus influencing TR jet velocity) and are exposed to drugs with vasoactive effects with frequent fluctuations from hyper- to hypovolaemia (perioperative fasting, fluid shift, haemorrhage, sepsis, etc.). Moreover, increasing levels of positive end-expiratory pressure (PEEP) may reduce septal and lateral *e'* values, suggesting possible impaired LV relaxation [8–10].

Finally, when evaluating acute changes in LV diastolic function, the assessment of LA size is probably unreliable because although its remodelling can happen over a relatively short period of time (i.e. months) it cannot occur over hours to days, as in the case of critically ill patients [6–8].

7.4 Assessment of the left atrium

Assessment of the LA, often referred to as the 'HbA1c of the heart' or the 'barometer of the LV', forms an important part of the assessment of the left heart. Changes in the dimensions of the LA reflect the chronicity of the underlying condition, either due to increased intra-chamber pressure or increased flow.

The LA has three important functions:

- **as a reservoir** during LV systole and the isovolumetric relaxation phase; this represents LA relaxation and compliance

- **as a conduit** during early LV filling; this depends on LV diastolic function, suction and stiffness

- **as a booster** of LV filling, due to its own contraction in the late diastolic stage (this is lost in patients with atrial fibrillation); this represents intrinsic LA contractility and LV diastolic compliance.

There are several causes of LA dilatation, including: mitral valve disease, dilated cardiomyopathy, LV diastolic dysfunction, atrial fibrillation or flutter, and high-output states (e.g. anaemia).

Assessment of the LA is performed through the combination of a visual assessment and specific measurements (e.g. diameter, area, volume and volume index). To begin with, an overall eyeballing of the LA for size, any intrachamber tumours or thrombi, presence of any spontaneous contrast ('smoke' in patients with longstanding AF or mitral valve disease), and position of the interatrial septum (e.g. bulging of the septum throughout the cardiac cycle) is made.

The TTE imaging windows that allow for the best visualization of the LA include:

- PLAX view (measurement of LA diameter)
- PSAX at aortic level
- A4Ch, A2Ch and A3Ch
- SC4Ch.

The LA appendage is best visualized using TOE imaging. However, it can be visualized using TTE in some individuals using the A2Ch view.

7.4.1 Left atrial dimensions

Measurement of the following LA dimensions should be part of a comprehensive TTE exam.

LA diameter
This is measured using the PLAX view at the end-systolic frame. Any value >40mm is abnormal.

LA size and volume
Volumetric methods are preferred and account for variations in the shape of the LA. This can be done by two methods:

1. Area–length method
2. Simpson's biplane.

For both methods, tracing of the endocardial border of the atrium is required in end-systole just before the mitral valve opens. Simpson's rule uses the methods of discs (similar to LV volumes) and requires tracing of the endocardial border of the atrium in the A4Ch and A2Ch views.

It is worth noting that an LA volume index (indexed to body surface area) above 34ml/m^2 is an independent risk factor for death, ischaemic stroke, heart failure and onset of atrial fibrillation.

LA strain
More recently, LA myocardial deformation or strain using speckle tracking has provided more insights into LA structural and functional parameters. LA strain is superior to LA volume index in certain circumstances; for example, when predicting the need for surgery in patients with mitral regurgitation.

In summary, assessment of the LA is an essential part of any focused or comprehensive TTE exam, with a raised LA volume index acting as an important independent predictor of outcomes. LA strain is increasing being used as its ability to provide insights into LA structure and function are recognized.

7.5 Assessment of cardiac output and fluid responsiveness

7.5.1 Echocardiographic assessment of cardiac output

Cardiac output (CO) is the product of stroke volume (SV) and heart rate (HR). CO is a measure of flow (volume/time) and in healthy subjects the SV is about 70ml and the HR about 75bpm (CO about 5–5.5L/min).

Echocardiography allows the measurement of CO with estimation of the SV via the continuity equation; in the absence of valve dysfunction or shunting, this equation states that blood flow is constant throughout the heart chambers. For a given chamber, such an assumption will be invalid if there is significant valve regurgitation or if valve flow is influenced by a shunt. Another caveat is the presence of valvular stenosis, where pre-stenotic accelerated flow signals must be avoided.

SV calculations are performed by measuring forward flow across the LVOT, the AV, or, less commonly, the RVOT. Other methods have been proposed for measuring trans-mitral and trans-tricuspid flows, but the complex dynamic geometry of the orifices of these valves makes them unreliable, and assessment through the LVOT is the most adopted technique. If TTE is performed, the LVOT size is measured in the parasternal long-axis view, whilst if TOE is performed this measurement is performed in the mid-

Left ventricular outflow tract diameter measurement

Left ventricular outflow tract VTI measurement

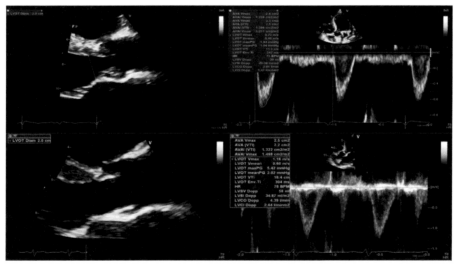

Figure 7.7. Left ventricular outflow tract (LVOT) velocity–time integral (VTI) measurements with stroke volume (SV) and cardiac output (CO) calculation. Top row – severely impaired left ventricular systolic function (VTI = 11.3cm, SV = 39ml, CO = 2.85L/min); bottom row – normal left ventricular systolic function (VTI = 18.4cm, SV = 58ml, CO = 4.39L/min). VTI – velocity–time integral.

oesophageal long axis (MELAX) view. In both cases, it is recommended to zoom in on the LVOT and the AV to maximize measurement accuracy. LVOT diameter should be measured in mid-systole, 3–10mm from the AV plane.

To obtain the SV, the size of the LVOT must be integrated with the assessment of the velocity–time integral (VTI) performed via measurement of the area under the curve of a pulsed wave Doppler spectrum placed at the LVOT level, as shown in *Figure 7.7* (A3Ch or A5Ch for the TTE route, or TGLAX or deep TG view in TOE). The VTI represents the length of a column of blood moving through the region sampled each heartbeat. VTI is expressed in units of distance (cm). The SV is finally obtained by multiplying the VTI by the area of the sampling site (LVOT), which is calculated using the formula for the area of a circle (πr^2, where r = the radius of the LVOT). The diameter should be measured at the same location as the VTI is sampled and particular attention should be made to accurately measure the LVOT diameter, because any error is squared (πr^2). Once the SV is calculated, its value is multiplied by the HR to obtain the CO.

Although indirect estimation of CO can also be performed by evaluating LV volumes at end-systole and end-diastole, this method is less reliable.

7.5.2 Assessing fluid responsiveness

Fluid responsiveness (FR) is a physiological condition whereby an increase in LV preload leads to an increase in CO. Conversely, fluid unresponsiveness defines a situation whereby further volume administration does not produce a significant increase in CO; in this latter case, the plateau of the Frank–Starling curve has been reached and fluid administration is unlikely to be indicated and may in fact be harmful.

Prediction of FR is a crucial step in the perioperative clinical evaluation and in the assessment of critically ill patients. The importance of predicting the haemodynamic response to fluid administration is based on the need to balance optimal organ perfusion with avoidance of unnecessary and potentially harmful fluid infusions. Indeed, an increase in the cardiac filling pressures and the consequent rise in hydrostatic pressures will contribute to the risk of pulmonary and/or systemic oedema. Importantly, fluid overload is associated with increased morbidity and mortality in critically ill and surgical patients. As a general principle, reaching supra-physiological CO values with the use of fluids or inotropic drugs has been proved to be harmful.

In light of this, the ability to predict FR and measure CO is crucial in order to identify those patients who might benefit from fluid loading, and those in whom the use of inotropes/vasopressors may be more beneficial. A patient is usually considered to have responded to a fluid challenge if there is an increase in CO of at least 10–15%, with the latter being the most adopted cut-off. Of note, variations in mean arterial pressure are not sensitive enough to describe changes in organ perfusion and oxygen delivery, and CO should be the clinical target [9,10].

Monitoring SV (and CO) is possible with advanced haemodynamic monitoring devices and/or with echocardiography. The latter has the advantages of being non-invasive and repeatable, but it does not provide continuous information. Another important consideration is that CO measurement with echocardiography will probably have some degree of inter- and intra-observer variability [9,10].

7.6 Summary

Echocardiography provides a rapid, non-invasive and effective way to assess both systolic and diastolic left ventricular function. The depth of this assessment may depend on the clinical question, time constraints and the ability of the user. It also allows the clinician to make dynamic assessments of cardiac function and rapidly evaluate the effects of interventions, such as a fluid bolus, at the bedside.

7.7 References

1.   Lang RM, Badano LP, Mor-Avi V, *et al.* (2015) Recommendations for cardiac chamber quantification by echocardiography in adults. *Eur Heart J Cardiovasc Imaging,* 16:233.

2.   Sanfilippo F, Huang S, Messina A, *et al.* (2021) Systolic dysfunction as evaluated by tissue Doppler imaging echocardiography and mortality in septic patients: a systematic review and meta-analysis. *J Crit Care,* 62:256.

3.   Sanfilippo F, Corredor C, Fletcher N, *et al.* (2018) Left ventricular systolic function evaluated by strain echocardiography and relationship with mortality in patients with severe sepsis or septic shock: a systematic review and meta-analysis. *Crit Care,* 22:183.

4.   Nagueh SF, Smiseth OA, Appleton CP, *et al.* (2016) Recommendations for the evaluation of left ventricular diastolic function by echocardiography. *Eur Heart J Cardiovasc Imaging,* 17:1321.

5.   Nagueh SF, Appleton CP, Gillebert TC, *et al.* (2009) Recommendations for the evaluation of left ventricular diastolic function by echocardiography. *Eur J Echocardiogr,* 10:165.

6.   Sanfilippo F, Scolletta S, Morelli A, Vieillard-Baron A (2018) Practical approach to diastolic dysfunction in light of the new guidelines and clinical applications in the operating room and in the intensive care. *Ann Intensive Care,* 8:100.

7.   Sanfilippo F, Corredor C, Fletcher N, *et al.* (2015) Diastolic dysfunction and mortality in septic patients: a systematic review and meta-analysis. *Intensive Care Med,* 41:1004. Erratum in: *Intensive Care Med,* 41:1178.

8.   Sanfilippo F, Corredor C, Arcadipane A, *et al.* (2017) Tissue Doppler assessment of diastolic function and relationship with mortality in critically ill septic patients: a systematic review and meta-analysis. *Br J Anaesth,* 119:583.

9.   Sanfilippo F, Di Falco D, Noto A, *et al.* (2021) Association of weaning failure from mechanical ventilation with transthoracic echocardiography parameters: a systematic review and meta-analysis. *Br J Anaesth,* 126:319.

10. Vieillard–Baron A, Millington SJ, *et al.* (2019) A decade of progress in critical care echocardiography: a narrative review. *Intensive Care Med,* 45:770.

CHAPTER 8

ASSESSMENT OF THE RIGHT HEART

Sam Clark

The right ventricle (RV), once described as the forgotten ventricle, has become increasingly important to cardiologists and intensivists alike. Originally thought to be a passive conduit, it is now understood to be a refined and complex vessel for pumping blood through the lungs, whilst adapting to significant changes in volume returning from the systemic circulation.

The adaptations required to achieve these tasks mean that assumptions based on Starling principles developed for the left-sided circulation are not always a perfect fit. This complexity has brought significant challenges in understanding its function, especially in the context of critical care with mechanical ventilation and other influences on the lungs present. At the same time, echocardiography has become the primary assessment tool for assessing, diagnosing and monitoring the right heart and RV haemodynamics.

Successful imaging and interpretation of either a focused or complete echocardiogram requires understanding of the anatomical and physiological differences between the right and left heart, alongside knowledge of the echocardiographic techniques used. Accordingly, this chapter covers three main areas: anatomy and physiology, imaging and the impact of pathology.

8.1 Right ventricular anatomy

The RV is located more anteriorly than the left ventricle (LV) almost immediately retrograde to the sternum. It shares its septal wall with the LV and is bound by the tricuspid valve upstream, pulmonary valve downstream and the pericardium circumferentially. The RV has a pyramidal triangular structure that wraps around the conical LV, giving it a crescent shaped cross-section (*Fig. 8.1*). It can be divided into three main areas:

1. The inlet, with tricuspid valve, chordae tendineae, and papillary muscles.

2. The trabeculated apical myocardium.

3. The infundibulum, which forms the smooth wall RV outflow tract (RVOT) proximal to the pulmonary valve.

The RV is inherently thin walled (3–5mm) with the fibres arranged into an inner longitudinal layer and a circumferential outer layer [1]. There is no third outer longitudinal layer, unlike the LV. The inner layer is responsible for longitudinal contraction and the outer layer for the inward/radial contraction. Importantly, these circumferential fibres maintain a continuum with the circumferential fibres of the left side. This means that the interaction between the ventricles is not solely through the pericardium, with both contributing to each other's function (or dysfunction).

Features distinguishing the RV from the LV include thick trabeculations, three or more papillary muscles, no fibrous continuity between the inlet and outlet valves and a moderator band. The multiple trabeculations can make several measurements challenging.

The RV arterial supply comes from three vessels:

1. **The right coronary artery** – suppling most of the free wall and base of septum.

2. **The posterior descending artery** – suppling the inferoposterior wall.

3. **The left anterior descending artery** – supplying most of the anterior septum.

Right ventricular coronary flow is dependent on the difference between RV pressure and aortic pressure (and the thickness of the muscle if RV hypertrophy is present). Therefore, under normal circumstances, coronary flow takes places during diastole and systole [2].

Acute RV failure with pressure overload can significantly reduce the coronary perfusion pressure, reducing systolic flow and promoting ischaemia. Chronic

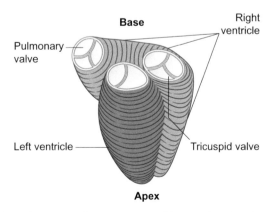

Figure 8.1. A three-dimensional visualization of the RV showing the orientation of the RV with regard to the LV.

pulmonary hypertension with RV hypertrophy can lead to a similar pattern with reduced flow in systole due to increased wall tension with increased contractility.

8.2 Right ventricular physiology and function

In order to assess, understand and distinguish normal RV function from pathological changes, it is important to understand the physiology of RV contraction, RV/LV interactions, RV haemodynamics and cardiopulmonary interactions. This allows the clinical echocardiographer to balance the different findings and possible interventions in pathological states affecting the cardiopulmonary system.

8.2.1 Right ventricular contraction

The RV is approximately 10–15% larger than the LV with a mass 3–6 times smaller, and its cardiac output must match the LV in a non-pathological state. Due to the lower afterload of the pulmonary circulation compared to the systemic circulation, the RV maintains this output with only ~25% of the stroke work of the LV.

Right ventricular contraction is peristaltic and takes place over a relatively prolonged period of time, lasting approximately 25–50msec from the first to the last phase [3]. These phases of RV contraction are:

1. Right ventricular circumferential oblique outer fibres contract, tightening the free wall and initiating its inward movement.

2. Longitudinal (inner) fibres contract, starting from the apex, pulling the tricuspid annulus towards the apex causing RV shortening. The inner anatomical location of the fibres allows them to shorten further than the outer radial fibres. Consequently, longitudinal contraction contributes more to RV contraction than LV contraction.

3. Left ventricular contraction occurs, which has two effects: traction on the RV free wall leading to inward movement and bulging of the septum causing compression of the RV cavity. Left ventricular co-ordinated contraction has been shown to contribute to 20–40% of RV contraction. As a result, LV impairment or RV dominance of septal contraction significantly affects the function of both ventricles.

4. Expansion of the infundibulum just prior to infundibular contraction.

5. The 'hangout' phenomenon, where the low pressures found in the wide vascular beds promote continued flow into the pulmonary circulation from the RV.

8.2.2 Right ventricular haemodynamics

Right ventricular function is a product of similar components to LV function: preload, contractility and afterload. In the case of the RV, these relate to systemic venous return, RV contraction (see above), afterload and pericardial compliance. However, there are important differences [4].

1. **Right ventricular preload:** the RV's thin wall works best at low pressures, making it sensitive to changes in preload and giving it the ability to significantly increase its volume relatively rapidly. This sensitivity to preload becomes more obvious with exaggerated changes in intrathoracic pressure or with an increase in pericardial pressure (e.g. cardiac tamponade).

2. **Right ventricular contractility:** described above.

3. **Right ventricular afterload:** unlike the systemic circulation, the pulmonary vascular bed is, under normal circumstances, a high capacity, low pressure system or in other words a low afterload high volume system. This combination gives rise to physiological differences in RV pressure–volume loops and the RV pressure over time graph. These include a lower but earlier peak RV pressure, a relative absence of isovolumetric contraction and relaxation, and the 'hangout' phenomenon (*Fig. 8.2*). The RV pressure–volume loops demonstrate a shallow end-systolic slope, with small changes in end-systolic pressure corresponding to large changes in end-systolic volume. The RV is therefore highly sensitive to changes in afterload, with even small changes potentially compromising RV stroke volume (SV). Afterload can therefore be considered the most influential factor of the three.

   Often thought of simply as pulmonary artery pressure, perhaps a better conceptualization for RV afterload is the stress on the RV wall

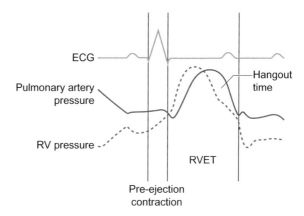

Figure 8.2. The hangout phenomenon. Comparing ECG (blue line) with pulmonary artery pressure (middle pink line) and right ventricular pressure (dotted pink line). Right ventricular pressure is lower than pulmonary artery pressure from mid to late systole. RV – right ventricle; RVET – right ventricular ejection time.

during systole. These stresses are a complex combination of resistive and pulsatile factors. Factors known to influence RV afterload beyond a direct effect on pulmonary vascular resistance (PVR) include retrograde flow caused by the anatomy of the lung vascular bed and, more relevant in echocardiographic terms, increases in left atrial pressure (LAP) or left ventricular end-diastolic pressure (LVEDP). Additionally, its complex pyramidal shape means that the afterload is not evenly distributed across the RV wall and thus the RV is prone to distort and fail in a non-uniform manner [5].

8.2.3 Right ventricular interdependence

The final piece in the RV function puzzle is ventricular interdependence. It is created through the combination of multiple factors, namely: the structure and function of the pericardium, the continuum of the muscle fibres and sharing of a ventricular wall, the serial nature of the blood flow from right to left, the difference in pressure between the two ventricles, and the contrasting impacts intrathoracic pressures can have on each ventricle. The fibrous pericardium prevents a rapid expansion in heart size so changes in pressure and volume in one ventricle will impact the other ventricle. It is a complex topic and a full up-to-date review was published by Naeije and Badagliacca [6].

It can be divided into two categories: serial versus parallel and diastolic versus systolic interdependence. Serial interdependence is part of normal physiology and refers to variations in RV and LV output that occur due to changes in cardiopulmonary interactions and are described in *Section 8.2.4*. Parallel interdependence is a pathological process that can be either diastolic or systolic.

Diastolic interdependence or volume overload occurs when the increase in volume of one ventricle has a direct relationship with the diastolic compliance of the other ventricle (see *Fig. 8.3*). This is seen on echocardiography as increased septal flattening throughout diastole as the increase in right ventricular end-diastolic volume (RVEDV) and right ventricular end-diastolic pressure (RVEDP) outweighs the simultaneous increase in LVEDP, leading to a reduction in LVEDV. *Figure 8.3* also demonstrates how a rapid increase in LVEDP (e.g. secondary to acute severe aortic regurgitation) can reduce RVEDV, though this is less visually overt on echocardiography.

Systolic interdependence or pressure overload occurs with a rapid increase in afterload. Increased afterload results in an increase in the strength and length of RV contraction to compensate for the reduction in cardiac output. This leads to an increase in pressure within the RV that 'overrides' the pressure in the LV towards the end of systole. Septal flattening occurs at end-systole and the beginning of diastole until the pressures re-equilibrate towards the middle of diastole. The combination of an impaired RV SV and compression of the LV at end-systole and early-diastole can lead to a small underfilled LV that is often hyperdynamic.

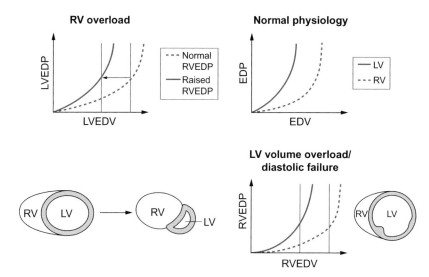

Figure 8.3. Demonstration of ventricular interdependence. LV – left ventricle; LVEDP – left ventricular end-diastolic volume; RV – right ventricle; RVEDP – right ventricular end-diastolic pressure; RVEDV – right ventricular end-diastolic volume.

8.2.4 Cardiopulmonary interactions

The anatomical location and layout of the heart and lungs has a significant impact on cardiac function. Changes in intrathoracic pressure affect the heart directly, alongside altering preload (through venous return) and afterload (through changes in the vasculature). As the pulmonary vasculature resides solo within the thorax, the impact of different types and levels of ventilation can be profound. Additionally, the serial layout means that changes occurring to RV output will alter LV output.

In spontaneously breathing patients, inspiration leads to an increase in venous return (therefore RV preload) and LV afterload. The former improves cardiac output, and the latter decreases it. The overall effect is small in healthy people. However, hypovolaemia or a rapid increase in LV afterload can greatly exaggerate these effects. Mechanical ventilation increases intrathoracic pressure during inspiration, reducing venous return and increasing RV afterload (through pressure being transmitted onto pulmonary vasculature, West's zones 1 and 2) [3,7]. Simultaneously, LV preload increases and LV afterload is reduced, leading to an increase in LV stroke volume. The decrease in RV output is transmitted to the LV during expiration, impairing LV output. The fibrous nature of the pericardium mitigates some of these effects, however, (parallel) ventricular interdependence can accentuate them as can hypovolaemia.

8.3 Viewing the right heart with echocardiography

The right heart can be seen in most of the standard views: parasternal long-axis (PLAX), parasternal short-axis (PSAX), the apical four-chamber (A4Ch) and subcostal views. A summary of the views that allow for either focused or comprehensive assessment of the RV can be seen in *Fig. 8.4*. The complex anatomy of the RV, with its non-uniform shape, means that it is easy to under- or overestimate both the size and function of the RV and RA. 3D imaging either by cardiac MRI or 3D echocardiography is becoming the gold standard, however, this is commonly not available or pragmatic in critical care. Therefore, critical care echocardiography relies on careful imaging, understanding commonly encountered pitfalls and interpretation in the clinical context.

8.3.1 Additional echo views

The standard echocardiographic views were described in *Chapter 5*. Below are descriptions of additional views demonstrated in *Figure 8.4* that are important when performing a more complex focused scan of the right heart:

1. **Right ventricular inflow view:** found by locating the standard PLAX view and tilting the probe to look caudally by bringing the tail up. A small anticlockwise rotation may help image alignment. It is often the best view for visualization of the inlet and tricuspid regurgitation (TR) jet Doppler alignment.

2. **Right ventricular outflow view**: found by locating the standard PLAX view and tilting the probe cranially with a small 10–30° tilt in a clockwise direction. Allows visualization of the pulmonary valve, and distal RVOT. It is useful for assessing pulmonary regurgitation (PR), RVOT velocity–time integral (RVOT VTI) and pulmonary stenosis (PS) especially if there are limited PSAX windows.

3. **Right ventricular focused apical four-chamber (RV A4Ch):** locate the standard A4Ch view and, keeping the apex of the LV in the centre of the image, perform a gentle anticlockwise rotation until the maximum width at the tricuspid annulus can be seen. Many patients will also need a small lateral slide and tilting of the probe in order to image more anteriorly and open up the RV. Studies have shown that most RV measures are more consistent in this view compared to the standard A4Ch [8].

4. **Modified right ventricular apical four-chamber (mod RV A4Ch):** located by sliding medially from the A4Ch and angling the probe more anteriorly. Should not be used for quantitative assessment because the RV is foreshortened but may provide a visual assessment of function if other images are limited and there is good TR jet alignment.

5. **Subcostal parasternal short-axis:** locate the standard subcostal view, rotate anticlockwise approximately 70–90° then angle the probe to look laterally towards the apex (left side). This allows visualization of the PSAX views at most levels. It can be particularly useful in patients with hyperinflated lungs or ventilated patients. This view is good for

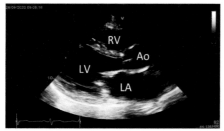

PLAX:

Measurement of RV wall thickness and RVOT diameter may be performed here.

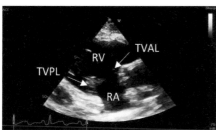

PLAX of RV inflow:

Allows assessment of the RV wall and tricuspid valve anterior and posterior leaflets. May also allow for TR jet measurements.

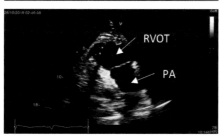

PLAX of RVOT and PA:

Allows assessment of the pulmonary valve.

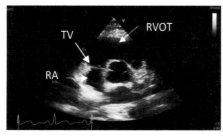

PSAX at basal RV:

Measurement of RVOT dimensions, TR jet parameters and assessment for interatrial shunts.

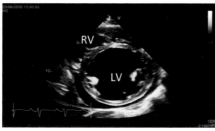

PSAX at mid-papillary muscle level:

The presence of septal flattening can be seen here in the context of RV pressure or volume overload. Good for initial RV size assessment but not for quantifying systolic function.

observing RV/LV interdependence and aligning the Doppler cursor with the PV.

8.4 Assessment of the right ventricle

Assessment of the right heart should be done in a systematic manner, considering size, shape and function, the clinical context and the likely chronicity of findings. Gaining experience through observing normal

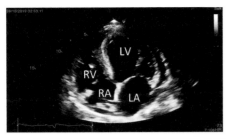

Apical four-chamber view:

Allows for RV size and functional assessment including measurement of basal, mid-level and long-axis distance, area and fractional area change, RA size and volume, and TR jet parameters.

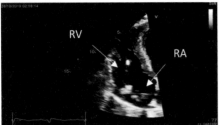

Apical four-chamber RV focused view:

Also allows for the same assessments of RA and RV shape, size and function as per the standard A4Ch view but with improved visualization of the RV free wall.

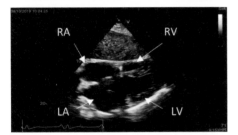

Subcostal four-chamber view:

Optimal view for RV wall thickness measurement. Allows for assessment of RA/RV in cardiac tamponade and interatrial shunts. Good to visualize RA/RV but not for measurements as foreshortened.

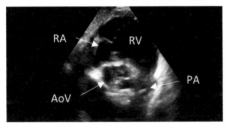

Subcostal basal RV short axis:

Measurement of RVOT dimensions are possible here alongside Doppler assessment of the pulmonary valve and artery.

Figure 8.4. Transthoracic echocardiography views used in the assessment of the right ventricle. A – aorta; AV – aortic valve; LA – left atrium; LV – left ventricle; PA – pulmonary artery; PLAX – parasternal long-axis; PSAX – parasternal short-axis; RA – right atrium; RV – right ventricle; RVOT – right ventricular outflow tract; TV – tricuspid valve; TVAL – anterior tricuspid valve leaflet; TVPL – posterior tricuspid valve leaflet.

findings in spontaneously breathing and mechanically ventilated patients can be helpful in differentiating clinically significant findings from normal adaptation. Detailed guidelines have been published by the American Society of Echocardiography, endorsed by the European Association in 2010, and the British Society of Echocardiography have also recently updated their guidelines [9,10]. More recent publications and guidelines have distinguished between males and females in the definitions of normal function and acknowledged that geographical differences may exist. It is also worth noting that there are currently no accepted normal criteria for mechanically ventilated patients. Numbers provided in this text are based on ASE/ECAVI guidelines [9].

8.4.1 Right ventricular dimensions and shape

As mentioned above, the size of the RV is dependent on the view and it is therefore important that both visual and quantitative assessments are based on the correct views (*Fig. 8.5*). This effect is exaggerated when dilation occurs because any increase in afterload is unevenly distributed across the complex RV shape leading to non-uniform dilation. However, similar images can also be found if the RV is assessed off-axis. The following techniques can be used to assess the size of the RV.

1. **Visual assessment**: should be performed using all the RV views and can provide a good impression of size and shape.

    i. **RVOT size:** comparison of the proximal RVOT with the LA and aorta, in the PLAX view, can give an indication of an increase in size if one is significantly larger than the other two. It can also be seen in the PSAX view.

    ii. **RV size:** best seen in the RV A4Ch, though the PSAX, RV inflow, A4Ch and subcostal views can add information. It should be smaller than the LV. A visual comparison of the RV area compared to the LV is a useful 'eyeball' technique, especially if the image quality precludes more detailed measurements (care should be taken with misinterpreting mirroring artefact if present). As it increases in size, the RV begins to dominate the apex, suggesting at least moderate dilation. The subcostal view slices the RV at an angle that often underestimates its size.

2. **RV/LV diameter ratio**: performed in the standard A4Ch view at end-diastole. This can and should be 'eyeballed' especially in emergency situations. However, it can also be quantified more formally through measurement of the width of the RV. A ratio of >1 is suggestive of significant RV dilation even if the dimensions are within normal ranges.

3. **RV dimensions**: measured in the RV A4Ch view at end-diastole aiming to capture the RV at its maximum diameter. RVD1 is measured at the maximal basal diameter; RVD2 is the mid RV maximal diameter and is measured at the level of LV papillary muscles; RVD3 is the RV length and is measured in a straight line from the RV apex to transect the tricuspid plane, though RVD3 is thought to be less clinically relevant than RVD1 and RVD2 (*Fig. 8.5*). Normal values are RVD1 <4.3cm, RVD2 <3.6cm and RVD3 <8.3cm.

4. **RV area (RVA):** measured in the RV A4Ch at end-diastole by tracing the endocardial border of the RV (*Fig. 8.5*). It is important to have clear definition of the RV free wall. An RVA >26cm^2 is consistent with RV dilation and >38cm^2 is suggestive of severe dilation [11].

5. **RVOT assessment**: the RVOT accounts for 20–30% of the RV volume and is often the first part of the RV to demonstrate signs of tamponade. RVOT is best viewed in the PLAX and PSAX, with subcostal and apical windows offering possible alternatives. Proximal RVOT (RVOT 1) is measured from the anterior aortic wall to the RV free wall in the PLAX or PSAX views, with a normal $RVOT_{prox}$ being <3.6cm. The distal RVOT can be seen in the RV outflow view, but is measured only in the PSAX and is found immediately proximal to the pulmonary valve. A normal $RVOT_{dist}$ is <2.8cm. Both are measured at end-diastole unlike the LVOT diameter.

6. **RV wall thickness**: best measured in the subcostal window.

7. **RV volume**: increasingly part of more comprehensive exams, using 3D probes. Rarely available as part of a focused critical care scan, though this may change as the technology improves. This correlates well with cardiac MRI with a normal 3D RVEDV being <90cm³ [3].

8.4.2 RV systolic function

RV systolic function, like LV function, is a product of its preload, contractility and afterload, but as described above, the influence of afterload on the RV is exaggerated and its shape and the peristaltic contraction add further complexity. Nevertheless, the standard measures to assess RV function correlate well with RV ejection fraction (RVEF) and are predictive of clinical outcome in the cardiac population [12]. Right ventricular function can be assessed in terms of longitudinal contraction and radial function (describing a bellows-like movement) as well as an overall assessment in the form of ejection fraction or stroke volume.

1. **Visual assessment**: a qualitative assessment of the area change and longitudinal contraction, as well as assessment of obvious deformation either in terms of the RV free wall becoming more trapezoid or septal flattening. One recent study demonstrated that there was reasonable correlation between visual estimation by echo-trained intensivists and quantitative measures of RV function, though the severity can be overestimated [11]. Additionally, areas of regionality should be considered.

2. **Tricuspid annular plane systolic excursion (TAPSE)**: measured in the RV A4Ch view. TAPSE is an angle-dependent measure of longitudinal contraction of the RV free wall. It is performed by placing the cursor through the tricuspid annulus when using M-mode and measuring the vertical distance that the base moves towards the apex from diastole to peak systole (*Fig. 8.5*). It is important to measure the same tissue at each time point. TAPSE has been demonstrated to correlate well with RVEF and has a high specificity but low sensitivity for detection of RV impairment. A normal TAPSE is >1.7cm.

3. **RV systolic velocity (RV S′):** whereas TAPSE measures the maximum distance the free wall travels in a longitudinal direction, RV S′ measures the maximum velocity of the movement. Again, it is a longitudinal measure of function, performed using tissue Doppler and pulsed wave Doppler on the tricuspid annulus in the RV A4Ch view (*Fig. 8.5*). The highest possible velocity during systole is measured. Like TAPSE, RV S′ is a relatively easy technique to perform (even with limited windows) and is well validated. Its disadvantage is that it will underrepresent impaired RV function. A normal RV S′ is >9.5cm/sec.

4. **RV fractional area change (RV FAC):** RV FAC is defined as:

   [(RV end-diastolic area − RV end-systolic area)/end-diastolic area] × 100

   It is a measure of longitudinal and radial function of the RV inlet and apex and is therefore less angle dependent than other measures of RV function. It is performed at end-diastole and end-systole, ideally using the RV A4Ch. As with RV area, the walls are traced ignoring the trabeculations. It is important to have clear definition of the entire ventricle throughout systole. RV FAC correlates well with RVEF from cardiac MRI and is an independent predictor of outcome in heart failure, myocardial infarction and pulmonary embolus. It is particularly sensitive to the effects of increased afterload on RV function. However, it is limited at accounting for regional variations in anatomy and can underestimate RV function by not including the RVOT's contribution to RV stroke volume (which can be up to 30%). A normal RV FAC is >35%.

5. **Interdependence/eccentricity index:** both pressure and volume overload can lead to deformation of the normal RV/LV geometry. Volume overload is generally associated with flattening of the septum during mid to late diastole with relative sparring at end-systole. Pressure overload, by contrast, has the greatest deformation at end-systole. Pressure overload can be accompanied by volume overload, especially with fluid loading. It is best assessed in the PSAX view at the level of the mitral valve but is also visible in apical views. The eccentricity index is a semi-quantitative measure of septal deformation, measured in the mid-level PSAX view at end-systole and diastole. It is defined as the ratio of D2/D1, where D1 is the diameter perpendicular to the septum and D2 is the diameter parallel to the septum. A ratio >1.1 is abnormal.

6. **Overall measures:** these include RVOT stroke volume, RVOT VTI as an easily measurable surrogate for stroke volume, RV index of myocardial performance and RV global longitudinal strain (GLS) (*Fig. 8.5*). A detailed description of the latter two are beyond the scope of this chapter. RVOT VTI is calculated using pulsed wave Doppler just behind the pulmonary valve and can be a used as an adjunct to describe RV function. However, it may be more useful as a mechanism to monitor

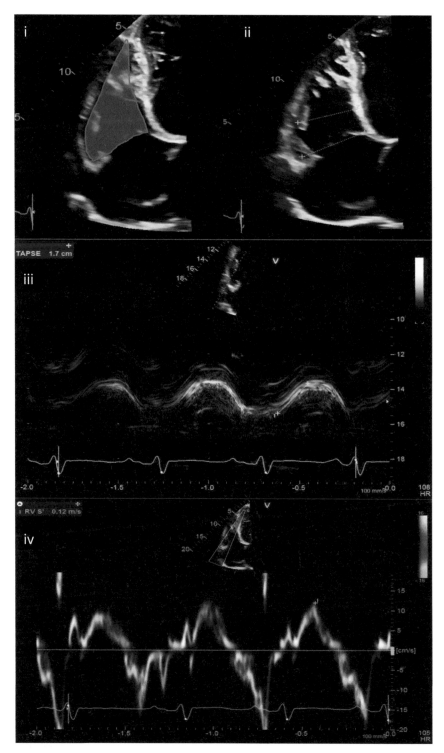

Figure 8.5. (i) Right ventricle (RV) focused apical four-chamber view with an example of RV area measurement in diastole; for fractional area change this would then be performed in systole and the percentage change calculated. (ii) RV basal and mid-chamber diameter measurement. (iii) Tricuspid annular plane systolic excursion (TAPSE) measurement. (iv) Tissue Doppler imaging measurement of RV S' wave velocity.

change in response to treatment. RVOT stroke volume is calculated using the following equation:

$$RVOT\ SV = RVOT\ area \times RVOT\ VTI$$

It is not recommended to calculate RVEF from 2D echocardiography. Calculation of RVEF using 3D echocardiography is more accepted, though shares similar issues to LVEF because it is load dependent and has a steep learning curve with a large variation in novice users.

ECHO TIP

Right ventricular strain

Right ventricular strain is becoming an increasingly common technique. It is less angle dependent and is a good predictor of RV function and outcome. It requires good endocardial wall definition and a high frame rate, and the normal values are vendor dependent. Right ventricular free wall strain is the most validated measure, though single view RV GLS and multiple view RV GLS have a growing evidence base in numerous disease states, if not yet in critical care.

Additional measures

Novel assessments of RV function are regularly proposed as clinical understanding and imaging techniques develop. The subcostal echocardiographic assessment of tricuspid annual kick (SEATAK), for example, is a proposed alternative to TAPSE in patients with inadequate apical windows [13].

Assessment of interdependence

Assessment of interdependence is best achieved with the adjuvant use of ECG monitoring to confirm the cardiac phase. Slowing the playback speed to review images or stopping the video and rolling the image backwards and forwards can also be helpful.

8.4.3 Right ventricular diastolic function

There is minimal data available regarding the assessment of RV diastolic function in critical care. Thus, critical care echocardiography is limited to employing techniques and ranges from cardiology, with diastolic assessment beyond the scope of a focused scan. However, given the importance impaired relaxation and raised LVEDP have in predicting outcome in critical illness, it is likely to become increasingly relevant. Right ventricular diastolic assessment is performed by evaluating similar parameters to the LV: TV *E*, TV deceleration time, TV *E/A* ratio, RV e′and E/e′. The pattern can demonstrate abnormal relaxation or a restrictive pattern, for example, an E/e′>6 suggests a raised RAP and an *E/A* <0.8 impaired relaxation. Current guidance suggests integrating several findings and largely limiting conclusions to normal or abnormal [10].

8.5 Assessment of the right atrium

Situated in the anterolateral region of the heart, the RA acts as reservoir, collecting the systemic circulation from the inferior vena cava (IVC) and the superior vena cava (SVC), and as an active conduit pumping blood into the RV [14]. Right atrial physiology has three phases:

1. A dominant systolic filling phase.

2. An early diastolic phase where blood flows down a pressure gradient passively into the RV.

3. A final active phase created by atrial contraction [14].

The atrial contraction phase is thought to contribute to up to 40% of RV filling, making avoidance of AF vital in severe right heart failure. Right atrial pressure shows a significant degree of variation over the respiratory cycle and can change by over 50%.

Seen predominantly in the apical, PSAX and subcostal view, it is best quantified in the A4Ch view. It can be measured either by RA area or by using Simpson's method to calculate RA volume from the single plane 2D images. RA area is measured by tracing around the inside of the RA and volume is calculated following RA length measurement. RA volume varies with gender and indexing it does not account for this variation. The RA will enlarge over time if subjected to increased pressure. RA enlargement and dysfunction appears to be predictive of adverse cardiovascular outcomes and death in heart failure and pulmonary hypertension. It is also associated with recurrent AF.

8.6 Anatomical masses seen in the right heart

There are several structures that can be seen in the right heart that may be confused for pathological masses such as thrombi or vegetations. These include:

- **Eustachian valve:** an embryonic remnant of the IVC valve, it can be large and is usually seen in the IVC inflow into the RA.

- **Chiari network:** a remnant of the eustachian valve, often appears mobile with thin filaments, found in the RA.

- **Thebesian valve:** a flap-like structure seen at the entrance to the coronary sinus.

- **Crista terminalis:** a bright ridge that runs across the posterior wall of the RA from the IVC to the SVC. Can appear like a thrombus, especially if only partially visualized.

8.7 Pulmonary hypertension and assessment of pulmonary pressures

Pulmonary hypertension is common in critically ill patients, for many reasons. It may occur acutely as a part of a clinical syndrome, a physiological response to hypoxia or as a response to organ support or, alternatively, secondary to an acute on chronic cause usually due to a respiratory or cardiac disorder. Liver failure, chemotherapy and autoimmune conditions can also present with pulmonary hypertension. It was previously defined as a mean pulmonary artery pressure >24mmHg though this has been revised to >20mmHg [15].

Morbidity and mortality from pulmonary hypertension are high, especially if left unnoticed or unaccounted for in mechanically ventilated patients. The gold standard for measuring pulmonary pressures is right heart catheterization, or in critical care possibly through a pulmonary artery catheter (although most pulmonary artery catheters measure the pressure in a segmental artery). Despite not being the gold standard, echocardiography has become the primary mode of assessment for pulmonary pressures both in acute and chronic settings.

Current echocardiographic guidelines take a probability approach to the diagnosis of pulmonary hypertension, based mainly on measurement of the RV–RA gradient through TR_{Vmax}, with the likelihood of pulmonary hypertension assessed as low, intermediate or high. This likelihood can increase if other indices suggestive of pulmonary hypertension are present, such as:

- RV / LV basal diameter ratio >1.0

- interventricular septal flattening

- RVOT Doppler acceleration time <105m/sec

- PR_{Vmax} >2.2m/sec

- pulmonary artery diameter >25mm

- distended and non-collapsing IVC (>2.1cm with <50% collapse on inspiration)

- RA area of >18cm^2.

Using both TR_{Vmax} and pulmonary hypertension markers in combination gives the following probability of PH:

- **Low echocardiographic probability of pulmonary hypertension:**

  o TR_{Vmax} <2.8m/sec with no other signs of pulmonary hypertension on echocardiography

- **Medium echocardiographic probability of pulmonary hypertension:**

  ○ TR_{Vmax} <2.8m/sec with other signs of pulmonary hypertension on echocardiography

or

  ○ TR_{Vmax} 2.9–3.4m/sec with no other signs of pulmonary hypertension on echocardiography

- **High echocardiographic probability of pulmonary hypertension:**

  ○ TR_{Vmax} 2.9–3.4m/sec with other signs of pulmonary hypertension on echocardiography

or

  ○ TR_{Vmax} >3.4m/sec.

Pulmonary hypertension can be considered in terms of its causes or its location in relation to the pulmonary capillaries. Both classifications can assist with understanding the prognosis and potential interventions, though the first ascribes an aetiology and the second helps define potential aetiologies.

Causes

- Idiopathic pulmonary arterial hypertension.

- Secondary to left heart pathology.

- Secondary to respiratory pathology or hypoxia.

- Chronic thromboembolic disease.

- Multifactorial or unclear aetiology.

Location

- Precapillary – inherently pulmonary arterial cause or respiratory cause with increased PVR.

- Postcapillary – often driven by left heart pathology, e.g. acute LV failure or heart failure with preserved ejection fraction (HFpEF).

- Combined pre- and postcapillary.

Acute pulmonary hypertension and the management of RV failure are discussed in more detail below.

8.7.1 Measuring pulmonary pressures

As with most RV haemodynamics, the assessment of pulmonary pressures is based on Ohm's law (which links pressure, flow and resistance) and the Bernoulli equation. The Bernoulli equation states:

$$\Delta P = 4\ (V_2^{\ 2} - V_1^{\ 2})$$

[V_1 is usually <1m/sec and therefore is negligible at clinically significant pressures]

Ohm's law is important when assessing pulmonary hypertension in critical care because it explains how an increased pressure can either be the result of increased PVR or an increase in cardiac output.

The assessment of pulmonary pressures and pulmonary hypertension is mainly based around TR_{Vmax} as a surrogate for pulmonary artery systolic pressure (PASP) [16]. This is because the challenges in correctly calculating RA pressure make PASP less reliable. Several methods can help in establishing the likelihood of significant pulmonary hypertension (*Figs 8.6 and 8.7*):

1. **Right atrial pressure (RAP)**: RAP is needed to calculate RV systolic pressure (RVSP) because the dominant driving force for TR jet pressure is the RV–RA gradient. Increasing RAP leads to a low TR jet pressure. Therefore, it is important to measure or estimate RAP. In spontaneously breathing patients, RAP can be estimated from IVC size and its collapsibility (see *Table 8.1*). In a mechanically ventilated patient, the only reliable method is to measure the central venous pressure (CVP), though diastolic hepatic vein flow and an E/e´>6 have both been associated with raised RAP.

2. **Pulmonary artery systolic pressure**: RVSP can be estimated from the maximum velocity found in the TR jet. Continuous wave Doppler is placed over and parallel to the TR jet. Peak velocity corresponds to PASP using the Bernoulli equation plus RAP (see above). PASP and RVSP are essentially the same assuming no restriction at the pulmonary valve (e.g. RVOT obstruction or significant PS). Care should be taken to accurately align the jet and correctly calculate RAP, as it can be underestimated and overestimated [12] (see *Echo tip* box below). Current guidance suggests considering pulmonary hypertension to be likely if the TR_{Vmax} >3.4m/sec and possible if TR_{Vmax} 2.9–3.4m/sec. These correspond to PASP values of >50mmHg and >31mmHg, respectively (see start of *Section 8.7*).

3. **RVOT VTI and pulmonary acceleration time (PAT)**: pulsed wave Doppler placed immediately prior to the pulmonary valve in the RVOT provides RVOT VTI. It is a surrogate of RV stroke volume and can be used to calculate RV stroke volume; additionally its shape and the time to peak velocity can be used to assess for pulmonary hypertension. A short PAT correlates with raised pulmonary artery pressures. It is

measured from the beginning of flow to the peak velocity and is best measured at a sweep speed of 100m/sec. Mid-systolic notching of the RVOT trace is also indicative of raised pulmonary pressures. It has low sensitivity and high specificity. A normal PAT is >105m/sec.

4. **Mean pulmonary artery pressure (MPAP)**: this can be calculated using several methods:

   a. $MPAP = 4 \times PR_{Vmax}^{2} + RAP$

      Early PR_{Vmax}, measured by continuous wave Doppler in the PSAX view, can estimate MPAP using the Bernoulli equation; a PR_{Vmax} >2.2m/sec is considered significant in the assessment of pulmonary hypertension.

   b. $MPAP = 0.6 \times PASP + 2 \ (mmHg)$

   c. $MPAP = 90 - (0.62 \times PAT), \ (if \ PAT <120m/sec)$

   d. *TR jet VTI mean gradient + RAP.*

5. **Diastolic pulmonary artery pressure (DPAP)**: can be estimated from $PR_{endVmax}$.

$$DPAP = 4 \times PR_{endvmax}^{2} + RAP.$$

6. **Additional measures**: PVR can be estimated using Ohm's law by dividing the pressure gradient across the right heart by the flow across the PV. Studies have shown that if PVR ratio (TR_{Vmax}/RVOT VTI) is <0.275 then the following equation provides a good estimate of PVT:

$$PVR = [(TR_{Vmax}/RVOT \ VTI) \times 10] + 0.16$$

If the PVR ratio is >0.275 then the following equation should be used instead:

$$PVR = (TR_{Vmax}^{2}/RVOT \ VTI) \times 5$$

RV/PA coupling has been described by different formulae using different measures of RV function divided by PASP. Essentially, they describe the RV's ability to adapt to afterload. They each have their pros and cons but mostly have been shown to have prognostic value in pulmonary hypertension. The most commonly described compares TAPSE to the PASP:

$$RV–PA \ coupling = TAPSE \ (in \ mm)/PASP$$

A ratio <0.35 is associated with poor outcome in pulmonary hypertension patients.

Table 8.1. Estimating right atrial pressure from inferior vena cava diameter measurements

	Normal (3mmHg)	Intermediate (8mmHg)		High (15mmHg)
IVC diameter	<2.1cm	<2.1cm	>2.1cm	>2.1cm
Collapse on sniff	>50%	<50%	>50%	<50%
Secondary measures				E/e´>6 Hepatic flow mostly diastolic Restrictive filling

IVC – inferior vena cava.

ECHO TIP

Tricuspid regurgitation velocity measurement

Correctly estimating PASP requires good parallel alignment with the TR jet. It is therefore recommended that TR_{Vmax} is measured in multiple views and the highest value used. It is important not to include the ill-defined non-dense part at the edges of the trace (the 'beard'). It has been shown that TR_{Vmax} measured from a well-defined spectral trace shows excellent correlation with measured pulmonary artery pressure. Tricuspid regurgitation can be found in approximately 80% of critical care patients and the addition of agitated saline can increase this percentage, though there is a risk of overestimation.

Pitfalls in interpreting tricuspid regurgitation

TR_{Vmax} can only measure the RV–RA gradient; if RV function is significantly impaired then the resultant gradient may underestimate PVR. Additionally, severe or free-flowing TR does not appear to follow the Bernoulli equation and may again underestimate pulmonary pressures.

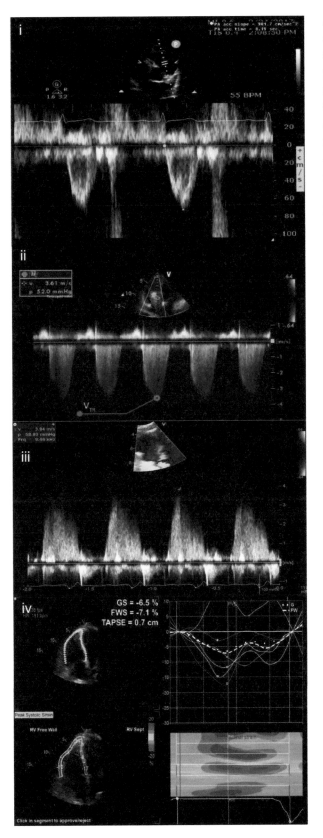

Figure 8.6. Examples of echocardiographic techniques used in the diagnosis of pulmonary hypertension. (i) Right ventricular outflow tract velocity–time integral. (ii) Tricuspid regurgitation maximum velocity (3.61m/sec). (iii) Pulmonary regurgitation maximum velocity (3.84m/sec). (iv) Right ventricular global longitudinal strain.

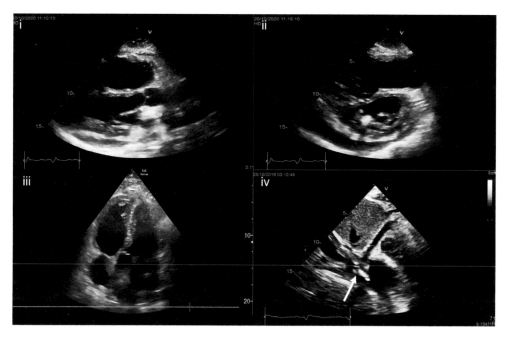

Figure 8.7. Echocardiographic signs of right ventricular strain / pulmonary hypertension. (i) Parasternal long-axis view with a dilated right ventricle. (ii) Parasternal short-axis view with septal flattening in a patient with pulmonary hypertension. (iii) McConnell's sign with right ventricular dilatation in a patient with an acute pulmonary embolus. (iv) A distended inferior vena cava in a patient with pulmonary hypertension with an ECMO cannula (arrow) visualized entering the right atrium.

8.8 Effect of clinical conditions on the right ventricle

8.8.1 Mechanical ventilation

The effects of positive pressure ventilation and negative pressure ventilation on intrathoracic pressures are exacerbated in disease states that impact the lungs or pulmonary vasculature. Positive pressure ventilation reduces venous return to the RV, increases RV afterload, and reduces LV afterload.

PVR changes depending on lung volume. At low lung volumes larger pulmonary vessels (normally supported by alveolar septal stretch) receive increasingly less support. Conversely, as alveoli expand with increasing lung volumes, smaller vessels are compressed. Consequently, pulmonary hypertension demonstrates a U-shaped distribution against lung volume, where pulmonary hypertension is at its lowest at functional residual capacity (FRC).

A similar effect is seen with changes in pulmonary vascular volume or filling. Hypovolaemia increases the proportion of type 1 and 2 West's zones and thus increases PVR. Hypervolaemia increases pulmonary capillary wedge pressure (increasing pulsatile PVR) and interstitial oedema (increasing static PVR).

The effects of PPV can be both beneficial and detrimental. These effects are amplified by fluid status and the interaction between fluid status and PEEP. Therefore, the management of ventilation and ventilator settings in RV failure also requires careful management of fluid balance. There needs to be sufficient fluid to maintain adequate CVP and systemic venous return to encourage appropriate cardiac output, whilst avoiding pulmonary congestion and RV dilation that further impairs RV function. Bedside echocardiography combined with lung ultrasound is an excellent clinical tool to assess fluid status and the cardiopulmonary response to PPV.

8.8.2 Acute right heart failure

Acute right heart failure occurs secondary to:

1. A relatively rapid increase in afterload leading to RV deformation. Common aetiologies include hypoxia (including acute respiratory distress syndrome (ARDS)), acidosis, and obstructive shock (e.g. pulmonary embolism) (see *Fig. 8.8*).

2. Reduced RV function or intrinsic impairment of contractility. This can be secondary to RV ischaemia, myocardial trauma including cardiopulmonary resuscitation, myocarditis and sepsis.

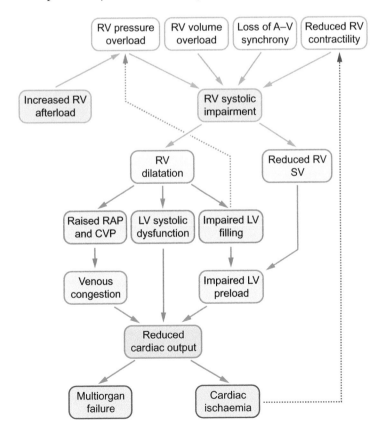

Figure 8.8. The pathophysiology of right ventricular failure. A–V – atrioventricular; CVP – central venous pressure; LV – left ventricle; RA – right atrium; RV – right ventricle; SV – stroke volume.

Both mechanisms can cause a reduction in RV stroke volume alongside RV dilation promoting annular dilation and increased TR, which then causes further RV dilation and reduction in RV stroke volume. This cycle can quickly lead to ventricular interdependence impairing LV diastolic and eventually LV systolic function. Impaired LV diastolic and systolic function increases pulmonary capillary wedge pressure, increasing PVR and leading to worsening RV function. This is further compounded by an increase in RAP pressure, leading to impaired venous return from the coronary sinus with increased RV (and potentially LV) ischaemia. Essentially, a complex of intertwining vicious cycles (see *Fig. 8.9*).

Management of acute right ventricular failure may be approached using the algorithm shown in *Figure 8.9*. Use of these steps is only supported by a small amount of published evidence, but they have biological plausibility and are in keeping with current expert opinion and guidance.

Note that acute RV strain rarely produces a PASP >60mmHg. Rapid onset of increased afterload initiates the cycle of RV impairment that inhibits RV function and flow, limiting the increase in pressure despite an increase in resistance.

Figure 8.9. Proposed flow chart for the management of a patient with right ventricular failure. CVC – central venous catheter; PAC – pulmonary artery catheter; PCI – percutaneous coronary intervention; PE – pulmonary embolus; RV – right ventricle.

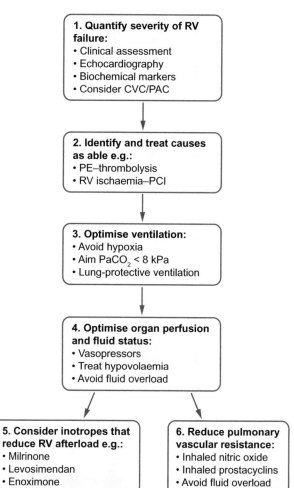

8.8.3 Chronic right ventricular failure

Chronic right ventricular failure is usually the result of a slow increase in RV afterload, allowing adaptation to take place. The commonest causes are LV systolic and diastolic failure or chronic volume overload (seen in severe TR). The indolent onset of pressure or volume overload promotes remodelling through myocyte hypertrophy. If left untreated then compensation eventually becomes overwhelmed and a decompensated pattern emerges, characterized by myocyte death and fibrosis.

As the heart muscle becomes thicker and stronger (right ventricular hypertrophy is defined as: mild 0.5–0.8cm, moderate 0.8–0.9cm and severe >1cm), the RV pressure–volume loop develops isovolumetric contraction and relaxation phases with increased RVSP and RVEDP. Decompensation can be seen as a rise in PVR and RAP followed by a fall in cardiac output and PASP. A falling PASP with ongoing high PVR is associated with extremely poor outcomes. Right ventricular dilation combined with biventricular diastolic failure reduces cardiac output impairing coronary perfusion. Management is complex: a high CVP may be needed, avoiding exacerbation with fluid overload and management of afterload.

8.8.4 Pulmonary embolism

Pulmonary embolism is a common and life-threatening condition with a reported mortality of 2–15%. At its most severe it can cause fatal obstructive shock with acute RV failure. The American Heart Association has characterized pulmonary embolism into three groups based on clinical effects and short-term mortality [17]:

- **Massive pulmonary embolism** – haemodynamic instability with a systolic BP <90mmHg for over 15min, need for inotropic support secondary to pulmonary embolism or loss of cardiac output. It has a short-term mortality of 25–65%.

- **Sub-massive pulmonary embolism** – no haemodynamic instability but RV dysfunction or myocardial necrosis present. This has a short-term mortality of 3%.

- **Low-risk pulmonary embolism** – no haemodynamic instability and no RV dysfunction or necrosis. This has a short-term mortality of <1%.

Computed tomographic pulmonary angiography (CTPA) remains the diagnostic gold standard for pulmonary embolism and can add information on RV dysfunction by comparing RV–LV ratios. Echocardiography is better equipped to assess RV dysfunction and pressure overload and provides information on the chronicity of findings. The latter can be important in risk stratifying catheter-directed thrombolysis because studies have shown that thrombolysis is not beneficial in chronic RV impairment. Echocardiography can also help in the diagnosis of other causes of shock in patients with a suspected massive pulmonary embolism and can be used to monitor response to therapy either through improvements in right heart indices or LVOT VTI.

Recent ESC guidelines recommend that, in a haemodynamically unstable patient, bedside TTE to assess for RV dysfunction should be the first line investigation [17]. If immediately available and feasible then CTPA should be performed after TTE before initiating treatment, but if not, then treatment should be based on clinical and TTE findings alone. If patients are haemodynamically stable, then CTPA is the first line investigation and further risk stratification is based on TTE and cardiac biomarkers.

Despite multiple studies searching for a sign with high sensitivity and specificity for high-risk pulmonary embolism, the answer remains elusive. Many of the findings in pulmonary embolism are a result of acute right heart failure, namely RV dilation, impaired RV function (global or regional), a short PAT, raised PASP, and septal flattening or paradoxical septal movement. These findings are non-specific for pulmonary embolism in the absence of an appropriate clinical picture or confirmatory CTPA. Additionally, absence of these signs does not exclude pulmonary embolism.

Occasionally, intracardiac thrombi can be seen trapped in the right heart; they are usually large, mobile and have a snake-like appearance (see *Fig. 8.10*) [18]. The 60/60 sign and McConnell's sign (see below) were previously thought to be specific for significant pulmonary embolism, but they more likely represent the RV's response to severe rapid onset afterload.

Paradoxical septal movement signifying pressure overload is an important finding because it clearly demonstrates RV dysfunction. If a pulmonary embolism's cardiovascular burden is sufficient then the combination of increased adrenergic response, impaired RV stroke volume and compression of the LV at end-systole and early-diastole leads to a small underfilled LV that is hyperdynamic despite having a reduced LVOT VTI or LV stroke volume.

Monitoring outcome should be based on assessing for improvements in RV function and dilation. An improvement in LV cardiac index or LVOT VTI is also associated with improved mortality. The ESC guidance also advises the use of echocardiography to help guide post-pulmonary embolism management in patients with ongoing dyspnoea at 3 months or at least one risk factor for chronic embolic pulmonary hypertension.

In summary, pulmonary embolism is the archetypal disease to describe the role of echocardiography in assessment and management of the RV. It can be useful in the diagnosis of massive pulmonary embolism, help stratify acute treatment and monitor the impact of treatment.

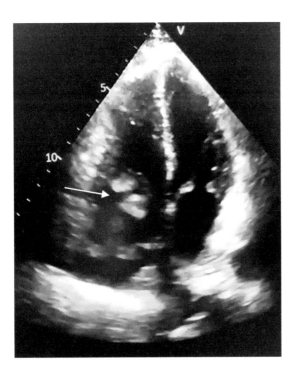

Figure 8.10. Large intracardiac thrombus (white arrow) mostly situated in the right atrium but pushing through the tricuspid valve in diastole. Also note right ventricular dilation and the small compressed left ventricular cavity.

ECHO TIP

McConnell's sign

Preserved kinesis of the apical RV free wall despite hypokinesis or akinesis of the rest of the free wall. The mid free wall is usually the first part to fail (*Fig. 8.11*).

60/60 sign

The 60/60 sign has been described as an indicator of RVF in acute pulmonary embolism, with a PAT <60m/sec and a TR jet maximum velocity suggesting a gradient of <60mmHg.

Both signs maintain some degree of specificity even if other cardiopulmonary diseases are present.

8.9 Summary

The right heart has a complex structure that operates as a high capacity, low pressure system. It is poorly adapted to adjust to rapid increases in afterload. Echocardiography is an excellent bedside tool for the assessment of right heart function and pulmonary hypertension. Due to its complexity, no single measure adequately describes RV function.

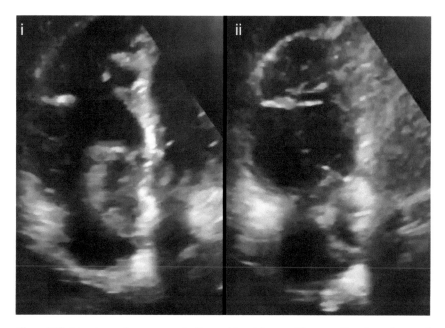

Figure 8.11. Massive pulmonary embolism with evidence of intracardiac thrombus and McConnell's sign. (i) The clot is mobile through the tricuspid valve with dilation of the right ventricle seen. (ii) A systolic image with the clot seen in the right atrium, a mid-wall regional wall motion abnormality visible and a good contracting apex present.

8.10 References

1. Ho S, Nihoyannous P (2006) Anatomy, echocardiography and normal right ventricular dimensions. *Heart,* 92(suppl 1):i2.

2. Mangion J (2021) Right ventricular anatomy. In: *ASE's Comprehensive Echocardiography,* 3rd ed (Eds Lang RM, *et al.*), p163. Elsevier.

3. Chew M (2020) Right ventricular function. In: *Oxford Textbook of Advanced Critical Care Echocardiography* (Eds McLean A, *et al.*), p119. OUP.

4. Markel TA, Wairiuko GM, Lahm T, *et al.* (2008) The right heart and its distinct mechanisms of development, function, and failure. *J Surg Res,* 146:304.

5. Konstam MA, Kiernan MS, Bernstein D, *et al.* (2018) Evaluation and management of right-sided heart failure. *Circulation,* 137:e578.

6. Naeije R, Badagliacca R (2017) The overloaded right heart and ventricular interdependence. *Cardiovasc Res,* 113:1474

7. Duke G (1999) Cardiovascular effects of mechanical ventilation. *Critical Care Resus,* 1:388.

8. Islam S, Khazan B, Keane MG (2021) Imaging the right heart: limitations and technical considerations. In: *ASE's Comprehensive Echocardiography,* 3rd ed (Eds Lang RM, *et al.*), p178. Elsevier.

9. Rudski LG, Lai WW, Afilalo J, *et al.* (2010) Guidelines for the echocardiographic assessment of the right heart in adults. *J Am Soc Echocardiogr,* 23:685.

10. Zaidi A, Knight DS, Augustine DX, *et al.* (2020) Echocardiographic assessment of the right heart in adults: a practical guideline from the British Society of Echocardiography. *Echo Res Pract*, 7:G19.

11. Orde S, Slama M, Yastrebov K, *et al.* (2019) Subjective right ventricle assessment by echo qualified intensive care specialists: assessing agreement with objective measures. *Critical Care*, 23:70.

12. Milan A, Magnino C, Veglio F (2010) Echocardiographic indexes for the non-invasive evaluation of pulmonary hemodynamics. *J Am Soc Echocardiogr*, 23:225.

13. Díaz-Gómez JL, Alvarez AB, Danaraj JJ, *et al.* (2017) A novel semiquantitative assessment of right ventricular systolic function with a modified subcostal echocardiographic view. *Echocardiography*, 34:44.

14. Galatas C, Grapsa J, Rudski LG (2021). The right atrium. In: *ASE's Comprehensive Echocardiography*, 3rd ed (Eds Lang RM, *et al.*), p198. Elsevier.

15. Yaghi S, Novikov A, Trandafirescu T (2020) Clinical update on pulmonary hypertension. *J Investig Med*, 68:821.

16. Augustine DX, Coates-Bradshaw LD, Willis J (2018) Echocardiographic assessment of pulmonary hypertension. *Echo Res Pract*, 5:G11.

17. Konstantinides SV, Meyer G, Becattini C, et al. (2020) 2019 ESC Guidelines for the diagnosis and management of acute pulmonary embolism developed in collaboration with the European Respiratory Society (ERS). *Eur Heart J*, 41:543.

18. Ahmed H, Aurigemma G (2021) Pulmonary embolus. In: *ASE's Comprehensive Echocardiography*, 3rd ed (Eds Lang RM, *et al.*), p202. Elsevier.

19. McConnell MV, Solomon SD, Rayan ME, *et al.* (1996) Regional right ventricular dysfunction detected by echocardiography in acute pulmonary embolism. *Am J Cardiol*, 78:469.

CHAPTER 9

FOCUSED
VALVULAR ASSESSMENT

Tim Keady & Sam Clark

Focused echocardiography most often refers to focusing either on major abnormalities in an urgent setting, or focusing on a particular aspect of the heart, for example, monitoring of left ventricle (LV) function [1].

In the focused assessment of cardiac valves, the priority of the practitioner is to detect a significant abnormality. Other aspects of echocardiography such as precise grading, determination of aetiology and longitudinal assessment are of secondary importance. Once a significant abnormality has been identified, a key step is referral to an appropriate expert for a more in-depth assessment.

To correctly identify any abnormality, awareness of normal anatomy is crucial for both expert and non-expert practitioners. This cannot occur without practice and every scan is an opportunity to hone skills in assessment of valve anatomy and function. Each valve should be considered in terms of its structure (e.g. thickening and calcification), its mobility and its flow.

If this is done regularly as part of normal practice then abnormal anatomy and function, such as significant valvular stenosis or regurgitation, can often be detected with simple 2D imaging and colour flow Doppler (CFD) [2]. Suspicions of significant abnormality may then be corroborated with some simple Doppler measurements. After adding associated findings, the final step is to evaluate all findings within the clinical context. This is true of all critical care echocardiography, but particularly so for valve assessment where haemodynamic fluctuations can radically impact echocardiographic findings.

9.1 The aortic valve

The aortic valve (AV) is trileaflet, consisting of right, left, and non-coronary cusps (RCC, LCC, NCC). The parasternal long-axis (PLAX) view allows visualization of the anterior RCC and NCC as well as the left ventricular outflow tract (LVOT) and aorta. The LVOT diameter (LVOTd) is measured in this view from inner edge to inner edge in mid-systole (up to 1cm) behind the AV. It is commonly 1.8–2.4cm. It is assumed to be circular, however, this is not always correct because it can be more ellipsoid, leading to errors in calculating its area. The LVOTd is useful when calculating LV stroke volume, the continuity equation and assessing aortic regurgitation (AR). CFD in the PLAX view can help assess AR or subvalvular stenosis. The apical five-chamber (A5Ch) view allows for good alignment of the Doppler signal and visualization of the extent of any AR present. The A5Ch view is found by locating the apical four-chamber (A4Ch) view and looking more anteriorly in the thorax by dropping the tail of the probe down, a gentle clockwise twist or a combination of both techniques.

9.1.1 Aortic stenosis

Aortic stenosis is characterized by obstruction of blood flow from the LV into the aorta. It is the most common valvular disease in Europe and North America. It should be suspected if the AV leaflets are thickened or calcified with restricted motion. *Figure 9.1* shows the normal anatomy and common valve pathologies seen in the parasternal short-axis (PSAX) view.

Assessment of aortic stenosis

Assessment of aortic stenosis relies on a number of key steps and principles.

1. **Valve characterization**: describes the thickening, calcification and mobility of the valve leaflets (*Fig. 9.2*). Valve planimetry (manual tracing of valve area) has not been shown to be accurate in transthoracic echo (TTE) but can be useful in transoesphageal echo (TOE). However, in a trileaflet valve, if only two leaflets are fixed, and a single leaflet opens well, then the aortic stenosis is mild at most. Planimetry of the AV is not recommended in calcific aortic stenosis but may be useful in aortic stenosis of other aetiologies, especially when using TOE.

2. **Peak velocity and mean gradient**: this may be assessed in the A5Ch or apical long-axis view, using CWD to ascertain the aortic maximum velocity and pulsed wave Doppler (PWD) for LVOT peak velocity. Alternatively, both traces may be visible simultaneously with CWD (*Fig. 9.3*). This technique uses the simplified Bernoulli equation to imply the severity of aortic stenosis. As with the continuity equation (explained below) it is important to find the highest peak velocity and mean gradient. This is best achieved by aligning the cursor accurately with the fastest part of the jet, not just the valve structure. Severe aortic stenosis may also be indicated by an AV peak velocity of >4m/sec or mean gradient >40mmHg [3].

3. **Continuity equation**: based on the conservation of mass principle, the continuity equation states that in a closed system, the volume of fluid passing through one part of the system must pass through the next

part of the system. Therefore, the velocity of the fluid must change if the orifice size changes. It relies on three assumptions:

i. The LVOT is circular.

ii. The LVOT velocity–time integral (VTI) represents the mean flow of all the blood within the LVOT (across time).

iii. The whole LVOT stroke volume leaves the heart via the AV. The calculated AV area is an effective, not an actual, area with severe being <1cm².

The continuity equation:

$$CSA_{(aorta)} = [CSA_{(LVOT)} \times VTI_{LVOT}]/VTI_{aorta}$$

where CSA = cross-sectional area, VTI = velocity–time integral.

4. **Dimensionless index** (aka Doppler velocity ratio): this measure compares the LVOT and aortic peak velocities (or VTIs). It avoids potential sources of error related to LVOT size and shape by simply comparing the maximum velocities through the valve and LVOT. If the ratio of the max LVOT velocity to AV velocity is less than 0.25, then severe aortic stenosis is likely.

Associated findings

Two-dimensional imaging of aortic stenosis may also reveal:

- concentric LV hypertrophy

- enlarged left atrium (LA)

- evidence of pulmonary hypertension.

Potential pitfalls when assessing aortic stenosis

There are several potential pitfalls. Most underestimate the severity of the aortic stenosis, but it is possible to overestimate its severity.

- Poor alignment of the cursor.
- Accidentally aligning with a mitral regurgitation or tricuspid regurgitation jet.
- Beat to beat variability in arrhythmia.
- Reduced left ventricular ejection fraction (LVEF) or significantly impaired systolic function.
- High output through LVOT VTI (limiting the use of simplified Bernoulli equations), either due to high cardiac output/inotropes or LVOT obstruction.

These last two may be common in the critical care setting, warranting caution and expert assessment particularly in low flow, low pressure severe aortic stenosis.

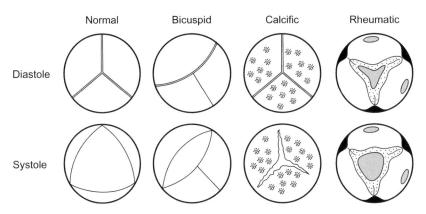

Figure 9.1. The parasternal short-axis view of the aortic valve is useful in detecting the presence and suggesting the aetiology of aortic stenosis. Common causes of valvular aortic stenosis are shown here. Redrawn from Brown J. & Morgan-Hughes N.J. (2005) *Cont. Ed. Anaes. Crit. Care & Pain*, 5:1, with permission from Oxford University Press, and from Baumgartner H. (2017) *J. Am. Soc. Echocardiog.* 30:372 with permission from Elsevier.

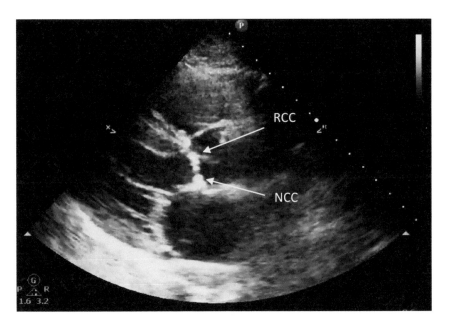

Figure 9.2. Parasternal long-axis view showing a heavily calcified and stenosed aortic valve. NCC – non-coronary cusp; RCC – right coronary cusp.

Dynamic LVOT obstruction

Subvalvular or supravalvular stenosis may also result in high Doppler peak velocities and subsequent misdiagnosis as valvular aortic stenosis. A common cause of subvalvular stenosis is dynamic LVOT obstruction. Fluid restriction, diuretics, use of inotropes or significant paradoxical septal shift can all cause or exacerbate LVOT obstruction. A small asymmetrically contractile LV with low preload and low afterload may cause flow acceleration in the

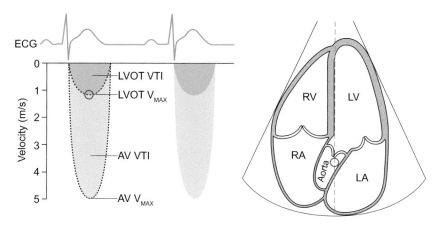

Figure 9.3. Apical five-chamber view showing continuous wave Doppler through the left ventricular outflow tract (LVOT) and aortic valve (AV). If there is aortic stenosis, you may see a 'double envelope' Doppler waveform as shown here. Tracing each envelope will calculate the velocity–time integral (VTI) as well as identify the maximum velocity (V_{max}). Alternatively, you may simply check the AV and LVOT V_{max} using the measurement cursor. In this figure, AV V_{max} is over 4m/sec indicating significant aortic stenosis. Furthermore, the Doppler velocity ratio (LVOT V_{max} / AV V_{max} = 1 / 4.5 = 0.22) is less than 0.25, again indicating severe aortic stenosis.
LA – left atrium; LV – left ventricle; RA – right atrium; RV – right ventricle.
Left part of image adapted from Brown J & Morgan-Hughes NJ (2005) *Cont. Ed. Anaes. Crit. Care & Pain,* 5:1, with permission from Oxford University Press.

LVOT. The resultant pressure drop can draw the anterior MV leaflet inwards during systole, obstructing the LVOT and causing mitral regurgitation. This is termed systolic anterior motion (SAM). Flow acceleration may be seen as turbulent flow during systole in the LVOT (variance on colour flow Doppler can be a useful guide). Unrecognized, it can lead to incorrect clinical assumptions about fluid and inotropic status. It often requires significant fluid challenge(s), despite possible pulmonary oedema, to correct afterload and preload conditions while limiting inotrope usage and treating the underlying cause, e.g. sepsis.

Clinical implications

The LV responds to deteriorating aortic stenosis with hypertrophy. This maintains a gradient across the valve without dilation or a reduction in cardiac output. However, this stiff hypertrophied muscle has an increased oxygen demand and lower oxygen supply due to impaired diastolic function, leading to impaired myocardial perfusion reserve [4,5]. A significant drop in aortic root pressure from sudden vasodilation (plus or minus negative inotropy) may result in severe LV ischaemia and a downward spiral of hypotension, reduced pressure recovery and reduced contractility. Anaesthetic techniques that reduce systemic vascular resistance must be used with extreme caution in the setting of severe aortic stenosis [4,5].

9.1.2 Aortic regurgitation

AR is caused by incompetence in the (trileaflet) AV. In more severe cases it can cause pressure and volume overload of the LV leading to significantly raised LV end-diastolic pressure (LVEDP) and LV failure, with few pharmaceutical options for its management in ICU. Important questions to be considered include:

- Is it severe?

- Is it likely acute or chronic?

- Is its cause integral to its management?

AR may be due to either aortic root or aortic valve pathology and may be detected using CFD in the PLAX, A5Ch or apical long-axis views. 2D imaging may reveal a dilated aortic root, excessive leaflet motion or LV dilation.

Common AV pathologies include calcification, rheumatic heart disease, bicuspid valve and infective endocarditis [6]. Common aortic root pathologies include Marfan syndrome, syphilis, collagen vascular disease and aortic dissection (*Fig. 9.4*). The LVOT, aortic annulus, sinus of Valsalva and sinotubular junction should be assessed carefully for abnormalities in the setting of AR [6].

Assessment for clinically significant AR may be carried out in several ways:

1. **Visual characterization**: a large central jet, or an eccentric jet may be noted (*Fig. 9.5*). Measurements of jet area and jet length are unreliable markers of severity because they are affected by multiple haemodynamic parameters including LV diastolic pressure gradient and LV compliance. Quantitative approaches are warranted if more than a small central jet is seen.

2. **Vena contracta**: this involves measuring the CFD trace to find the width of the jet at its narrowest point, often slightly below the valve. The use of zoom mode and a small colour Doppler box can help improve accuracy. This is the most reliable measure if the AR jet is eccentric. Multiple jets are not additive. A vena contracta of >6mm is suggestive of severe AR.

3. **Jet width/LVOT width >65%**: the width of the regurgitant jet is measured within 1cm of the AV and compared with the LVOT width.

4. **Pressure half-time <200msec**: this refers to the speed at which the pressure gradient of the AR jet within the ventricle drops. It is measured using CWD through the AR jet (ideally through the largest part of the jet), with a line drawn down the gradient of the slope starting at the peak velocity. The machine will automatically calculate pressure half-time. It is inversely proportional to the severity of AR. Pressure half-time is most sensitive in acute AR where the LV has not adapted to compensate for the volume overload. It requires a good CWD trace ideally with a peak velocity over 3m/sec. The density of

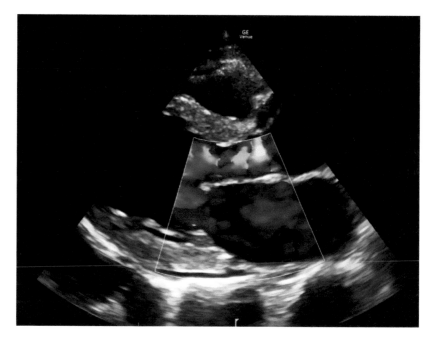

Figure 9.4. Severe aortic regurgitation from a Stanford Type A aortic dissection. Note turbulent flow the full width of the left ventricular outflow tract, a dilated aortic root, and a dissection flap extending from the root to the descending aorta.

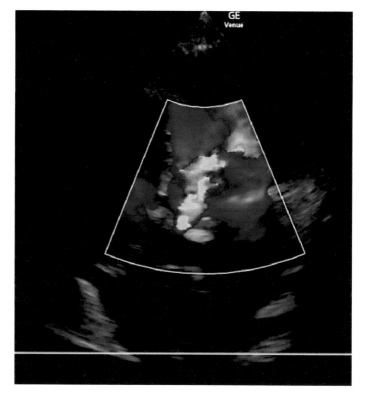

Figure 9.5. Apical five-chamber view showing severe aortic regurgitation on colour flow Doppler.

the CWD trace can also give an indication of severity, with increasing density suggesting increasing severity. A weak signal indicates mild and a dense signal indicates moderate or severe.

5. **Diastolic flow reversal in the descending aorta**: this is measured distal to the left subclavian artery in the suprasternal view. It is an important adjunct to assessment of AR severity. Some flow reversal in early diastole can be seen in mild AR, however, significant holodiastolic flow reversal with velocities over 20cm/sec are a sign of severe AR.

6. **Sequelae of AR**: assessment of LV end-diastolic diameter, LV systolic and diastolic function will help inform the chronicity and the impact of the AR.

7. **Other quantitative assessments for AR**: these include proximal isovelocity surface area (PISA) and regurgitant fraction which are beyond the scope of this text.

Haemodynamics in acute AR

The haemodynamic effects alter depending on the speed of onset of significant AR. This is due to adaptations in chamber mechanics that can take place if there is a slow onset. Chronic AR causes changes in LV size to accommodate the additional volume caused by the regurgitant volume, thereby initially maintaining cardiac output until the adaptation becomes overly pathological and LV failure sets in. Significant acute AR, on the other hand, does not allow time for these adaptive changes and LVEDP rises quickly leading to pressure and volume overload and rapid LV failure unless corrective action is taken. *Table 9.1* highlights some of the differences in findings seen between chronic and acute AR.

Table 9.1. Differences in findings between acute and chronic aortic regurgitation

	Acute aortic regurgitation	**Chronic aortic regurgitation**
Aetiology	Infective endocarditis, aortic dissection involving the root, trauma	Calcification and degeneration
Clinical presentation	Shock, heart failure, pulmonary oedema	Usually asymptomatic, presents with secondary cause to ICU
Systolic pressure	Normal or decreased	Increased
Pulse pressure	Normal or slightly decreased	Increased
Cardiac output	Impaired	Normal
Heart rate	Increased	Normal
Left ventricular size	Normal to slightly enlarged	Enlarged
LVEDP	Significantly raised	Mildly raised

Adapted from Flint *et al.* [7]. ICU – intensive care unit; LVEDP – left ventricular end-diastolic pressure.

Aortic dissection

In acute severe AR of any cause, the abrupt increase in backward blood flow may result in elevated LVEDP and pulmonary oedema. A dissection flap can be seen in several views, especially the PLAX, either near or in the aortic root or in the descending aorta below the LA. Compensatory tachycardia may preserve cardiac output initially but eventually shock will also develop. In the setting of aortic dissection with AR and hypertension it may be tempting to commence beta blockade. However, this may diminish the compensatory tachycardia and hasten the development of shock. Alternative anti-hypertensive agents should therefore be considered [6].

9.2 The mitral valve

The mitral valve (MV) is a complex of structures comprising an annulus, leaflets, chordae and papillary muscles. The LA wall and the LV myocardium play an important role in its successful function. There are two leaflets, anterior (AMVL) and posterior (PMVL), though they have also been described as aortic and mural. Each leaflet has three scallops, a detailed description of which is beyond the scope of this book [8]. MV area is normally 4–6cm² with little to no measurable gradient across it when open. Echocardiographic assessment can be complex and focused assessment is often a prelude to a more experienced assessment. Due to the impact that LA and LV size, function and filling status have on its function, its appearance can change significantly depending on cardiac state, fluid status and clinical management.

9.2.1 Mitral stenosis

Though definitive diagnosis is outside the remit of focused echocardiography (it is complex and requires integration of multiple parameters and clinical context), mitral stenosis may be suspected if the mitral leaflets are thickened or calcified with restricted motion. Rheumatic heart disease is the most common cause, with other causes (congenital, inflammatory/infiltrative) occurring only rarely. Critical illness directly due to mitral stenosis is uncommon. It usually presents either having been precipitated by another condition which necessitates an increased cardiac output (e.g. sepsis or pregnancy), or related to sequelae associated with mitral stenosis (e.g. arrhythmias, thromboembolic events or right ventricular failure). Occasionally, mitral stenosis can lead to significant LV failure. Maintaining sinus rhythm and preventing tachycardia to improve LV filling time can be vital. Severe mitral stenosis is often not well tolerated in critical illness and consideration for urgent intervention should be considered, but requires expert assessment.

Assessment of mitral stenosis

1. **Visual characterization**: a description of the various components, their shape, thickening and movement. Here particular focus should be on the presence and degree of commissural fusion, change in chordae and the extent and distribution of calcification. Rheumatic disease

is associated with thickening of commissures and chordae. This can result in the classic 'hockey stick' appearance of the AMVL when open (*Fig. 9.6*).

2. **Planimetry**: performed in the PSAX view during mid-systole. The image must be on axis and have optimal gain. Trace the inner edge to measure MV area. In experienced hands, this technique is the gold standard. However, challenges with calcification, orientation and subvalvular stenosis limit its use in focused echocardiography.

3. **Mean pressure gradient**: tracing the CWD through the MV in the A4Ch view for a VTI measures the mean gradient using the simplified Bernoulli equation and estimates MV area. However, it is susceptible to variations in heart rate and cardiac output (both of which can significantly vary in critical illness), so is a guide at best. A mean gradient of >10mmHg suggests severe mitral stenosis.

4. **Pressure half-time**: like pressure half-time (PHT) in AR, it is measured from the peak *E* wave on CWD down the gradient of the mid-diastolic descent (ignore any early rapid slope).

$$MV\ area = 220/PHT$$

Caution is advised with atrial fibrillation and other arrhythmias.

5. **Sequelae of mitral stenosis**: severe LA enlargement is common, as is pulmonary hypertension (*Fig. 9.6*).

Potential pitfalls when assessing mitral stenosis

There are several potential pitfalls when assessing mitral stenosis, these include:

- low cardiac output states with subsequent low transvalvular velocities
- the presence of arrhythmias
- high cardiac output states leading to overestimation of the severity of stenosis
- an atrial-septal defect or patent foramen ovale offloading the left atrium, leading to underestimation of severity
- significantly raised LVEDP or aortic regurgitation leading to pressure half-time shortening and underestimation.

9.2.2 Mitral regurgitation

Mitral regurgitation (MR) is caused by incompetence in the complex two leaflet valve. It is associated with volume overload of the LV leading to significantly raised LVEDP and LV failure. MR can be detected with CFD in multiple views. It can be primary (inherent valve issue) or secondary (functional) and it can be acute or chronic. Like AR, there are differences in

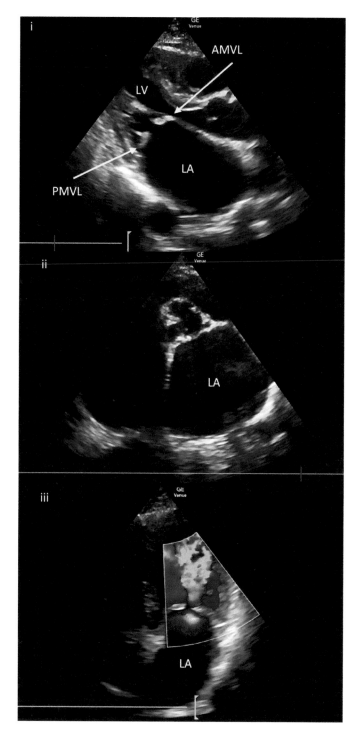

Figure 9.6. Mitral stenosis. (i) Parasternal long-axis view demonstrating the hockey stick sign and a dilated left atrium in a patient with mitral stenosis secondary to rheumatic heart disease. (ii) Parasternal short-axis view showing a severely dilated left atrium secondary to mitral stenosis. (iii) Apical four-chamber view showing turbulent flow through a stenosed mitral valve.

AMVL – anterior mitral valve leaflet; LA – left atrium; LV – left ventricle; PMVL – posterior mitral valve leaflet.

the acute and chronic findings. The size of the MR CFD trace is determined by the size of the defect, the direction of the jet and the LV–LA gradient. The LV–LA gradient is influenced by LV afterload, contractility, LVEDP, LA pressure, fluid status and mechanical ventilation (where relevant).

Common causes of primary MR include myxomatous degeneration (non-inflammatory progressive disarray), Marfan syndrome, rheumatic disease, infective endocarditis, and papillary muscle or chordae tendineae rupture. Additionally, the direction of the jet of MR in combination with the mobility of the MV leaflets can help determine the mechanism of MR, according to the Carpentier classification:

- **Type I**: normal mobility of leaflets with annular dilation that causes a central jet (secondary MR) or perforation of a leaflet.

- **Type II**: excessive mobility with ruptured chords or severe prolapse, causing a jet directed to the opposite side of the affected leaflet.

- **Type III**: restricted mobility due to shrinkage of the subvalvular apparatus and tethering of the papillary muscle causing a jet directed to the same side as the affected leaflet.

Assessment of mitral regurgitation

1. **Visual characterization**: this should consist of a description of the valve apparatus, LV and LA. There should be particular focus on leaflet prolapse or flail, vegetations, calcification, chordae, and for LV dilation causing distortion of the mitral annulus and functional (secondary) MR. There may a dilated LV or LA.

2. **Semi-quantitative assessment**: CFD – this is an excellent screening tool to rule in or out significant MR. A large central jet, or an eccentric jet may be noted (*Fig. 9.7*). There are multiple pitfalls. The size of the jet can be smaller if eccentric (the Coanda effect) or if the MR is acute (due to a rapid and significant rise in LA pressure, see *Echo Tip* below). Despite these challenges, a small central jet corresponds well with mild MR. Signs of likely significant MR include:

- a jet area of >8cm^2

- jet area / LA area >40%

- large eccentric jet reaching the inferior/posterior wall of the LA.

3. **Vena contracta**: this involves measuring the CFD trace to find the width of the jet at its narrowest point, often slightly below the valve. The use of zoom mode and a small colour Doppler box can help improve accuracy. Its predictive capacity relies on the incompetence being circular, but this is not always the case. 3D assessment may be more accurate than 2D. Multiple jets are not additive. A vena contracta of >7mm is indicative of severe MR.

4. **Quantitative assessment**: advanced techniques include the PISA method to measure effective orifice area, and Doppler volumetric methods for regurgitant volume and fraction. Additional supportive measures include assessment for systolic flow reversal in the pulmonary veins, and signal intensity of the continuous wave jet envelope.

Acute versus chronic MR

Acute MR (e.g. papillary muscle rupture): results in a reduction in forward stroke volume and acute pulmonary oedema. Compensatory tachycardia may initially be enough to preserve cardiac output but eventually shock will develop. Surgical intervention is indicated after initial stabilization.

Chronic MR: as the regurgitant fraction increases, the LV gradually dilates, ejection fraction increases, and a normal stroke volume is maintained. However, the LV diastolic pressure eventually rises, leading to a downward spiral of worsening MR with subsequent pulmonary hypertension. This is also an indication for surgical repair.

MR in critical illness

Dynamic variation can be significant in critical illness. Several factors may influence the severity of the MR. Factors that worsen MR are associated with increased LV afterload or workload and impaired LV performance; these include sepsis, myocardial ischaemia, raised systemic vascular resistance, tachycardia, arrhythmia and significant shock and volume overload.

Factors that can reduce the severity of MR include those that reduce cardiac workload and afterload such as negative inotropes, vasodilation and fluid removal. Mechanical ventilation and the administration of PEEP may reduce the severity of MR (though it can recur on reduction of the PEEP). This is due to a reduction of LV preload and afterload. In these situations, haemodynamic data from other sources such as a pulmonary artery catheter may be required [9,10].

Overall, this means that quantification of MR may change significantly during ICU admission and is worthy of reassessment, both if the clinical state changes rapidly and after discharge from ICU.

ECHO TIP

Colour flow Doppler

CFD is a measure of turbulent flow within a chamber. It includes the jet that created the turbulent flow and blood that was already in the chamber. An analogy would be if a showerhead was placed in a bath of water, the moving water seen is greater than the size of the shower jet and the amount of additional water entrained is influenced by the speed and velocity of the jet.

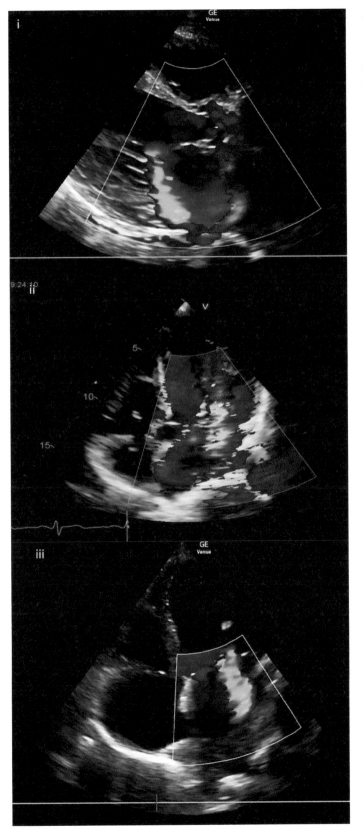

Figure 9.7. Examples of mitral regurgitation. (i) Parasternal long-axis view showing an eccentric regurgitant jet. (ii) Apical five-chamber view showing severe mitral regurgitation secondary to papillary muscle rupture. (iii) Apical four-chamber view showing an eccentric regurgitant jet.

9.3 The tricuspid valve

The tricuspid valve is a trileaflet valve with a complex anatomy leading to variation in naming of the leaflets. The commonest used naming system is anterior (largest), septal and posterior (smallest) with papillary muscles often supporting two leaflets. It can easily be visualized in multiple views including the RV inflow, PSAX, RV centred A4Ch and subcostal. The tricuspid valve is located apically when compared to the anterior leaflet of the MV. If this distance is significant then it is known as Ebstein's anomaly (*Fig. 9.8*).

9.3.1 Tricuspid stenosis

Tricuspid stenosis is rare. It may be suspected where there is leaflet thickening, calcification, doming or restriction. It may be associated with tricuspid regurgitation (TR), and most commonly occurs due to rheumatic heart disease. Other causes include carcinoid syndrome, pacemaker-associated stenosis, and obstruction by a tumour. An enlarged right atrium and dilated IVC are supportive, with further Doppler assessments requiring expert involvement. This will include pressure gradients averaged over a respiratory cycle, pressure half-time and valve area by continuity equation (calculated using similar methods to the MV). Indications that stenosis may be clinically important can include a pressure half-time of >190m/sec, a mean gradient of >5mmHg and a valve area of <1cm^2 [6].

9.3.2 Tricuspid regurgitation

Trace or mild 'physiological' TR occurs in approximately 70% of normal individuals [10,11]. Most pathological TR in adults is 'secondary', due to RV dilation from pulmonary or left heart disease.

Primary TR is uncommon but can occur due to a variety of disease processes: carcinoid, rheumatic disease, endocarditis (especially in intravenous drug abuse), myxomatous degeneration, congenital (Ebstein anomaly), and trauma (including blunt non-penetrating trauma to the precordium). Iatrogenesis may also be a factor with guidewires, catheters, and pacemakers sometimes causing damage to valvular apparatus.

Assessment of TR

1. **Visual characterization**: 2D imaging should be used to inspect for RV dilation, excessive leaflet motion and tricuspid annular dilation. TR can be detected using CFD in the RV inflow view, PSAX view at the level of the aorta or the A4Ch view (*Fig. 9.8*). In severe TR, the RV and RA are often dilated but RV function may be hyperdynamic, normal, or reduced depending on the cause. A large central jet (>10cm^2) reaching the posterior wall is also suggestive of severe TR, a small jet (<5cm^2) is suggestive of mild TR.

2. **Continuous wave Doppler**: this is mainly used to estimate pulmonary artery systolic pressure (PASP). The shape of the Doppler trace also provides information about severity of TR in the density, shape and timing of the peak velocity (*Fig. 9.8*). An early peaking, full envelope triangular trace suggests significant TR.

3. **Vena contracta**: this is measured in relation to the TR jet using the same method described in the AR and MR sections, with a vena contracta of >7mm suggestive of severe TR.

4. **Hepatic vein flow**: blunting or reversal of flow can indicate increasing severity, though this is a non-specific sign to TR.

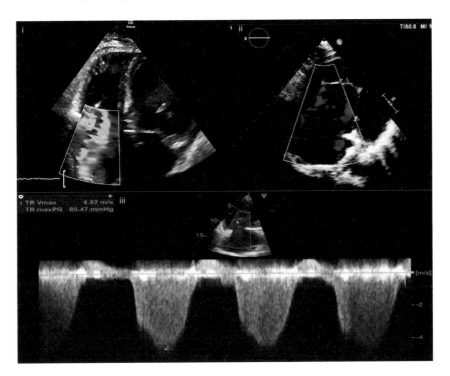

Figure 9.8. Examples of tricuspid regurgitation. (i) Right ventricular focused apical four-chamber view demonstrating severe tricuspid regurgitation. (ii) Apical four-chamber view demonstrating Ebstein's anomaly with tricuspid regurgitation. Note the atrialization of most of the right ventricle and the distortion of the left side of the heart. (iii) Continuous wave Doppler trace of regurgitant jet with a max velocity of 4.62m/sec suggestive of severe pulmonary hypertension.

Haemodynamics and management of tricuspid regurgitation

Worsening TR can lead to RA and RV dilation through volume overload in a progressive vicious cycle with worsening TR and subsequent hepatic venous congestion. Forward flow from the RV can be increasingly impaired, and at the same time severe RV dilation can impact LV diastolic filling. Both together can reduce LV cardiac output. Medical management is often the mainstay of treatment even in severe cases. Volume management is key because volume overload will lead to progressive regurgitation, venous congestion and cardiac-induced cirrhosis. Factors increasing pulmonary pressures such as hypoxia, hypercarbia and acidosis must be treated aggressively. Where mechanical ventilation is required, the complex interplay of factors may necessitate the placement of a pulmonary artery catheter to optimize treatment. Isolated tricuspid valve repair is uncommon, probably due to an absence of evidence for survival benefit [11,12]. However, repair during left-sided surgery may help with heart failure symptoms.

9.4 The pulmonary valve

The pulmonary valve is a tricuspid structure, similar to the aortic valve. The cusps are thinner, however, and the valve can be difficult to visualize. The PSAX (angled just above the aortic valve), or a superiorly tilted PLAX view (RVOT view) may be used.

9.4.1 Pulmonary stenosis

Isolated pulmonary stenosis is uncommon; however, it can be associated with syndromes such as Noonan syndrome. Subvalvular, valvular or supravalvular pulmonary stenosis can also be seen post Tetralogy of Fallot repair or, less commonly, due to endocarditis, carcinoid, rheumatic disease, myxomatous degeneration or trauma.

2D imaging may show features such as RV hypertrophy, valve thickening, systolic doming, or post-stenotic dilation. CWD is the mainstay of assessment, with a peak pressure gradient of >64mmHg being the cut-off for severe stenosis [12,13].

9.4.2 Pulmonary regurgitation

A trace of PR is present in up to 75% of normal individuals. Trace PR can be useful in establishing the precise location of the valve if imaging is challenging. Severe PR is most commonly seen post repair of congenital lesions, such as Tetralogy of Fallot. However, acquired mild to moderate PR mostly occurs due to pulmonary hypertension causing pulmonary artery dilation [12,13]. Other acquired causes mirror those associated with pulmonary stenosis, i.e. post Tetralogy of Fallot repair, endocarditis, carcinoid, rheumatic disease, myxomatous degeneration or trauma.

2D imaging may reveal annular dilation, or distorted, absent or flail leaflets. The absence of RV dysfunction suggests milder PR. Colour flow imaging will show a small spindle-like jet in physiological PR. Pathological PR is characterized by a wide, holodiastolic jet. Similar to AR, a jet width/RVOT ratio of >65% indicates severe disease (*Fig. 9.9*). Other markers of severity are not well established.

Chronic severe PR is often well tolerated for many years. However, RV volume overload does occur over time and RV function should be monitored.

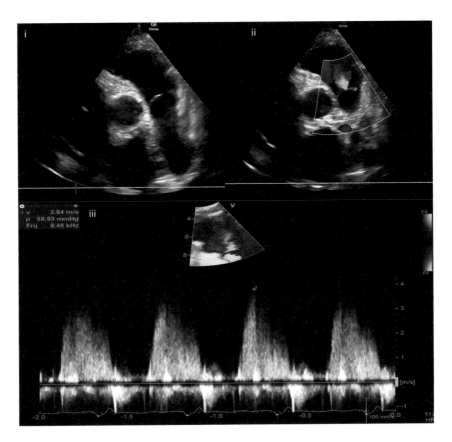

Figure 9.9. (i) Parasternal short-axis view at the level of the pulmonary and aortic valves. (ii) Pulmonary regurgitation jet visible from the parasternal short-axis view. (iii) Continuous wave Doppler of pulmonary regurgitation jet in the right ventricular outflow view in a patient with pulmonary hypertension.

9.5 Prosthetic valves

Prosthetic valves can be challenging to image. Metallic components produce signal drop-out and the normal expected findings are dependent on the particular valve and size used (*Fig. 9.10*). Mechanical and bioprosthetic valves are inherently stenotic compared with normal tissue. It can be difficult to distinguish between obstruction from valve design, pathological obstruction, and patient–valve mismatch. So, their routine assessment should be carried out by experts.

Each valve has its own reference ranges that can be looked up and so knowledge of the size and type of valve can be extremely useful (access to operation notes or clinical letters are often helpful). Many valves are associated with trivial or mild regurgitation. This is either inherent in the design (to prevent thrombus or pannus) in mechanical valves (known as 'washing' jets) or perivalvular, which is now increasingly common with percutaneous valves. Detailed guidelines on the assessment of prosthetic valves and perivalvular leak can found in the American Society of Echocardiography guidelines [14].

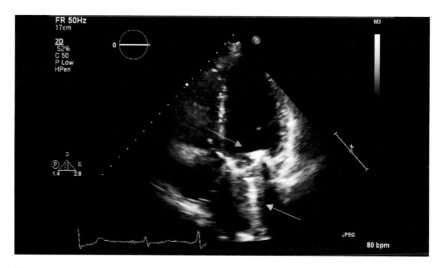

Figure 9.10. Apical four-chamber view demonstrating acoustic shadowing (orange arrow) caused by a metallic mitral valve (green arrow).

Description of a prosthetic valve focuses on several areas:

- Is it well positioned?

- Is it rocking?

- Is it dehisced?

- Is there new or significant perivalvular leak?

- Is there thrombosis or pannus on the valve?

- Is there a suspected vegetation?

- Is the valve unexpectedly stenotic?

- Is there prosthetic–patient mismatch?

Dimensionless index (see *Section 9.1.1*) can be used to help determine abnormal valve stenosis because it avoids the challenges of measuring outflow tracts.

Haemodynamic instability in the presence of a prosthetic valve should be regarded as prosthetic valve malfunction until proven otherwise and urgent expert review sought. Additionally, in the setting of haemodynamic instability, focused bedside echo should identify other contributing factors such as a low cardiac output [2]. It is worth noting that high cardiac output states can increase the flow across the prosthetic valve and mimic stenosis.

9.6 Endocarditis

Diagnosis of infective endocarditis by major Duke's criteria requires a combination of positive microbiology and typical findings on echocardiography (see Duke's criteria box below) [15].

Echocardiography only has 50–70% sensitivity (prosthetic/native) for the presence of a lesion consistent with infective endocarditis. False positives can occur with nodules, ruptured chordae or fibroelastomas. Vegetations can be located 'off-axis' of standard imaging and therefore can be missed if the scan is focused or rapid. Additionally, lesions can be flat, making them impossible to see on TTE. Infective endocarditis, therefore, cannot and should not be ruled out with TTE. However, due to several pragmatic reasons, TTE is the standard first line investigation and there are a number of typical features and tips that can help in finding and identifying vegetations (see infective endocarditis *Imaging Tips* box below).

Vegetations may be seen on native valves or foreign materials such as pacemaker leads and prosthetic valves. However, infection may also present as an abscess, or prosthetic valve dehiscence. TOE may be required if TTE is inconclusive and there is a high index of suspicion of infective endocarditis, especially if there is potential prosthetic valve involvement or technical challenges related to TTE, e.g. limited views due to mechanical ventilation.

IMAGING TIP

Infective endocarditis

Focused infective endocarditis echocardiography includes scanning 'on and off axis' across the valves in the different standard views.

Appropriate use of zoom required to examine valves clearly.

Be wary of artefacts and attempt to find anomalies in more than one view.

New regurgitation should raise suspicion of infective endocarditis when performing a scan.

Typical features of a vegetation include:

- a texture similar to the myocardium (not overly bright)
- usually upstream of the valve
- lobulated shape that can have an oscillating motion.

Report the location, maximum size, mobility and any regurgitation (or stenosis with large lesions).

Echocardiographic criteria as part of modified Duke's criteria for endocarditis

Echocardiographic evidence of endocardial involvement:

1. Oscillating intracardiac mass on a heart valve, on supporting structures, in the path of regurgitant jets, or on implanted material without another anatomical explanation.
2. Cardiac abscess.
3. New dehiscence of a prosthetic valve.
4. New valvular regurgitation.

9.7 Summary

The ability to perform a focused valvular assessment refers to an ability to detect clinically significant valvular dysfunction. Findings should be interpreted in the context of clinical history, examination and haemodynamics. Discovery of suspected significant valvular pathology should prompt referral for an advanced echocardiographic assessment.

9.8 References

1. Wharton G, Steeds R, Allen J, *et al.* (2015) A minimum dataset for a standard adult transthoracic echocardiogram. *Echo Res & Pract,* 2:G9.

2. Levitov A, Frankel HL, Blaivas M, *et al.* (2016) Guidelines for the appropriate use of bedside general and cardiac ultrasonography in the evaluation of critically ill patients – Part II: cardiac ultrasonography. *Crit Care Med,* 44:1206.

3. Bradley SM, Foag K, Monteagudo K, *et al.* (2019) Use of routinely captured echocardiographic data in the diagnosis of severe aortic stenosis. *Heart,* 105:112.

4. Irvine T, Kenny A (1997) Aortic stenosis and angina with normal coronary arteries: the role of coronary flow abnormalities. *Heart,* 78:213.

5. Brown J, Morgan-Hughes NJ (2005) Aortic stenosis and non-cardiac surgery. *Cont Ed Anaes Crit Care & Pain,* 5:1.

6. Akinseye OA, Pathak A, Ibebuogu UN (2018) Aortic valve regurgitation: a comprehensive review. *Curr Prob Cardiol,* 43:315.

7. Flint N, Beigel R, Siegel RJ (2021) Aortic regurgitation: pathophysiology. In: *ASE's Comprehensive Echocardiography,* 3rd ed (Lang R, Goldstein SA, Kronzon I, Khandheria BK, Saric M, Mon-Ani V, eds), pp 487. Elsevier.

8. Ho SY (2002) Anatomy of the mitral valve. *Heart,* 88:iv5.

9. McLean A, Huang S, Hilton A (2020) *Oxford Textbook of Advanced Critical Care Echocardiography.* OUP.

10. Zoghbi WA, Adams D, Bonow RO, *et al.* (2017) Recommendations for noninvasive evaluation of native valvular regurgitation. *J Am Soc Echocardiogr,* 30:303.

11. Zack CJ, Fender EA, Chandrashekar P, *et al.* (2017) National trends and outcomes in isolated tricuspid valve surgery. *J Am Coll Cardiol,* 70:2953.

12. Baumgartner H, Hung J, Bermejo J, *et al.* (2009) Echocardiographic assessment of valve stenosis. *J Am Soc Echocardiogr,* 22:1.

13. Zaidi A, Oxborough D, Augustine DX, *et al.* (2020) Echocardiographic assessment of the tricuspid and pulmonary valves. *Echo Res & Pract,* 7:G95.

14. Zoghbi WA, Chambers JB, Dumesnil JG, *et al.* (2009) Recommendations for evaluation of prosthetic valves with echocardiography and doppler ultrasound: a report From the American Society of Echocardiography's Guidelines and Standards Committee and the Task Force on Prosthetic Valves. *J Am Soc Echocardiogr,* 22:975.

15. Li JS, Sexton DJ, Mick N, *et al.* (2000) Proposed modifications to the Duke criteria for the diagnosis of infective endocarditis. *Clin Infect Dis,* 30:633.

CHAPTER 10

ASSESSMENT OF THE PERICARDIUM AND PERICARDIOCENTESIS

Alejandra Ceballos, Julian Rios Rios & Pradeep Madhivathanan

The pathophysiology of pericardial disease and the consequent haemodynamic changes often represent a challenge for clinicians. POCUS assessment of the pericardium is an invaluable, non-invasive diagnostic tool that can be performed at the bedside. In addition to aiding diagnosis and directing management, POCUS can also provide procedural guidance for the drainage of pericardial effusions [1].

10.1 Anatomy of the pericardium

The pericardium is a two-layer membranous structure that encircles the heart, proximal portions of the great vessels, distal venae cavae and pulmonary veins. Classically, these two layers are described as the parietal (fibrous) and visceral (serous) pericardium [2]. The visceral pericardium is the layer adhered to the epicardium covering the heart and it extends to the proximal portion of the great vessels where it merges to the parietal pericardium. The pericardial cavity normally contains 15–50ml of pericardial fluid, composed essentially of plasma ultrafiltrate and a small quantity of lymph [2]. At the base of the heart the pericardium forms two sinuses arising from the pericardial reflections around the great vessels.

- **The oblique sinus** – located between the pulmonary veins and the inferior vena cava. This is visible on echocardiography if the volume of fluid in the pericardial cavity increases.

- **The transverse sinus** – located posteriorly to the ascending aorta and pulmonary trunk. The transverse sinus can be visualized in the parasternal long-axis (PLAX) view.

10.2 Functions of the pericardium

The pericardium has several functions: it protects the heart from overdistension, decreases friction, facilitates free movement and ensures that the heart has enough support to remain in the mediastinum. In addition, the pericardium plays metabolic, immunological and fibrinolytic roles alongside modulation of neurotransmission and contractility of ligaments [3,4].

10.3 Normal echocardiographic features of the pericardium

The pericardium is seen on echocardiography as an hyperechogenic line surrounding the heart, with a thickness of 1–2mm, and should be visible in all standard POCUS windows. The small amount of pericardial fluid normally found in the pericardial space can be visualized as a thin anechoic line separating the two layers of the pericardium (*Fig. 10.1*).

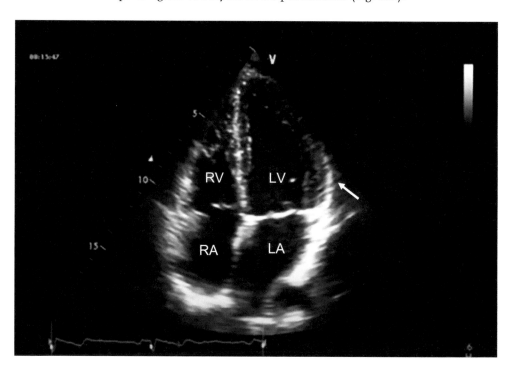

Figure 10.1. Apical four-chamber view showing a normal pericardium (arrow). LA – left atrium; LV – left ventricle; RA – right atrium; RV – right ventricle.

10.4 Pericardial pathology

Despite the 'simple' structure of the pericardium, it can be affected by congenital abnormalities and several pathological processes including infectious, neoplastic, inflammatory, traumatic, metabolic and idiopathic [3]. The focus of this chapter is to review the most common pathologies associated with the pericardium:

- acute pericarditis

- pericardial effusions (with or without cardiac tamponade)

- constrictive pericarditis.

10.4.1 Acute pericarditis

Pericarditis refers to inflammation of the pericardial layers and is divided into acute (<4–6 weeks), recurrent (new signs and symptoms after a symptom-free interval of 4–6 weeks), and chronic (>3 months) [3,5].

The potential causes of acute pericarditis are numerous. In developed countries the most common cause is viral infection, whilst in developing countries it is tuberculosis [3,5]. The diagnosis is confirmed by the presence of a minimum of two of the following four criteria:

1. chest pain

2. pericardial rub

3. ECG changes

4. a new or worsening pericardial effusion.

Accordingly, echocardiography is the initial tool of choice as it plays an important role in diagnosis, assessment of physiological and haemodynamic effects, evolution and response to therapies. However, echocardiography may be normal in up to 40% of cases.

To identify patients at high risk of complications, such as large pericardial effusions with haemodynamic compromise and cardiac tamponade, it is essential to quantify the pericardial effusion. This is done by measuring the size of the echo-free space between the parietal and visceral pericardium at the end of diastole.

Findings on echocardiography may include a pericardial collection, increased echogenicity, pericardial thickening, septal bounce and segmental wall abnormalities [5].

10.4.2 Pericardial effusions (with or without tamponade)

Pericardial effusions vary in size (from small to very large) and in their haemodynamic effects (*Fig. 10.2*). Effusion sizes may be classified as follows:

- trivial (only seen during systole)

- small (<10mm)

- moderate (10–20mm)

- large (21–24mm)

- very large (>25mm).

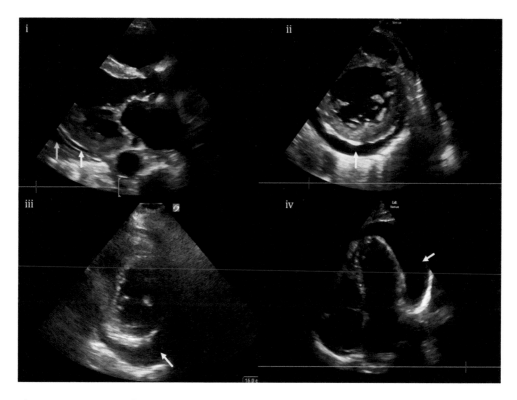

Figure 10.2. Examples of pericardial effusions. (i) Trivial pericardial effusion (yellow arrow) seen in the parasternal long-axis window in systole and a pleural effusion (blue arrow). (ii) Small pericardial effusion seen in the short-axis window (yellow arrow). (iii) Moderate pericardial effusion seen in the short-axis window (yellow arrow). (iv) Very large pericardial effusion seen in the apical four-chamber window (yellow arrow).

In the context of cardiac surgery, post-surgical bleeding may be the cause of a pericardial effusion with cardiac tamponade (*Fig. 10.3*). Other common causes of effusions include malignancy, tuberculosis and immune-mediated illnesses such as systemic lupus erythematosus [6,7]. Pericardial effusions caused by these pathologies frequently accumulate slowly producing a large amount of fluid, sometimes greater than 500ml, with minimal symptoms due to cardiac adaptation. Conversely, small collections in the pericardial space that accumulate rapidly can cause severe haemodynamic instability [6,7]. This is explained by the J-shaped pressure/volume curve of the healthy pericardium (*Fig. 10.4*) [7,8].

Pathophysiology of cardiac tamponade

It is paramount to understand the effects of respiration on the heart's diastolic filling dynamics. Ventricular filling occurs during diastole when the atrioventricular valves open. During the diastolic phase, there are two echocardiographic identifiable inflow waves in both the right and left ventricles:

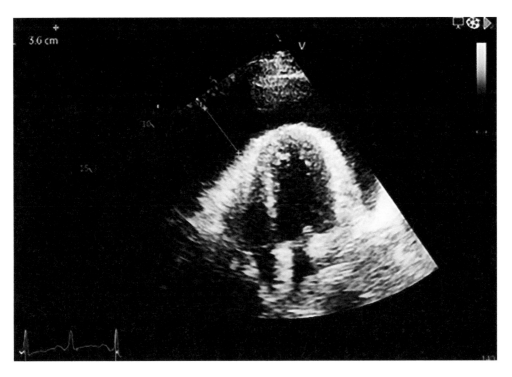

Figure 10.3. Cardiac tamponade in a patient with a very large pericardial effusion (3.6cm).

Pericardial pressure-volume relationship

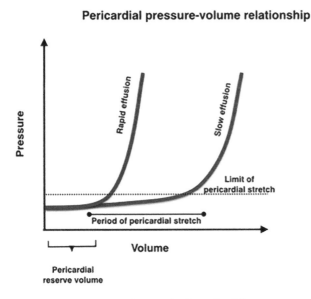

Figure 10.4. When pericardial fluid accumulates rapidly in the case of acute or 'surgical' tamponade (blue line), the limit of pericardial stretch is reached early causing tamponade. Slow accumulation of fluid such as in chronic or 'medical' tamponade (red line), allows a longer period of pericardial stretch before reaching a state of tamponade. Image reproduced from Madhivathanan *et al.* [8].

- the *E* wave – related to early diastolic filling

- the *A* wave – related to atrial contraction or late diastolic filling.

Normally, during spontaneous inspiration, the decrease in intrathoracic and intrapericardial pressures leads to an increase in the trans-tricuspid inflow, which results in augmented right ventricle (RV) diastolic filling and stroke volume. However, during this phase of the cardiac cycle the combination of ventricular interdependence (where the interventricular septum is shifted towards the left ventricle (LV)) and limited pericardial space, results in a compensatory decrease in LV stroke volume in early inspiration.

During expiration, the opposite occurs. There is an increase in intrathoracic and intrapericardial pressures resulting in a mild reduction in RV diastolic filling alongside an increase in LV diastolic filling, aided by shifting of the interventricular septum towards the RV.

Under physiological circumstances the intrapericardial pressure is below the intracardiac pressures. However, once the volume of fluid in the pericardial sac exceeds pericardial stretch, there is an increase in the intrapericardial pressures resulting in compression of cardiac chambers and a decrease in normal diastolic filling. In cardiac tamponade, the excessive pericardial fluid accumulation causes elevation and equalization of diastolic and pericardial pressures in the cardiac chambers [7,8]. Consequently, there is inhibition of ventricular filling and a decrease in cardiac output. Initially, the lowest pressure cardiac chamber is most affected by the raise in the intrapericardial pressure. Therefore, the right atrium (RA) collapses during systole which can be seen on echocardiography [8,9].

In more severe cases, the intrapericardial pressures become equal to the diastolic RV pressure resulting in compression and collapse of the ventricle during diastole. Once intrapericardial pressures overcome intraventricular pressures, pulsus paradoxus will ensue; this refers to a systolic pressure drop of more than 10mmHg during inspiration. Pulsus paradoxus occurs due to an exaggerated decrease in LV filling during inspiration because of an increase in RV filling, or a stiff or tense free wall. This leads to RV distension with shifting of the interventricular septum further towards the already underfilled LV. In cardiac tamponade the normal effects of respiration on the filling of cardiac chambers are accentuated [8,9].

Clinical features of a pericardial effusion

Symptoms may vary depending on the speed of fluid accumulation. Common signs and symptoms include shortness of breath on exertion, orthopnea, chest pain, nausea, fatigue, palpitations and sinus tachycardia. Symptoms associated with compressive effects include dysphagia, hoarseness and hiccups due to oesophageal, recurrent laryngeal nerve and phrenic nerve compression, respectively. Beck´s triad in cardiac tamponade describes the combination of hypotension, raised jugular venous pressure and muffled heart sounds [7].

Key points when assessing a pericardial effusion

- Obtain multiple different views of the effusion (*Fig. 10.5*).

- The rate of accumulation of the effusion is more important than its estimated size in predicting tamponade.

- Be aware of false positives such as a left-sided pleural effusion or a pericardial fat pad.

- Identify the descending aorta in the PLAX view – if the effusion lies adjacent or posterior to this structure, it is a pleural effusion. If the effusion lies anterior to the descending aorta, it is a pericardial effusion.

- The pericardial fat pad is seen on ultrasound as an echogenic structure that moves together with the myocardium. It is usually specular or granular in appearance.

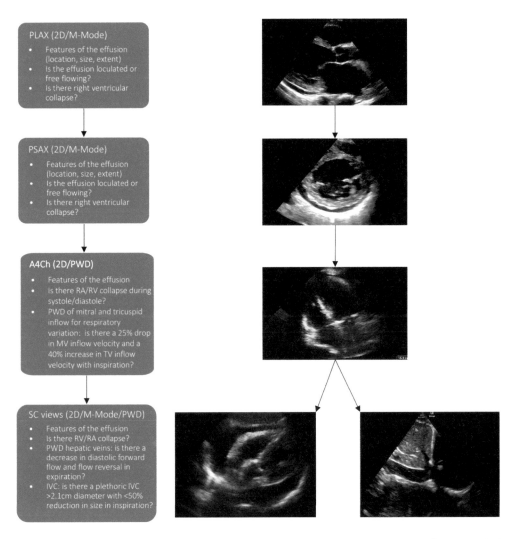

PLAX (2D/M-Mode)
- Features of the effusion (location, size, extent)
- Is the effusion loculated or free flowing?
- Is there right ventricular collapse?

PSAX (2D/M-Mode)
- Features of the effusion (location, size, extent)
- Is the effusion loculated or free flowing?
- Is there right ventricular collapse?

A4Ch (2D/PWD)
- Features of the effusion
- Is there RA/RV collapse during systole/diastole?
- PWD of mitral and tricuspid inflow for respiratory variation: is there a 25% drop in MV inflow velocity and a 40% increase in TV inflow velocity with inspiration?

SC views (2D/M-Mode/PWD)
- Features of the effusion
- Is there RV/RA collapse?
- PWD hepatic veins: is there a decrease in diastolic forward flow and flow reversal in expiration?
- IVC: is there a plethoric IVC >2.1cm diameter with <50% reduction in size in inspiration?

Figure 10.5. Flowchart for a focused transthoracic echocardiographic assessment of a pericardial effusion. A4Ch – apical four-chamber; IVC – inferior vena cava; MV – mitral valve; PLAX – parasternal long-axis view; PWD – pulsed wave Doppler; RA – right atrium; RV – right ventricle; SC – subcostal; TV – tricuspid valve.

10.4.3 Constrictive pericarditis

The typical feature of constrictive pericarditis is obliteration of the pericardial cavity due to thickened, fibrous, and adherent visceral and parietal pericardium layers, causing a significant reduction in compliance of the pericardial sac (*Fig. 10.6*). These changes lead to impairment of diastolic ventricular filling and elevated intracardiac pressures alongside an increase in the systemic venous pressures and exaggerated ventricular interdependence. The most common cause of constrictive pericarditis in developed countries is recurrent pericarditis, post cardiac surgery and radiotherapy. Tuberculosis remains the most frequent cause in developing countries [3,5].

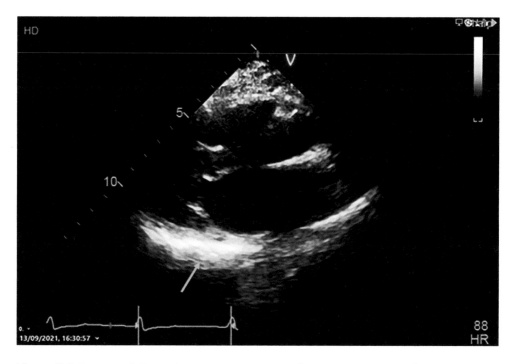

Figure 10.6. Parasternal long-axis view in a patient with constrictive pericarditis. Note visible pericardial thickening (blue arrow).

Echocardiographic features of constrictive pericarditis

Using 2D echocardiography:

- Pericardial thickening (>4mm): the thickening may have an asymmetrical distribution, hence a careful assessment from different views is essential.

- Abnormal interventricular septum motion: leftward septal bounce in early diastole (transient RV pressure > LV pressure).

- Atrial dilation.

- Dilated extra-pericardial venae cavae and hepatic veins with loss of respiratory variation in diameter (elevated RA pressures).

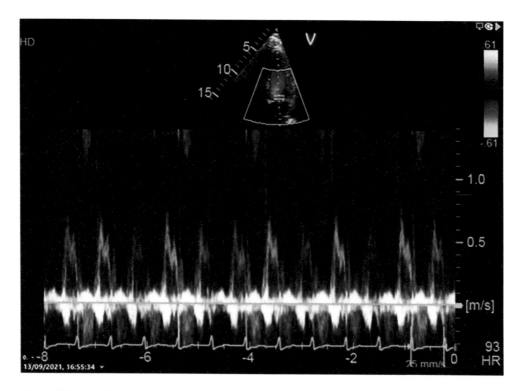

Figure 10.7. Apical four-chamber view assessing mitral valve inflow using pulsed wave Doppler. Here we see a high *E* wave velocity, a short *E* velocity deceleration time and a small *A* wave velocity.

Using M-mode:

- Useful for measuring pericardial thickening.

- In the PLAX and PSAX views, it shows an increased echogenic area posterior to the LV epicardium.

Using Doppler: the blood flow velocity across the tricuspid and mitral valve, in spontaneously breathing healthy patients, varies during inspiration and expiration because of the respiratory cycle's effect on systemic and pulmonary venous return and intrathoracic pressure (respirophasic variation).

- Tricuspid valve:
  - **inspiration:** increase of trans tricuspid inflow velocity up to 20%
  - **expiration:** decrease of inflow velocity.

- Mitral valve:
  - **inspiration:** decrease of trans mitral inflow velocity up to 5%
  - **expiration:** increase of inflow velocity.

In spontaneously breathing patients with constrictive pericarditis, the respirophasic variation is markedly increased, normally to >40% for tricuspid inflow and >25% for mitral inflow.

Doppler recordings may also show:

- High *E* wave velocity, short deceleration time of the *E* wave velocity and a very small *A* wave velocity (*Fig. 10.7*).

- A >20% increase in LV relaxation time in inspiration.

- A pulmonary vein systolic to diastolic inflow ratio (S/D) of >1 and systolic flow reversal in the hepatic veins.

- Normal or increased *E'* wave velocity on TDI.

- 'Annulus reversus' on TDI: higher *E'* wave velocity at the septal mitral annulus compared to the lateral mitral annulus.

Differentiating constrictive pericarditis and restrictive cardiomyopathy

These entities are clinically similar with impairment of cardiac filling a common finding in both conditions. As a result, the diagnosis can sometimes be challenging and other investigations such as cardiac catheterization,

Table 10.1. Clinical and echocardiographic differentiation between constrictive pericarditis and restrictive cardiomyopathy

Clinical and echo findings	Constrictive pericarditis	Restrictive cardiomyopathy
Cardiac muscle	Normal	Rigid
Conduction disturbances	Uncommon	Common
Ventricular filling	Impaired	Impaired
Ventricular size	Normal	Near-normal, but there may be LVH and a small LV in later stages
LV function	Preserved	Diastolic and/or systolic dysfunction
Septal motion	Respiratory shift	Normal
Pericardium	Thickened	Normal
Atria	Normal	Enlarged
Transmitral inflow respirophasic variation	Increased	Normal
TDI	Normal velocities Septal e' >7cm/sec	Reduced velocities Septal e' <7cm/sec
E/e' ratio	<15	>15
Pulmonary vein flow	Expiratory diastolic flow reversal	Inspiratory diastolic flow reversal
Hepatic vein flow	Expiratory diastolic flow reversal	Inspiratory diastolic flow reversal

LV – left ventricle; LVH – left ventricular hypertrophy; TDI – tissue Doppler imaging.

magnetic resonance imaging (MRI) or endomyocardial biopsy may be required. However, the medical history, clinical presentation, haemodynamic variables and the use of Doppler echocardiography velocities are key in helping differentiate the two diagnoses (*Table 10.1*). The differentiation is crucial because the clinical impact, treatment and prognosis may differ dramatically.

10.5 Echocardiographic guided pericardiocentesis

Pericardiocentesis is a procedure that can be performed in an elective or urgent manner. Elective pericardiocentesis is more of a diagnostic technique whilst urgent pericardiocentesis is mainly a therapeutic technique which is indicated when a pericardial effusion is causing haemodynamic compromise, usually manifested as hypotension [10,11].

Studies have found the use of echocardiography to guide pericardiocentesis results in fewer complications (<2%) and a higher success rate (>95%) [10,11]. There are two approaches to echo-guided pericardiocentesis:

1. **The echo assisted method:** here the operator memorizes the required needle trajectory using pre-procedural echocardiography, but the advancement of the needle towards the pericardial space is not under live guidance.

2. **The echo guided method:** here the advancement of the needle is monitored in real time with ultrasound.

The pericardial space can be accessed from three different anatomical aspects:

1. apical

2. subxiphoid

3. parasternal.

Pericardiocentesis should be performed in a room with resuscitation equipment and emergency drugs available. Electrocardiography, pulse oximetry and invasive arterial pressure monitoring are strongly recommended alongside access to a large peripheral cannula for rapid fluid administration. Sometimes, central venous access is needed to facilitate administration of inotropic and/or vasoactive drugs. It is important to check the platelet count and coagulation state of the patient and have red blood cells ready in case transfusion is needed. Informed consent should be obtained if possible. The patient is positioned in a semi-reclined position at 30–45° with mild leftwards rotation [10,11].

Equipment:

- echocardiography probe

- sterile ultrasound probe cover

- sterile gel

- 16–18G 9cm Teflon-sheathed needle (16cm needle if subxiphoid approach)

- J-tipped guidewire

- 6–8Fr dilator and introducer sheath

- pericardial drainage set

- antiseptic agent swabs

- sterile gloves and gown

- local anaesthetic for subcutaneous and needle trajectory infiltration

- size 11 blade scalpel.

Major complications – it is important to remain cognisant of:

- ventricular arrhythmias

- pneumothorax

- pneumopericardium

- abdominal viscera puncture

- laceration of coronary arteries

- laceration of intercostal vessels

- pericardial decompression syndrome (paradoxical haemodynamic worsening with pulmonary oedema and cardiogenic shock)

- injury of cardiac chambers

- death.

Minor complications:

- vasovagal signs with bradycardia and hypotension

- supraventricular arrhythmias

- pleuro-pericardial fistulas.

Technique for drain insertion – a suggested technique for pericardial drain insertion is as follows:

1. The most common approach is the subxiphoid.

2. The area should be prepared in a sterile fashion.

3. The area and needle trajectory should be infiltrated with local anaesthetic.

4. A 16cm sheathed needle attached to a saline-filled syringe is inserted between the xiphisternum and left costal margin with an angulation of 30–45° advancing carefully towards the left shoulder with continuous aspiration applied.

5. The needle position within the pericardial cavity should be confirmed with ultrasound and by aspiration of blood or pericardial fluid.

6. The sheath is then advanced and the needle is withdrawn.

7. Using the Seldinger technique, the catheter is then inserted into the pericardial sac and the effusion is drained using syringe suction.

10.6 Top tips when assessing the pericardium

- Eyeball the general anatomy of the heart and estimate its function.

- Look for evident pathology and integrate this with the clinical context.

- Describe the appearance of the pericardium (thickened, calcified, masses, etc.).

- Identify anechoic structures outside the LV and RV that become circumferential and try to differentiate these from artefact or fat.

- Assess whether the fluid surrounding the heart is causing compression of the LV or the free walls of the RA or RV.

- It is important to visualize the pericardium in multiple POCUS sonographic windows.

- Ascertain whether the effusion is pericardial or pleural (a pericardial effusion may appear above the descending aorta in the PLAX view).

- Remember that you are doing a focused rapid exam. Identify if a pericardial effusion is present and describe its appearance as a small, moderate or large effusion and its haemodynamic impact.

- Not all pericardial effusions cause cardiovascular compromise. However, a small amount of fluid may lead to cardio-circulatory collapse if the accumulation is rapid or the patient is hypovolaemic.

- It is paramount to correlate what you are seeing on echo with the clinical status of the patient.

- A rapid estimation of the severity of a pericardial effusion is feasible. If the fluid measures >1cm it is at least a moderate pericardial effusion.

10.7 Summary

POCUS has evolved into a vital tool for both diagnostic assessment of the pericardium and to guide therapeutic intervention. When assessing pericardial effusions, clinical context is crucial because the speed of accumulation of an effusion is often more important than its size. Differentiating between conditions such as constrictive pericarditis and restrictive cardiomyopathy can be challenging but is significantly aided by echocardiography.

10.8 References

1. Klein AL, Abbara S, Agler DA, *et al.* (2013) American Society of Echocardiography clinical recommendations for multimodality cardiovascular imaging of patients with pericardial disease. *J Am Soc Echocardiogr*, 26:965.

2. Hoit BD (2017) Anatomy and physiology of the pericardium. *Cardiology Clinics*, 35:481.

3. Hoit BD (2017) Pathophysiology of the pericardium. *Prog Cardiovasc Diseases*, 59:341.

4. Rodriguez ER, Tan CD (2017) Structure and anatomy of human pericardium. *Prog Cardiovasc Diseases*, 59:327.

5. Chiabrando JG, Bonaventura A, Vecchié A, *et al.* (2020) Management of acute and recurrent pericarditis. *J Am Coll Cardiol*, 75:76.

6. Imazio M, Adler Y (2013) Clinical update: management of pericardial effusion. *European Heart J*, 34:1186.

7. Appleton C, Gillam L, Koulogiannis K (2017) Cardiac tamponade. *Cardiology Clinics*, 35:525.

8. Madhivathanan PR, Corredor C, Smith A (2020) Perioperative implications of pericardial effusions and cardiac tamponade. *Br J Anaes Edu*, 7:226.

9. Kaplan JA, Cronin B, Maus T (eds) (2017) *Essentials of Cardiac Anesthesia for Cardiac Surgery*. Elsevier.

10. Chiara De Carlini C, Maggiolini S (2017) Pericardiocentesis in cardiac tamponade: indications and practical aspects. *e-Journal Cardiol Pract*, 15:no.19.

11. Flint N, Siegel R (2020) Echo-guided pericardiocentesis: when and how should it be performed? *Curr Cardiol Reports*, 22:71.

CHAPTER 11

FUNDAMENTALS OF POINT-OF-CARE LUNG ULTRASOUND

Hatem Soliman-Aboumarie & Luna Gargani

Sonographic assessment of the thorax has been increasingly utilized in daily medical practice. Until the end of the 20th century, the lungs were considered unsuitable for ultrasound assessment due to the presence of air which theoretically limits the visualization of the parenchyma. However, several artefacts generated by ultrasound interactions with thoracic structures (tissues, air and fluid) have since been analyzed and increasingly utilized to assess and understand pulmonary pathologies [1]. Lung ultrasound (LUS) relies on assessing various patterns of artefacts or real images. LUS has shown superior sensitivity and specificity when compared to chest radiography and/ or physical examination in the diagnosis of various respiratory pathologies [2].

11.1 Anatomy

The chest wall is composed of skin, subcutaneous tissue and then muscles covering the thoracic cage. At the inner side of the rib lies the outer layer of the pleura which is separated from the inner layer (visceral pleura) by a thin microfilm of pleural fluid. This pleural fluid helps to lubricate movement between the two layers during respiration. Both layers of the pleura are around 5μm in thickness and are normally seen as one hyperechoic bright line on LUS.

The alveoli are located deep to the visceral pleura and form millions of airspaces within lobules which are divided by interlobular septa. These are not normally visible because their resolution is well below the ultrasound threshold. Thickening of the interlobular septa is the hallmark of LUS in the diagnosis of interstitial syndrome (B-lines). However, it is important to note that LUS provides regional assessment of each lung as opposed to CXR which provides a global assessment of both lungs. Therefore, a systematic approach to LUS scanning is crucial to increase the diagnostic accuracy of the scan.

11.2 What is LUS and the semiotics?

The use of thoracic ultrasound relies on detecting and analyzing both artefacts and real images. Most thoracic disorders involve the pleura; clear identification of the pleura is therefore crucial for accurate analysis of artefacts that may arise from it. The ribs are important landmarks for identifying the pleural line; in the longitudinal transducer position, the pleural line will connect both anterior ends of the rib shadows forming the so-called 'bat sign' (*Fig. 11.1*). The pleura is visualized as a horizontal bright line that moves synchronously with respiration and the appearance of this 'shimmering' movement between the visceral and parietal layers of the pleura is described as 'lung sliding'. When using M-mode, visualization of the 'seashore sign' confirms the presence of pleural sliding at the area of scanning (*Fig. 11.2*); the anterior horizontal lines represent the chest wall; the middle bright horizontal line represents the pleura; then the distinctive heterogeneous sand-like pattern represents the lung parenchyma.

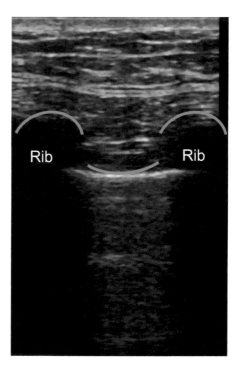

Figure 11.1. The 'bat sign' demonstrating anterior rib shadows separated by the pleural line.

The presence of air in between both layers of the pleura, as in the context of pneumothorax, extensive pleural fibrosis, adhesions, or reduced lung ventilation, can lead to loss or reduction of the lung sliding.

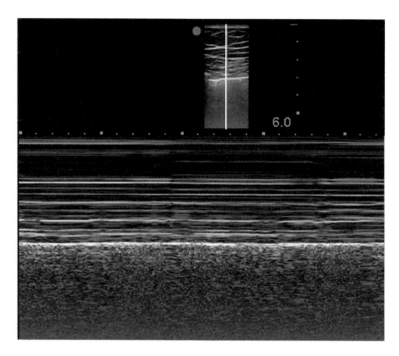

Figure 11.2. The 'seashore sign' visualized secondary to lung sliding when using M-mode.

A-lines are horizontal reverberation artefacts of the pleural line (*Figure 11.3*). They are visualized at equal distances from each other, as reflections of the distance between the pleura and the transducer. The presence of A-lines and lung sliding together represent preserved aeration at the area of scanning. When interstitial or alveolar air is replaced partially by fluid (exudate,

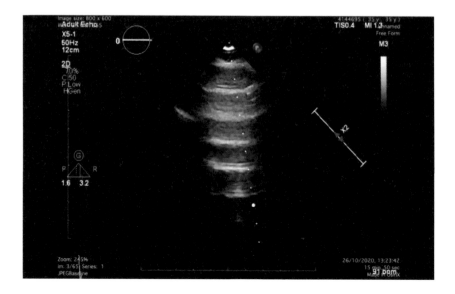

Figure 11.3. A-lines, representing horizontal reverberation artefacts of the pleural line.

transudate, blood, etc.), vertical reverberations start to develop [3]. These reverberations are due to the reduced acoustic mismatch between the lung and the surrounding structures. These vertical artefacts are named B-lines, and are characterized as being:

- hyperechoic

- well-defined

- laser-like beams starting from the pleural line and extending all the way until the ultrasound sector far-field

- synchronously moving with lung sliding.

B-lines are considered the sonographic marker of partial deaeration of the pulmonary parenchyma and their number correlates well with the degree of lung water and the increase in lung density [4]. In a normal healthy lung up to two B-lines may be seen in a single intercostal space, more than that is considered abnormal.

Non-pathological vertical artefacts that arise from the pleural line also exist and are called 'Z-lines'. They are characterized as:

- ill-defined and non-discrete beams

- not moving with the pleural line

- clearly not reaching the far-field of the ultrasound sector.

When the lungs become further deaerated, the parenchyma develops a 'hepatization' pattern. Here lung becomes visualized as a solid structure that is similar in appearance to parenchymal organs (e.g. liver or spleen) and is termed consolidation. This could be of infectious (pneumonia), obstructive or compressive (atelectasis), ischaemic (infarction), traumatic (contusion) or malignant aetiology.

The rhythmic motion of the pleura secondary to transmitted cardiac pulsations can be seen particularly well in deaerated lungs (e.g. atelectasis) and is known as a 'lung pulse'. This can be seen on both 2D and M-mode scanning as a synchronized lung pulsation with every heartbeat and reflects the apposition of the parietal and visceral layers of the pleura.

The visualization of a curtain-like shadow at the base of the lungs, that obscures the lateral part of the diaphragm and moves synchronously with respiration, is referred to as the 'curtain sign'. This reflects full aeration of the lung bases [5].

11.3 How to perform lung ultrasound

11.3.1 Transducers

Low frequency transducers (the phased array 'cardiac' transducer and convex 'abdominal' transducer) are useful for scanning the parenchyma because they enable scanning of deep structures, while high frequency transducers (the linear 'vascular' transducer) can better assess the pleura and subpleural space (*Fig. 11.4*). The universal transducers for parenchymal assessment are the convex and the microconvex transducers; these have intermediate frequency so they can visualize both the pleura and the lung parenchyma. Thus, low frequency transducers are useful for assessment of pleural effusions, pneumonia, atelectasis, pulmonary interstitial oedema, and empyema. High frequency transducers are better at assessing for the presence of a pneumothorax, and for performing a detailed assessment of the pleural line and subpleural abnormalities that may provide clues to the diagnosis of non-cardiogenic pulmonary oedema. Of note, any of these transducers could be utilized to assess both the pleura and the parenchyma. The lack of the ideal recommended probe should not preclude the clinician from trying to use the available probe and optimizing the image whilst remaining cognisant of the limitations. All transducers can assess B-lines except the linear transducer.

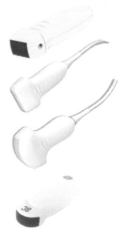

Cardiac transducer – 2-7.5MHz
lung sliding, consolidation, pleural effusion

Linear transducer – 2-15MHz
lung sliding, subpleural consolidations

Curvilinear transducer – 2-10MHz
consolidation, pleural effusion

Microconvex transducer – 2-22MHz
lung sliding, subpleural consolidation

Figure 11.4. Ultrasound probes that may be used for sonographic assessment of the lungs.

11.3.2 Machine settings

The examination should start by adjusting the machine on the lung pre-set (or abdominal pre-set with convex probes if lung pre-set is not available, or soft tissue or similar with linear probes). Depth should be set to 8–16cm, dependent on the size of the patient (less for slim subjects, more for obese subjects). Gain should be optimized for the whole image, and the focus should be adjusted to the area of interest (e.g. the pleural line). The probe can be placed either vertically, perpendicular to the ribs (longitudinal approach), or horizontally along the intercostal spaces (transverse/oblique approach). A phased array transducer can also be used to visualize the parenchyma, albeit with more limited visualization of the pleura. Each point should be examined for at least one complete respiratory cycle (5–6 seconds).

11.3.3 Scanning protocol

Different scanning protocols are available ranging from simple to comprehensive depending on the available time (acute versus chronic patient). Whenever possible, a comprehensive and systematic approach is recommended. The first suggested in the context of acute respiratory distress syndrome (ARDS) monitoring is the 12-zones protocol (*Fig. 11.5*) dividing each lung into anterior, lateral, and posterior zones so each lung will have six zones. The nipple line separates the upper from the lower zones and vertically the zones are defined by the parasternal line, anterior axillary, posterior axillar line and the paraspinal line. It is often challenging to mobilize supine critically ill patients to scan the posterior zones, however, we recommend scanning the most posterolateral zones possible. This is because pleural effusions, pneumonia or atelectasis often appear in these zones in supine patients. A more universal scanning protocol is the 8-zones protocol (*Fig. 11.6*) which doesn't involve assessment of the posterior zones and is more standardized in patients with heart failure and more universal for the differential diagnosis of respiratory failure/acute dyspnoea [6]. Of note the UK's Focused Ultrasound in Intensive Care (FUSIC) lung protocol consists of a 6-zones protocol: anterior upper and lower zones and the posterolateral regions bilaterally.

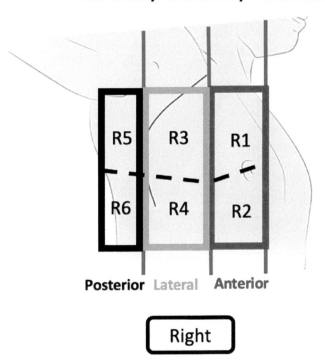

Figure 11.5. 12-zones lung scanning protocol with the thorax divided into anterior, lateral and posterior segments (six zones demonstrated here on the right hemithorax). Reproduced from Gargani *et al.* [15] with permission from Oxford University Press.

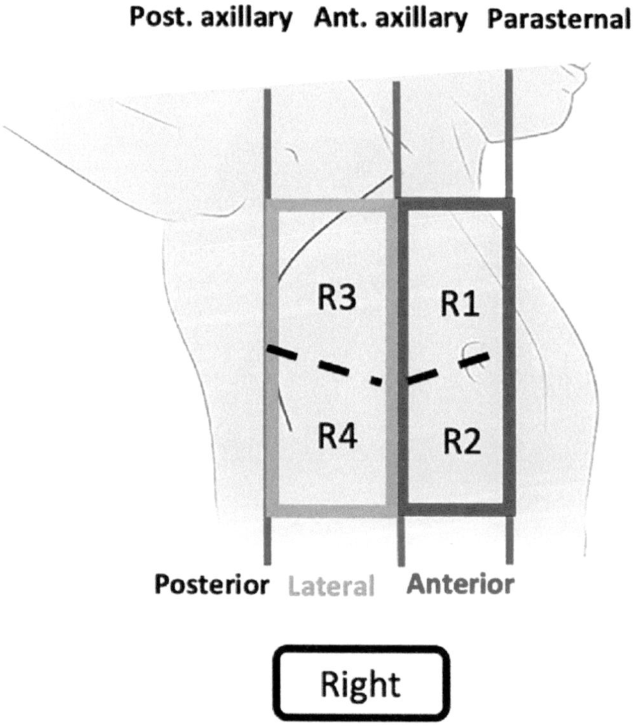

Figure 11.6 8-zones scanning protocol (four zones on the right hemithorax demonstrated). Adapted from Gargani *et al.* [15] with permission from Oxford University Press.

11.4 Uses of lung ultrasound

We will cover a few of the common uses and limitations of LUS in this section, with pulmonary and pleural pathology covered in more depth in *Chapter 12*.

11.4.1 Pneumothorax

Air accumulation between the parietal and visceral layers of the pleura precludes the ability of ultrasound to visualize the visceral pleura and therefore lung sliding will be lost. Absence of lung sliding has a high sensitivity for pneumothorax and specificity depends mostly on the patient's clinical condition. This loss of sliding leads to the appearance of repeated horizontal lines all over the ultrasound screen on M-mode and this is known as the 'barcode sign' or 'stratosphere sign' (*Fig. 11.7*). Whilst several pathologies other than pneumothorax could lead to loss of lung sliding (see list below), the presence of lung sliding can definitively exclude a pneumothorax with 100% specificity [7].

Potential causes of absent lung sliding on lung ultrasound:

- pneumothorax
- right mainstem intubation (loss of sliding contralateral lung)

- extensive pleural thickening

- adhesions

- fibrosis

- post-pleurodesis

- pneumonectomy

- cardiac arrest

- ultraprotective ventilation such as during veno-venous extracorporeal membrane oxygenation (VV-ECMO).

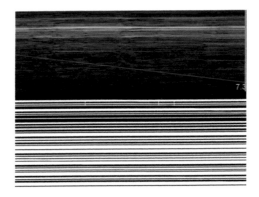

Figure 11.7. The stratosphere or barcode sign.

The transition zone between an area of lung sliding and an area with no lung sliding is the most specific sign for pneumothorax and is known as a 'lung point' and it has 100% specificity for pneumothorax [7]. An algorithmic approach in patients suspected of having pneumothorax could be lifesaving when applied at the point of care (*Fig. 11.8*) [7].

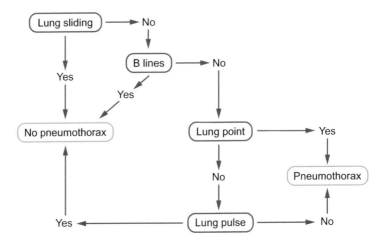

Figure 11.8. Algorithm for the sonographic assessment for the presence of a pneumothorax.

11.4.2 Atelectasis

Atelectasis of the basal zones of the lungs is commonly encountered in mechanically ventilated patients either due to proximal mucous plugging (resorption atelectasis) or due to external compression by pleural effusion (compressive atelectasis) especially in the most dependent lung zones. In atelectasis 'static air bronchograms' can be seen as hyperechoic punctiform particles that don't move with respiration. Static air bronchograms can be seen in almost half of patients with pneumonia, clinical correlation is thus always advisable when interpreting such findings.

The appearance of the solid lung floating within a pleural effusion is characteristic of compressive atelectasis with simple pleural effusion and is known as the 'jellyfish sign'. The presence of a complex or exudative pleural effusion could lead to loss of the floating movement of the lung tip within the effusion.

11.4.3 Pulmonary embolism

Integrated cardiopulmonary ultrasound can assist the clinician in diagnosing pulmonary embolism by providing indirect clues and excluding other causes of shortness of breath. For example, the combination of a patient presenting with dyspnoea, reduced oxygen saturation, dry lungs pattern (predominant A-lines), bilateral lung sliding, and evidence of deep vein thrombosis would be suggestive of pulmonary embolism [8]. Dilation of the right ventricle at echocardiography is usually seen in more severe forms of pulmonary embolism, often with haemodynamic instability.

In pulmonary infarction, LUS findings may include:

- focal B-lines around the infarcts
- multiple subpleural consolidations – usually small and 'wedge-shaped'
- localized effusion and more frequent involvement of the lower parts of the lungs [9].

Such abnormalities were seen frequently in patients with Covid-19 pneumonia and suggested as evidence for the presence of associated thromboembolism [10].

11.4.4 Pleural effusion

LUS can reliably evaluate the presence, quantity and complexity of a pleural effusion. The presence of an anechoic extraparenchymal collection in the chest cavity indicates a simple pleural effusion, often seen in the most dependent parts of the lungs. Normally, the thoracic spine is not visible because the aerated lungs hinder the transmission of ultrasound beams, therefore, the visualization of the hyperechoic shadow of the spine (the spine sign) beyond the edge of the liver denotes loss of aeration at the lung base which can be seen with pneumonia, atelectasis and/or pleural effusion. LUS can characterize the complexity of a pleural effusion:

- a simple anechoic pleural effusion is often transudative

- the presence of turbid fluid with fibrinous strands could indicate an exudative process

- the presence of multiple echogenic dots (air bubbles) within turbid pleural effusion suggests exudate, haemothorax, or empyema ('plankton sign').

The use of LUS in guiding pleural drainage has been associated with reduced procedural complications (see *Chapter 13*). LUS can also be used to monitor for residual effusion after thoracentesis and to exclude iatrogenic pneumothorax. The presence of hyperechoic fluid could raise suspicion for an empyema or a haemorrhagic effusion.

The estimation of pleural effusion size could be performed qualitatively (small, moderate or large), semi-quantitatively or quantitatively [11]. Balik *et al.* suggested an equation to estimate pleural effusion quantitatively [12]:

Amount of effusion (ml) = 20 × viscero-parietal pleural separation (mm)

11.4.5 Hydrostatic (cardiogenic) pulmonary oedema

LUS has a much higher sensitivity than CXR or clinical examination in the evaluation of hydrostatic oedema [13]. B-lines could be considered the sonographic biomarker of increased extravascular lung water (EVLW). Therefore the appearance and the pattern of B-lines could be used alongside other clinical and echocardiographic signs to diagnose patients with cardiogenic pulmonary oedema. Such patients usually have a bilateral symmetrical B-line distribution, with more present in the dependent zones. These B-lines are separated during the earlier phases of pulmonary congestion and later become more coalescent. The pleural line is usually thin, even in elderly patients, with preserved lung sliding and the presence of spared areas rare unless a co-existing pneumonia is present.

A semi-quantitative approach can be used to estimate the degree of interstitial oedema by dividing the percentage of the 'white' screen by 10, producing an estimate for the number of B-lines (i.e. 50% white screen equals to five B-lines). Pleural effusions are also frequently seen in patients with cardiogenic pulmonary oedema and can be unilateral (more frequently on the right side) or bilateral.

11.4.6 Non-cardiogenic pulmonary oedema

Patients with non-cardiogenic pulmonary oedema also have increased EVLW, however, the pattern of distribution is different from that seen in cardiogenic pulmonary oedema. In mild and moderate ARDS, B-lines are usually seen in a patchy, asymmetrical, non-gravity related distribution with spared areas of preserved aeration and the presence of pleural abnormalities such as pleural irregularities with subpleural small consolidations. The presence of B-lines denotes the partial deaeration of that area of the lung (as interstitial–alveolar air is replace by fluid). Vertical artefacts arising from consolidation and not the pleural line, are not considered B-lines. Nevertheless, vertical artefacts arising from the pleural line around an area of consolidation are considered B-lines and they represent peri-consolidation oedema. In severe ARDS, large consolidations can be seen. Pleural effusions of variable sizes may also be present.

11.4.7 Pneumonia

LUS has a much higher sensitivity for the diagnosis of pneumonia than CXR (93% compared to 54%) with chest CT considered the gold standard diagnostic modality [14]. In the early stages of pneumonia, LUS can show focal B-lines with preserved lung sliding, then subpleural small consolidations and/or large lobar consolidation can be visualized. The consolidation is an area of deaerated lung that becomes visible as a tissue-like echogenic structure. 'Shred sign' is the appearance of the irregular and shaggy edge of the deaerated lung separated from the partially deaerated lung. A specific sign for pneumonia is the presence of 'dynamic air-bronchograms' which appear as mobile hyperechogenic small particles (air bubbles) moving back and forth within the bronchioles with respiration.

11.4.8 Intrapulmonary shunt

The presence of intrapulmonary shunt could be demonstrated by the evidence of arterial flow within the consolidation with colour flow Doppler and or/pulse wave Doppler with distinctive patterns described for the pulmonary arterial, central bronchial and peripheral bronchial arterial flows (*Fig. 11.9*). Further studies are needed to assess the potential benefit of Doppler characterization, quantification of intrapulmonary shunting and assessing the response to therapies [16].

11.4.9 Chronic interstitial lung disease

Patients with pulmonary fibrosis have multiple, bilateral B-lines which are more diffuse at the lung bases. The pleural line is usually spared and thin in the early stages and in the late phases it becomes irregular and fragmented. It is noteworthy that the pleural line changes don't reflect anatomical changes in the pleura which may not be directly affected. The presence of small sub-pleural consolidations or pleural effusion is rare in chronic interstitial lung disease.

11.5 Lung ultrasound in Covid-19 pneumonia

The SARS CoV-2 pandemic has produced a challenging syndrome of respiratory failure known as Covid-19 pneumonia. This form of respiratory

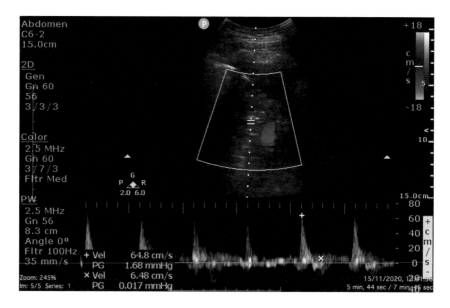

Figure 11.9. Doppler assessment of bronchial artery flow.

failure was different from other well-known forms of acute respiratory illnesses. A significant proportion of patients had a dissociation between clinical and radiological findings (i.e. asymptomatic yet with gross LUS abnormalities). In a theoretical model, two phenotypes have been described. One of these is phenotype L, denoting relatively preserved lung compliance albeit with a disproportionate level of hypoxaemia which was attributed to possible virus-induced diffusion abnormality and alveolar flooding. The other is the H phenotype, with reduced lung compliance and evidence of lobar consolidation on chest CT (similar to classic ARDS). The LUS findings are the same as seen generally in non-cardiogenic pulmonary oedema, yet more patients with Covid-19 pneumonia have a distinctive patchy alveolar oedema pattern (coalescent curtain-like B-lines with spared areas of A-lines) with pleural abnormalities frequently seen. This pattern of shiny white patchy B-lines correlates with ground-glass opacification and crazy paving on chest CT [14]. The 'light beam' artefact has been described as an early sign of Covid-19 pneumonia; this is a large band-like lucent artefact appearing and fading with respiration and arising from a usually thin pleural line [17].

11.6 Using ultrasound to monitor lung recruitment

Experimental studies, both *in vitro* and *in vivo*, have demonstrated that progressive worsening of aeration correlates with the following sonographic changes:

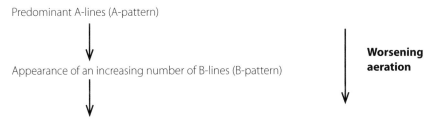

Predominant A-lines (A-pattern)

Appearance of an increasing number of B-lines (B-pattern)

Worsening aeration

Coalescent B-lines until complete deaeration which correlates with tissue-like consolidation.

This dynamic change leads to the sonographic appearance of variable shades of white/grey on the screen (see *Fig. 11.10*), and represents the ability of LUS to monitor progression of aeration/deaeration at the bedside in response to various therapeutic manoeuvres (positive pressure ventilation, recruitment, physiotherapy, bronchoscopy, etc.). Different LUS aeration scores have been studied in attempts to semi-quantify the changes in aeration/deaeration.

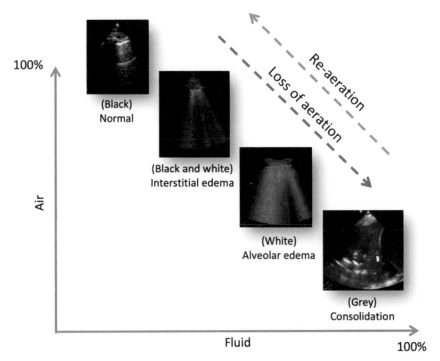

Figure 11.10. *Demonstration of lung ultrasound changes seen with increasing loss of lung aeration.*

The most frequently used scoring system in critically ill patients distinguishes four grades of loss of aeration each represented by a score from 0 to 3:

- A-lines or less than three B-lines (normal aeration, score 0)

- three or more B-lines (moderate loss of aeration, score 1)

- coalescent B-lines (severe loss of aeration, score 2)

- consolidation (complete loss of aeration, score 3) (*Fig. 11.10*).

Estimating the score regionally for each of the 6 zones on each hemithorax bilaterally (12 zones) and then summing all to a global aeration score provides a score from 0 (best aeration) to 36 (complete deaeration).

In ARDS, both regional and global LUS aeration scores strongly correlate with tissue density as measured by quantitative chest CT scan. Additionally, global LUS aeration scores correlate with EVLW assessed by transpulmonary thermodilution. Daily monitoring using the LUS aeration score could be useful in the following circumstances:

- to assess readiness of patients for weaning from mechanical ventilation

- to predict failure of extubation

- to assess for excessive fluid administration with the potential for pulmonary congestion

- to assess progression of aeration in patients with respiratory failure on VV-ECMO as an alternative to CXR.

However, LUS information should always be interpreted within the clinical context and integrated with clinical, laboratory and other available imaging findings.

11.7 Limitations of LUS

Like any other imaging modality, LUS requires training. However, it is relatively easy to learn when compared with other ultrasound modalities such as echocardiography. It has a high sensitivity but low specificity for the diagnosis of pulmonary diseases and its power is thus mainly reliant on the ability to rule out, rather than rule in, specific diseases. It also has recognized limitations in detecting deep structural abnormalities of diseases sparing the pleura. Diseases with peri-bronchial involvement may therefore not be well assessed by LUS and it is unable to recognize lung hyperinflation.

11.8 Summary

Lung ultrasound is a valuable bedside imaging tool. It can assist in the diagnosis of various causes of respiratory and cardiac failure and it can help the clinician in the diagnosis and monitoring of the response to heart failure management as well as monitoring the oxygenation/recruitment of critically ill patients. We recommend integrating LUS into the daily assessment of critically ill patients and performing it as an extension of the bedside physical examination. A proper assessment of LUS's advantages and limitations, and the limited yet evolving evidence for its use in critical care, is needed to fully benefit from this undoubtedly game-changing bedside imaging approach.

11.9 References

1. Gargani L (2019) Ultrasound of the lungs: more than a room with a view. *Heart Fail Clin*, 15:297.

2. Xirouchaki N, Magkanas E, Vaporidi K, *et al*. (2011) Lung ultrasound in critically ill patients: comparison with bedside chest radiography. *Intensive Care Med*, 37:1488.

3. Gargani L, Volpicelli G (2014) How I do it: lung ultrasound. *Cardiovasc Ultrasound*, 12:25.

4. Gargani L, Picano E, Caramella D, *et al*. (2013) Lung water assessment by lung ultrasonography in intensive care: a pilot study. *Intensive Care Med*, 39:74.

5. Lee FCY (2017) The curtain sign in lung ultrasound. *J Med Ultrasound*, 25:101.

6. Volpicelli G, Mussa A, Garofalo G, *et al*. (2006) Bedside lung ultrasound in the assessment of alveolar-interstitial syndrome. *Am J Emerg Med*, 24:689.

7. Volpicelli G (2011) Sonographic diagnosis of pneumothorax. *Intensive Care Med*, 37:224.

8. Nazerian P, Vanni S, Volpicelli G, *et al*. (2014) Accuracy of point-of-care multiorgan ultrasonography for the diagnosis of pulmonary embolism. *Chest*, 145:950.

9. Reissig A, Kroegel C (2003) Transthoracic ultrasound of lung and pleura in the diagnosis of pulmonary embolism: a novel non-invasive bedside approach. *Respiration*, 70:441.

10. Boccatonda A, Ianniello E, D'Ardes D, *et al*. (2020) Can lung ultrasound be used to screen for pulmonary embolism in patients with SARS-CoV-2 pneumonia?. *Eur J Case Rep Intern Med*, 7:001748.

11. Prina E, Torres A, Carvalho CR (2014) Lung ultrasound in the evaluation of pleural effusion. *Bras Pneumol*, 40:1.

12. Balik M, Plasil P, Waldauf P, *et al*. (2006) Ultrasound estimation of volume of pleural fluid in mechanically ventilated patients. *Intensive Care Med*, 32:318.

13. Soliman-Aboumarie H, Miglioranza MH (2020) The sound of silence. *JACC: Case Reports*, 2:1550.

14. Ye X, Xiao H, Chen B, Zhang S (2015) Accuracy of lung ultrasonography versus chest radiography for the diagnosis of adult community-acquired pneumonia: review of the literature and meta-analysis. *PLoS ONE*, 10:e0130066.

15. Gargani L, Soliman-Aboumarie H, Volpicelli G, Corradi F, Concetta Pastore M, Cameli M (2020) Why, when, and how to use lung ultrasound during the COVID-19 pandemic: enthusiasm and caution. *European Heart J - Cardiovascular Imaging*, 21:941.

16. Soliman-Aboumarie H (2022) Doppler demonstration of ventilation–perfusion mismatching due to intrapulmonary shunting. *European Heart J - Cardiovascular Imaging*, 23:e89.

17. Volpicelli G, Gargani L (2020) Sonographic signs and patterns of COVID-19 pneumonia. *Ultrasound J*, 12:22.

CHAPTER 12

LUNG AND
PLEURAL PATHOLOGY

Ashley Miller, Marcus Peck & Jonny Wilkinson

Lung ultrasound (LUS) is now an essential tool for answering key clinical questions in critically ill patients. Not only does it have a high diagnostic accuracy, but it is relatively easy to learn and quick to perform. LUS is non-invasive, done at the point of care, readily repeatable for monitoring, and avoids ionizing radiation. It is superior to chest radiography and for many pathologies is nearly as good as computed tomography (CT) scanning. This chapter will go through the most important of these clinical questions, describing and explaining the various pathologies that can be assessed with ultrasound. As with all diagnostic tools in medicine, pretest probability is very important and ultrasound findings should always be taken in context.

Fundamentally, lung ultrasound answers the question 'why does this patient have respiratory failure?'. But it can also answer more specific questions which this chapter will cover in turn. All these questions can usually be answered rapidly with a simple three-point examination of each hemithorax consisting of upper and lower anterior points, and then a posterolateral point (*Fig. 12.1*).

First the pleural line is identified and inspected to look for lung sliding. Secondly, examination under the pleural line will reveal either A-lines, B-lines, consolidation/collapse or effusion. Applying the sonographic findings, at each point, to a decision tree known as the BLUE protocol (combined with DVT scanning in some instances) has been shown to have an extremely high diagnostic accuracy in acute respiratory failure (see *Fig. 12.1*). The diagnoses from this protocol may need to be altered outside of the context of *acute* respiratory failure, but examining at only these points has been shown to demonstrate most lung pathologies, even if the conclusions drawn are different. Greater experience allows a more comprehensive examination of the whole thorax, but the same sonographic signs are looked for. Each lung pathology has characteristic appearances which leads us on to our clinical questions.

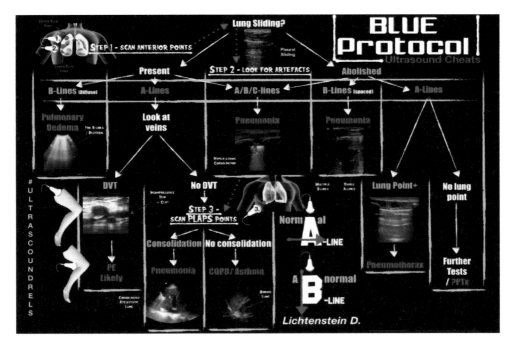

Figure 12.1. Daniel Lichtenstein's bedside lung ultrasound in emergency (BLUE) protocol.

12.1 Is there a pneumothorax?

The visceral and parietal pleura are usually closely opposed to one another with a small amount of fluid in between them. These two pleural layers can be seen with ultrasound to slide over one another with respiration. This sign, known as lung sliding, can be subtle and measures should be taken to improve its visualization. These include shallow depth, low gain, high frequency and placing the focus point at the same depth as the pleura. Using a high frequency linear probe will improve the image further if there is any doubt. Small imperfections in the pleural line will be seen to move to and fro in a horizontal plane. Any B-lines (see below) will also move with sliding. In a deeper view the subpleural space will be seen to shimmer.

Seeing lung sliding immediately rules out a pneumothorax at the examination point. Pleural air will collect in the most nondependent area, so if the patient is sat up slightly, examining the upper anterior point will allow exclusion of a pneumothorax. Absent sliding does not necessarily mean a pneumothorax is present. Respiratory arrest, one lung intubation, pleural effusion, atelectasis, and the pleural layers being stuck together from an inflammatory process (e.g. pneumonia) can all cause absence of sliding. Low tidal volumes, lung hyperinflation and severe parenchymal disease that limit expansion will *reduce* lung sliding. Fortunately, there are other ways to rule a pneumothorax in or out.

The presence of B-lines, consolidation or an effusion means there can be no air in the pleural space and so exclude a pneumothorax at that point.

Transmitted cardiac pulsations, known as the lung pulse, can also be detected in 2D or M-mode, but only if the pleural layers are not separated (*Fig. 12.2*). It is worth noting that while the presence of lung sliding is easy to confirm, the absence of lung sliding can be more difficult, particularly when the stakes are high. Making every effort to optimize the image with your probe choice, shallow depth, low gain, high frequency and focus point positioned at the pleura will help your decision making.

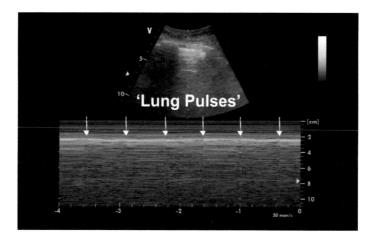

Figure 12.2. The lung pulse seen on M-mode.

If a pneumothorax is present, depending on its size, there will be a dependent point where the pleural layers come together – a transition point between no sliding and sliding. This will move with respiration as the inflating lung moves upwards. Examining the anterior chest and moving the probe laterally will identify this point at which lung sliding appears; this sonographic sign is known as the lung point. A rough estimation of the size of the pneumothorax can be performed by measuring the distance between the sternum and the lung point and can be utilized to monitor the progress of a pneumothorax. This combined with absent sliding has a 100% specificity for a pneumothorax. It is usually easy to find (as long as the pneumothorax is not massive).

Small pneumothoraces do not usually need to be treated, even in ventilated patients. Repeated LUS helps allow safe monitoring of a pneumothorax size by noting where the lung point is each time. Migration of the lung point towards the more dependent areas means the pneumothorax is expanding.

12.2 Is there pulmonary oedema?

When ultrasound hits the interface between soft tissue and air, it is virtually all reflected back to the transducer. Some sound then bounces back and forth between the probe and pleura causing repeating artefacts below the pleura known as A-lines. As lung water increases, the interstitium engorges and sound waves will then reverberate between the air in the alveoli and the thickened alveolar septae causing artefacts below the pleural line called B-lines (*Fig. 12.3*). These B-lines arise from the pleural line, are laser like, move with lung sliding, reach the depths of the image and obliterate A-lines where they cross them. They become more numerous as oedema increases until they fuse together as the alveoli flood. These coalesced B-lines can progress to a 'white-out' appearance.

Whilst cardiogenic pulmonary oedema is a common cause of B-lines, these can be seen in any condition that leads to septal thickening, such as fibrosis, lymphangitis carcinomatosis or inflammation (contusions, bacterial or viral pneumonia), as was demonstrated so well by the Covid-19 pandemic, the characteristic feature of which was B-lines. In fact, Covid-19 brought with it an exponential rise in the uptake of LUS as an indispensable modality for clinical examination and disease monitoring. The pattern of B-line distribution can help in diagnosis, as do other features. If B-lines are caused by pneumonia, they will only be present at the site of infection. In inflammation or fibrosis, B-lines will be scattered in between 'spared areas' of normal-looking pleura. Pretest probability is, as ever, important in establishing the diagnosis.

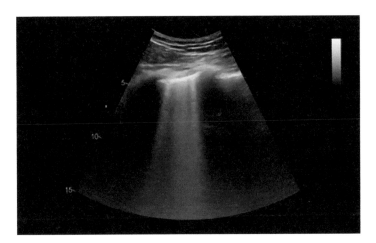

Figure 12.3. B-lines arise from the pleural line, are laser like, move with lung sliding, reach the depths of the image and obliterate A-lines.

12.3 Is there pneumonia?

In pneumonia, air in the lung is replaced by inflammatory fluid to varying degrees, allowing sound waves to penetrate the lung instead of being reflected. As above, pneumonia can manifest as localized B-lines. However, the most common feature is consolidation and there is a spectrum of appearances between these entities.

When there is a partial lobar consolidation, the interface between consolidation and air can be seen. Artefacts resembling B-lines will arise from this interface because they are always seen when air and fluid are next to each other. Technically speaking these are not classified as B-lines (because they do not arise from the pleura), although this can be confusing in very small (millimetric) consolidations where these lines arise just below the pleura. In such instances it is really semantics as to whether they are called

B-lines or not (further consensus is needed on this terminology). The degree of aeration may also appear to change with respiration, as different areas of aerated and non-aerated lung come into the plane of the beam and move in and out of view.

A fully consolidated lobe will allow that whole area of lung to be seen. The density of the lung here, and therefore its echogenicity, will be similar to the abdominal organs and the appearance is therefore sometimes described as hepatization (*Fig. 12.4*). Fluid (black) and air (white) bronchograms may be seen within the lung and are highly specific signs of pneumonia. These will be linear if parallel to the beam and punctiform if perpendicular. Air may even be seen to move in and out of the airways, a sign referred to as 'dynamic air bronchograms'.

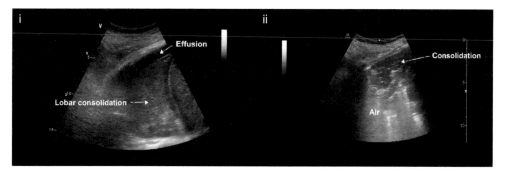

Figure 12.4. (i) A fully consolidated right lower lobe surrounded by a small effusion. (ii) Partial consolidation showing the interface between fluid and air.

12.4 Is there collapse?

Lung collapse/atelectasis is very similar in appearance to consolidation because a feature of both is that air has been displaced from the lung. A large lobar collapse from an obstructed airway will cause a significantly raised hemi-diaphragm. Air bronchograms can be discriminators – they will not be present in collapse, except in the early stages after which distal air will be absorbed. Collapse caused by extrinsic pressure from a pleural effusion can be difficult to distinguish from a pneumonic consolidation with an associated effusion. The size of the effusion will make one more likely than the other. The only way to absolutely distinguish them is to drain the effusion and see if the lung re-expands. Significant effusions nearly always compress the lung and it is very unusual for the lung not to re-expand after drainage of a moderate to large effusion.

12.5 Is there pleural disease?

A pleural effusion is perhaps the easiest lung pathology to see on ultrasound. Fluid allows transmission of sound waves, as does the compressed lung which is usually present within an effusion. Instead of artefact interpretation, the sonographer can now visualize the anatomy beneath the pleura. Fluid appears black (anechoic) on ultrasound although there can be echogenic material within it (pus, clotted blood, etc.). There may also be fibrin strands and loculations. The diaphragm is easy to see when there is an effusion, and this is an important reference point for identifying the location of the fluid (do not confuse ascites and pleural effusion which may both be present). There are several formulae for estimating the size of an effusion by taking various measurements. None is particularly accurate, and it is only really necessary to know if an effusion is small, medium or large, experience of which comes from scanning patients. As a rough rule of thumb, if the distance between the pleural layers measures more than 5cm at any point there is likely to be >1L of fluid. Scanning in the posterior axillary line with the probe parallel to the floor, rather than angled into the thorax, can slice through the dependent effusion, and miss the lung, making it appear bigger than it actually is. Always bear in mind the 3D structures you are scanning with ultrasound and fan the probe through the area of interest.

Pleural thickening is easy to see with ultrasound and in some instances can be dramatic. It can be confused with a pleural effusion because the thickened pleura appears black like fluid. The two can be distinguished by the fact that when an effusion is present the visceral pleura will move towards and away from the parietal pleura with respiration (generating a sinusoidal pattern if viewed with M-mode), whereas the pleural thickness will remain the same throughout the respiratory cycle (see *Fig. 12.5*).

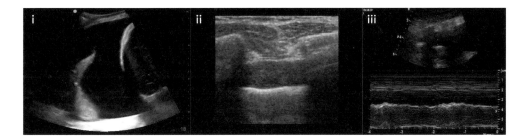

Figure 12.5. (i) A large pleural effusion compressing the lung; the diaphragm is clearly seen. (ii) Pleural thickening which can easily be mistaken for an effusion. (iii) Placing M-mode through the anechoic space shows it to be changing width, with respiration confirming it is an effusion rather than pleural thickening.

12.6 Is there a lung contusion?

Blunt chest wall trauma can cause lung contusions which appear on ultrasound as B-lines or small areas of consolidation at the site of trauma (*Fig. 12.6*). The size and number of lesions correlate with the severity of the injury. Without knowing the clinical context, contusions are indistinguishable in appearance from lung inflammation due to other causes.

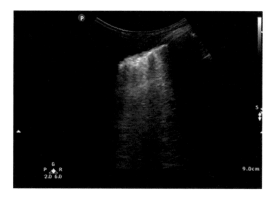

Figure 12.6. A small lung contusion in a trauma patient resembling a small area of consolidation.

12.7 Is there a pneumonitis?

The features of a pneumonitis (including viral) are widespread scattered B-lines which often fuse together to form wide B-lines (light beams has been suggested as a name for them). Millimetric consolidations make the pleural line appear thickened and, as explained above, it can be difficult to work out if the B-line type artefacts are arising from the pleura or these consolidations. The nomenclature is irrelevant though – their presence indicates inflamed lung tissue and increased lung water. These features can sometimes be dramatic even in patients who are not critically unwell. There is some evidence that sonographic features mirror clinical severity, but this has yet to be fully established. There are often spared areas with a more normal-looking pleural line (*Fig. 12.7*). Effusions are uncommon and will reflect fluid balance. Dense consolidations are only seen later in the illness and are associated with super-added bacterial infection, collapse, or fluid overload. Any cause of acute respiratory distress syndrome (ARDS) will result in this type of appearance. It is becoming increasingly recognized that much of what used to be thought of as ARDS was iatrogenic fluid overload. The presence of pleural fluid is a useful discriminator here, as are fluid balance, weight, echocardiographic and venous congestion parameters.

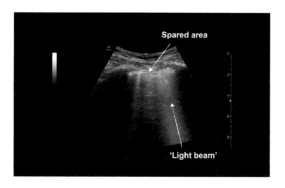

Figure 12.7. Pneumonitis with B-lines (including a 'light beam') and a spared area with a normal-looking pleural line and A-lines below.

12.8 Is there a pulmonary embolus?

Similarly to chest radiography, the hallmark of LUS in pulmonary embolism (PE) is that it is usually normal. The combination of a normal LUS and hypoxia should always put PE at the top of the list of differential diagnoses. Ultrasound of the leg veins, to look for a deep venous thrombosis, and ultrasound of the heart, to look for pressure overload of the right heart, will provide important additional information. Emboli can cause small peripheral infarcts which can sometimes be seen with lung ultrasound and look like areas of small peripheral consolidation. Contrast-enhanced ultrasound has recently been proposed as a method of discriminating whether these small abnormal areas are avascular infarcts or simple consolidation. Further studies are awaited.

12.9 Is there a source of infection?

The source of infection can often be difficult to pin down, especially in critically ill patients who may have multiple organ dysfunction. Consolidation reaches the pleura 90% of the time so if present it will usually be seen with ultrasound. Consolidation and collapse can be distinguished as above. Air and fluid bronchograms are very specific to pneumonia. If pleural fluid is infected there may be echogenic particles swirling in the effusion, fibrin strands or frank loculation (*Fig. 12.8*). Ultrasound has a better resolution than CT and can reveal septations that cannot be seen with a CT scan. Sonographic features may raise suspicion of infected pleural fluid but not diagnose it. Ultrasound does, however, guide pleural aspiration or drainage from which a sample can be tested (see *Chapter 13*).

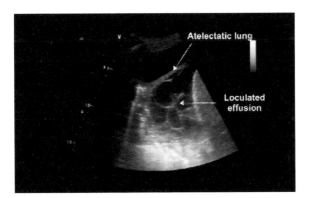

Figure 12.8. A complicated pleural effusion due to infection with septations.

12.10 Is this patient fluid overloaded?

Pulmonary capillaries, like in muscle and connective tissue, are non-sinusoidal and non-fenestrated which allows easy escape of fluid when capillary pressures increase. The lung interstitium becomes engorged and the alveolar septae widen causing reverberation artefacts (B-lines) because of their juxtaposition with alveolar air. As pulmonary oedema worsens, B-lines become more numerous until the alveoli flood and at which point a white lung appearance ensues from confluent B-lines. Fluid collects by gravity, so B-lines from fluid overload are usually more severe in dependent areas. Pleural effusions are also a common feature.

LUS is only a small part of the answer to this question of fluid overload. History, fluid balance, peripheral oedema, weight, and other ultrasound features (right heart size, left atrial and pulmonary artery pressures, inferior vena cava size and venous flow patterns) are all key elements. The presence of B-lines though, if not due to fibrosis, means the lungs are wet or inflamed. There are some clues to distinguish simple cardiogenic pulmonary oedema from acute lung injury (see *Table 12.1*), but the two often overlap, especially in critically ill and ventilated patients. Whatever the cause, there is increased extravascular lung water, and a fluid bolus is only likely to worsen respiratory function.

Table 12.1. *Ultrasound findings in fluid overload versus an inflamed lung*

Cardiogenic oedema / fluid overload	Pneumonitis
Thin, well-defined pleural line	Thickened pleural line
Signs more prominent in dependent areas	No dependent predominance
Bilateral, homogenous	Scattered, spared areas, juxtaposed normal and abnormal areas
Effusions common	Effusions uncommon
Basal lobar consolidation	Small, scattered areas of consolidation

12.11 Is the lung recruitable?

As the lung goes from aerated to de-aerated, the sonographic signs progress from a few B-lines to multiple fused B-lines, then to partial consolidation and finally to full lobar consolidation (*Fig. 12.9*). The reverse process can be demonstrated with lung recruitment or pleural effusion drainage. This has been quantified for research purposes into lung scoring systems which were discussed in *Chapter 11*. Another approach is to see how these patterns change with treatment, whether that be antibiotics, pleural effusion drainage or increased positive end-expiratory pressure. It is important to note that ultrasound cannot reveal overdistension. Aerated lung shows an A-line pattern that does not change with increased lung volume. Safe ventilatory practices should always be employed.

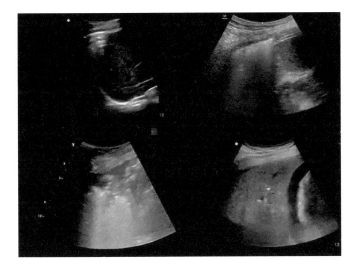

Figure 12.9. Varying degrees of aeration from air filled in the top left to fully consolidated in the bottom right.

12.12 Why is there weaning failure?

Weaning failure may be due to respiratory pathology, muscle weakness, heart failure or central nervous system pathology. As outlined above, most lung pathologies which can contribute to weaning failure are easy to see with ultrasound. Lung scoring systems have shown good correlation with weaning, although these quantitative methods are time-consuming and probably best left to research. The diaphragm can also be assessed. The direction of movement, distance travelled and muscle thickening are easily interrogated (during spontaneous breathing), although the clinical utility of this is yet to be determined (see *Chapter 27* for more details on this). Integration with heart ultrasound is important. The combination of a rounded, dilated left atrium and B-lines means that left atrial pressure (LAP) is almost certainly high. Left ventricular failure and mitral valve regurgitation may each be revealed as the cause of the raised LAP and pulmonary oedema. So, combined with heart ultrasound, LUS is a valuable tool to help the clinician decide why a patient may not be weaning.

12.13 Summary

LUS is a powerful instrument to assess and monitor patients. Combined with a pretest probability synthesized from history, examination, and ancillary testing, it allows a clinician to answer a series of vital clinical questions with great accuracy. It can thus help guide patient management, from diagnosis to monitoring of treatment response.

CHAPTER 13

ULTRASOUND-GUIDED THORACENTESIS

Chuen Khaw, Luke Flower & Jim Buckley

The growing availability of POCUS over recent years (both in terms of equipment and the requisite skill set) has led to an increase in ultrasound-guided procedures. This has improved both procedural success and safety. This chapter will work through the technique for inserting an ultrasound-guided chest drain and highlight some important points to remain cognisant of when performing such a procedure.

13.1 Scanning the patient

The primary aim of lung ultrasound (LUS) when performing chest drain insertion is to:

- confirm the presence of an effusion or a pneumothorax

- determine the size and nature of an effusion to guide decision making (i.e. whether aspiration or drain insertion would be most appropriate)

- allow the clinician to identify a safe drain insertion site and minimize the risk of visceral injury.

13.1.1 Which probe to use?

The curvilinear transducer is the most used probe for scanning pleural effusions. It enables examination of a comparatively large area of the pleural surface and has good penetration, allowing the user to look deeper into the thoracic cavity. The linear transducer operates at a higher frequency and is useful for assessing fine details, such as the pleural surface and sub-pleural pathology.

13.1.2 Patient positioning

Optimal patient positioning prior to commencing a scan is extremely important to image acquisition. The optimal position is patient and scenario dependent, and influenced by several factors including the following.

- The site of pathology based on chest radiograph or computed tomography (CT) scan findings:

  o the posterior chest is best scanned with the patient sitting upright and leaning forward with their arms elevated resting on a table (*Fig. 13.1i*)
  o the lateral and anterior chest wall is best examined with the patient in a supine position with their arm abducted (*Fig. 13.1ii*)

- Operator preference.

- Patient factors, i.e. the scan may have to be performed supine if the patient is unable to sit upright.

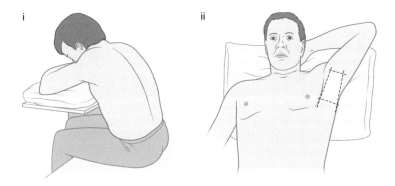

Figure 13.1. (i) Patient sitting upright leaning forwards – the preferred position when scanning the posterior chest wall. (ii) Supine patient with arm abducted – the preferred position when scanning the lateral or anterior chest.

13.1.3 Where to start scanning?

If scanning for a pleural effusion, begin in the long-axis below the diaphragm, either from mid-posterior axillary line (when in the supine position) or posterior (when upright). Try to identify a reference organ (the liver if on the right or spleen on the left) and move the probe cephalad in the long-axis plane until lung movement becomes apparent.

13.2 Normal thoracic ultrasound appearance

This is discussed in more depth in *Chapters 11* and *12*. In this chapter we will briefly revisit some of the common ultrasound findings seen in pleural effusions and pneumothoraces.

The anatomical relationship of the thorax with the abdomen creates a demarcated leading edge of the lung air artefact giving the impression of a lung curtain. As a result, the lateral diaphragm is hidden under the curtain and the costophrenic angle is not visualized [1]. The first sign of a small pleural effusion is when the costophrenic angle is visualized (*Fig. 13.2*).

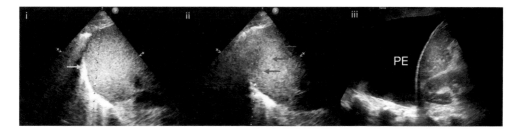

Figure 13.2. (i) and (ii) Demonstration of the curtain sign with the diaphragm (orange arrow) obscured by lung (red arrows) on inspiration. (iii) A large pleural effusion (PE) with no curtain sign present.

13.3 Pleural effusions on ultrasound

Thoracic ultrasound has a better sensitivity and specificity than chest radiography and CT when diagnosing pleural effusions.

13.3.1 Types of pleural effusion

Identifying the likely aetiology of an effusion is important when deciding management strategies [2]. There are four main ultrasonographic characteristics of pleural fluid that are determined by its internal echogenicity (*Figure 13.3*):

1. **An anechoic effusion** – a totally echo free, free flowing effusion. This may be seen in a transudative effusion, acute haemothorax and some malignant effusions.

2. **Homogenously echogenic** – this may be seen in an exudative effusion or a subacute haemothorax.

3. **Complex non-septated** – an echogenic effusion with swirling densities present. This may be seen in an exudative effusion, a malignant effusion and, on rare occasions, a transudative effusion.

4. **Complex septated** – describes the presence of fine strands within the effusion. This may be seen in an exudative or malignant effusion.

13.4 When to intervene?

Once you have confirmed the presence of an effusion and its characteristics, the next step is to identify those that require aspiration or drain insertion. As a general rule, there are two indications for aspiration or drainage:

1. The effusion is large enough to cause respiratory compromise.

2. Suspicion of an exudative effusion.

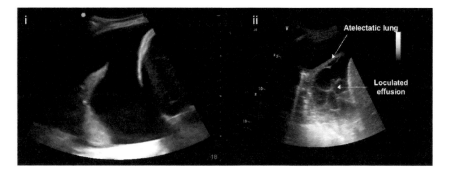

Figure 13.3. (i) Anechoic effusion. (ii) Complex septated effusion.

The clinical risks and benefits of the procedure should of course also be considered. These include:

- Patient consent.

- Likely benefits the patient will experience because of successful aspiration/drainage.

- The presence of coagulopathy or any contraindications.

Although anechoic effusions are mostly transudates, they may also be exudative (not uncommonly a malignant effusion) or an acute haemothorax. Echogenic effusions are usually exudates. Research looking into the use of an effusion's echogenicity to distinguish exudative from transudative effusions found a specificity of only 57%, thus it has been suggested that the echogenic qualities of an effusion should not influence clinical decision making [3].

Therefore, the decision to aspirate an effusion depends on clinical suspicion and the likelihood of an alternative diagnosis. Thoracic ultrasound is certainly useful to support such clinical decision making and to ensure aspiration/drainage is performed safely [4].

An echogenic effusion which correlates with clinical suspicion should prompt a simple pleural aspiration first before proceeding to chest drain insertion. Pleural aspiration of up to 50ml of pleural fluid is useful to differentiate between simple and complicated parapneumonic effusion or empyema. The latter requires chest tube drainage and appropriate antimicrobial treatment.

13.4.1 Determining the size of an effusion

Some effusions are too small or too complex to tap and may need referral to a more experienced operator. There are many ways to quantify the size of an effusion, some of which were discussed in previous chapters. One other practical way to do this is to classify the volume of an effusion in relation to the curvilinear probes range:

- Minimal: effusion confined to the costophrenic angle.

- Small: effusion greater than the costophrenic angle but within a single probe range.

- Moderate: an effusion spanning between one and two probe ranges.

- Large: an effusion bigger than two probe ranges.

The size of an effusion is also important when considering the choice of procedure: simple aspiration versus Rocket aspiration versus insertion of chest drain.

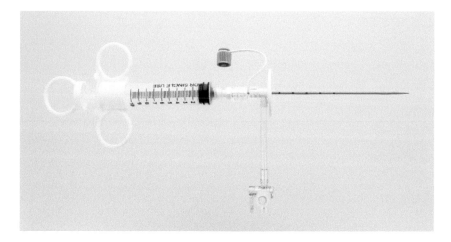

Figure 13.4. Rocket aspiration catheter. Reproduced with permission from Rocket Medical.

The Rocket aspiration catheter (size 6Fr) is normally used for both diagnostic and therapeutic aspiration of up to 1.0–1.5L of fluid (*Fig. 13.4*). The catheter should be removed after the procedure.

Simple aspiration is suitable for the diagnostic assessment of an effusion. This can be performed with a simple needle and syringe. Chest drain insertion will be discussed in depth later in the chapter.

13.5 Optimal site for safe drain insertion

Identifying a safe and effective site for drain insertion is important to reduce the risk of visceral injury (e.g. lung, liver, spleen, heart). The site chosen should have the following features.

- Sufficient depth of pleural fluid, usually at least 1cm measured between the pleural layers (depending on experience). Aspiration of effusions of less than 1cm carries increased risk of visceral injury (*Fig. 13.5*).

- No intervening lung at maximal inspiration.

- Minimal risk of laceration of the intercostal neurovascular bundle. To do this the needle should be inserted into the intercostal space, just above the inferior rib, preferably in the safe triangle. Sometimes in the case of posterior lying pleural fluid, it may be necessary to insert the needle more posteriorly. The intercostal neurovascular bundle is normally covered by the costal groove of the rib above. However, it may have a tortuous course posterior-medially to the angle of the rib. To avoid risk of injury, it is safer to insert the needle 5–10cm lateral to the spine or lateral to the mid-scapular line (*Fig. 13.1i*).

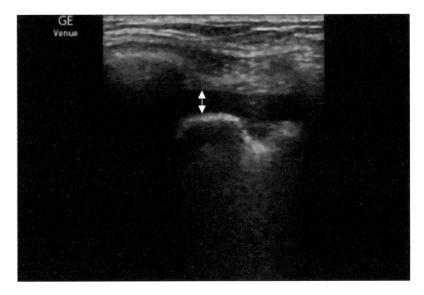

Figure 13.5. A small pleural effusion <1cm in depth (double headed arrow) in a patient with Covid-19.

13.6 Pleural effusion mimics

Before undertaking an aspiration or drainage it is important to consider potential effusion mimics, including the following.

- **Pleural thickening:** anechoic or hypoechoic pleural thickening can easily be mistaken for a small pleural effusion. In a patient with a pleural effusion, you should expect to see a positive colour Doppler sign both from respiratory and cardiac movement. The absence of the fluid colour sign is in favour of pleural thickening.

- **Abdominal ascites:** the reflection of abdominal fluid above the diaphragm may mimic a pleural effusion. To avoid this, patients with abdominal fluid should be scanned from several alternative angles.

13.7 Small bore chest drains insertion – the Seldinger technique

Probably the most common technique used for non-surgical chest drain insertion is the Seldinger technique. This will be familiar to many readers who are versed in the insertion of central venous catheters and other similar procedures. We have broken the procedure down into the following 12 steps.

1. Identify the optimal site for drain insertion using ultrasound as discussed above. The drain may either be inserted under real-time guidance or after prior marking of the point of insertion (if this approach is used, it is important that once the site is marked there is no alteration to the patient's position, and the procedure is performed with minimal delay).

2. Select the desired drain size. Small bore drains (12Fr size) are generally used as first line. Sizes up to 18Fr are available and can be considered in patients with empyema.

3. The complete drain pack should be open and prepared (*Fig. 13.6*) and a full aseptic technique used including sterile gown and gloves.

4. The skin should be cleaned and draped.

5. The marked spot should be infiltrated with local anaesthetic; lidocaine is commonly the anaesthetic of choice (maximum dose without adrenaline 3mg/kg: ~20ml 1% lignocaine or 10ml 2% lignocaine in a 70kg patient). A small gauge needle (e.g. a 25-gauge orange needle) should be used first to inject subcutaneous tissue and raise a bleb. Subsequent deeper infiltration of the intercostal muscles and pleura can then be performed with a larger needle (e.g. 21-gauge green). You should expect to aspirate fluid with the green needle (although this may not be possible in patients with thicker chest walls), giving you further confirmation of your initial ultrasound findings.

6. Attach a syringe to your introducer needle and advance it slowly through skin and subcutaneous tissue, superior to the inferior rib, whilst drawing back on the syringe until fluid is aspirated. It is helpful to remember the depth fluid was aspirated at during anaesthetic infiltration to help guide your needle insertion here.

7. A J-tip guidewire should then be passed through the needle, which can be gently used to guide the wire to the apex (pneumothorax) or base (pleural effusion) of the pleural cavity as required. Then remove the introducer needle whilst holding the guidewire steady. Some clinicians scan the chest again here to confirm correct positioning of the wire.

8. A small incision should then be made with a scalpel at the insertion site adjacent to the guidewire. The dilator is then advanced over and in the same plane as the guidewire using a gentle advancing and rotating motion. The dilator is usually advanced only 1cm beyond the depth of the pleura as measured with the introducer needle in step 6.

9. The pleural catheter, with its internal stiffener *in situ*, should be advanced over the guidewire whilst ensuring the proximal tip of the guidewire is visible throughout. The drain is usually inserted to at least 8–14cm depending on chest wall thickness.

10. The guidewire and internal stiffener are then to be removed together.

11. Attach a 3-way stopcock and Luer lock connector with a tube to the pleural catheter (*Fig. 13.6*). This is then connected to the connecting tubing for the chest drain bottle, which should be pre-filled with water to the marked level.

12. Secure the drain in position. This is usually performed using a non-absorbable silk suture, followed by the application of a drain fixator dressing if available.

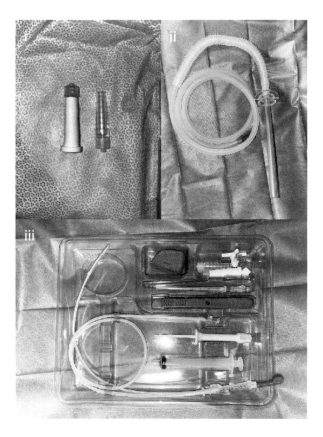

Figure 13.6. (i) Luer lock connector. (ii) Chest drain bottle connection tube. (iii) Seldinger chest drain kit.

13.8 Chest drain insertion for a pneumothorax

The use of ultrasound to diagnose a pneumothorax may be invaluable in cases where chest radiography is not readily available and rapid diagnosis is required [5]. It can also be beneficial in diagnosis of small pneumothoraces that may be missed on chest X-ray (CXR), although a small pneumothorax, not visible on CXR, is unlikely to cause symptoms or change immediate management.

Ultrasound may also play a role in differentiating a pneumothorax from a subpleural bulla or even skinfolds artefact, although this is highly operator and experience dependent [5,6]. In clinical practice, the next logical step would be to request a radiology review or a CT chest if there is any suspicion of subpleural bulla mimicking a pneumothorax.

Certain sonographic signs will point you towards a diagnosis of a pneumothorax (discussed in detail in *Chapters 11* and *12*), but some key findings include:

- Absence of pleural sliding.

- Absence of B-lines.

- Presence of a lung point.

- Absence of a lung pulse.

- M-mode image consistent with the absence of lung sliding (the 'barcode' or 'stratosphere' sign).

Although it is often safe to insert a blind drain into the 'safe triangle' in a large pneumothorax with no lung adherent to the chest wall, the adjuvant use of ultrasound can help minimize any visceral damage. In patients with a small or localized pneumothorax, referral to an experienced operator is advised, because ultrasound will be needed to map the location of the pneumothorax to ensure the drain is inserted away from the lung point.

13.9 Some peri-procedure safety points

- All individuals inserting a chest drain must be trained and competent or supervised by someone who is competent in drain insertion.

- Non-urgent chest drain insertion should be avoided in anticoagulated patients until their international normalized ratio (INR) is <1.5 / sufficient time has passed since their last dose.

- A recent CXR should ideally be available prior to the procedure commencing.

- Written consent should be obtained where possible. Complications include pain, infection, haemorrhage, pneumothorax, drain dislodgment, and visceral injury.

- Chest drain insertion should be in the 'safe triangle' unless indication for another position is present.

- Analgesia should be given preprocedure where possible alongside intraprocedure lidocaine.

- A high level of force should never be used to insert drains.

- Once inserted, a chest drain should be connected to a drainage system that contains a valve mechanism to prevent fluid or air from entering the pleural cavity. This may be an underwater seal, flutter valve or other recognized mechanism.

- A CXR should normally be performed post drain insertion to review position.

- After insertion, a drain should never be advanced further if thought to be malpositioned, due to the risk of infection, however, it may be withdrawn if necessary.

- If a chest drain is bubbling, it should **not** be clamped.

- Post drain insertion no more than 1.5L should be drained within the first hour and drainage of large effusions should be done in a controlled fashion due to risk of re-expansion pulmonary oedema.

- Drains should be checked at least daily for signs of infection, volume drained and whether they are swinging or bubbling.

13.10 Summary

Thoracocentesis can be a vital diagnostic and therapeutic technique in patients with pleural effusions or a pneumothorax. The use of POCUS either statically or dynamically can improve procedural success and safety.

13.11 References

1. Lee FCY (2017) The curtain sign in lung ultrasound. *J Med Ultrasound*, 25:101.

2. Yang PC, Luh KT, Chang DB, Wu HD, Yu CJ, Kuo SH (1992) Value of sonography in determining the nature of pleural effusion: analysis of 320 cases. *AJR Am J Roentgenol*, 159:29.

3. Asciak R, Hassan M, Mercer RM, *et al.* (2019) Prospective analysis of the predictive value of sonographic pleural fluid echogenicity for the diagnosis of exudative effusion. *Respiration*, 97:451.

4. Groote-Bidlingmaier F, Koegelenberg CFN (2019) A practical guide to transthoracic ultrasound. *Breathe*, 9:131.

5. Tsai TH, Jerng J-S, Yang P-C (2008) Clinical applications of transthoracic ultrasound in chest medicine. *J Med Ultrasound*, 16:7e25.

6. Chen C-T, Chang S-Y (2014) Giant pulmonary bullae mimicking spontaneous pneumothorax. *QJM*, 107:681.

CHAPTER 14

BASIC HEPATIC AND BILIARY ULTRASOUND

Jonny Wilkinson, Marcus Peck & Ashley Miller

14.1 Liver ultrasound

This section focuses on basic sonoanatomy of the liver and discusses vascular supply, anatomical segments, and basic measurements of relevance to POCUS.

The liver's anterior to posterior (A–P) dimension, at the mid-clavicular line, should be no more than 14.5cm in males and 13.5cm in females (when measured from a mid-point along the diaphragm, to the most lateral tip seen). A line drawn through the gallbladder, the main lobar fissure and the inferior vena cava (IVC) separates right and left lobes of the liver (*Fig. 14.1*).

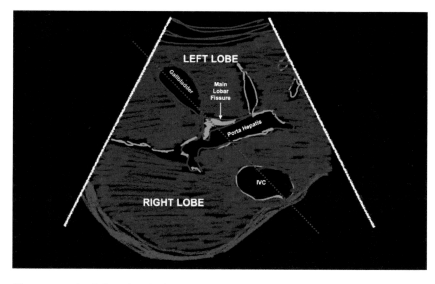

Figure 14.1. The left and right lobes of the liver with anatomical relations. A crude line drawn through the gallbladder and the IVC acts as a dividing line. IVC – inferior vena cava.

14.1.1 Liver lobes

The liver is arbitrarily divided into three lobes:

- right lobe – this is divided into anterior and posterior segments

- left lobe – this is divided into medial and lateral segments

- caudate lobe – this is not well visualized and sits on the posterior aspect of the liver; the IVC forms its posterior border, whilst the fissure from the ligamentum venosum forms its anterior border (*Fig. 14.2*).

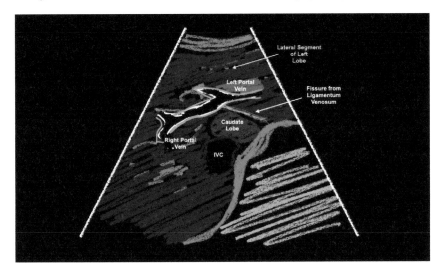

Figure 14.2. The posteriorly lying caudate lobe with its anatomical relations, as well as the portal vein with its branches. IVC – inferior vena cava.

14.1.2 Blood vessels

Hepatic veins
There are three main hepatic veins, viewed best whilst scanning the superior liver (*Fig. 14.3*). They run an **inter** segmental and **inter** lobar course:

- right hepatic vein – runs within the right intersegmental fissure, it divides the right lobe into anterior and posterior segments

- middle hepatic vein – this separates the right anterior lobe from the left medial lobe

- left hepatic vein – this divides the left lobe into medial and lateral segments.

Portal veins
The main portal vein takes supply from the intestinal veins, the splenic vein, the pancreatic vein, and the veins from the gallbladder. It runs upwards and obliquely towards the liver hilum, accompanying the hepatic artery and common bile duct, forming the portal triad. It divides into left and right branches at the porta hepatis and runs an **intra** segmental course (see *Fig. 14.2*):

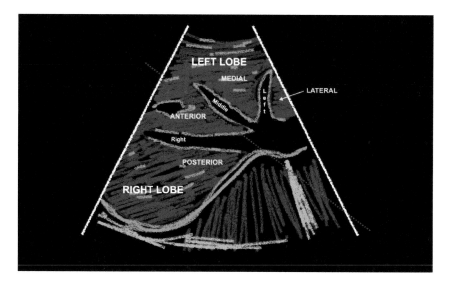

Figure 14.3. Superior scan of the liver showing the hepatic veins and their relationship with the lobes of the liver.

- main portal vein – divides into right and left

- left portal vein – divides into medial and lateral

- right portal vein – divides into anterior and posterior.

There are clear sonographic differences between the portal veins and the hepatic veins:

- portal veins:

  - bright echogenic (white walls)
  - route of travel = **intra** segmental only

- hepatic veins:

  - no hyperechoic walls, appearance like tree trunks
  - route of travel = **inter** segmental and **inter** lobar.

14.1.3 The Couinaud classification

This classification divides the liver into eight functionally distinct segments. Each has its own arterial supply, venous supply and biliary drainage. Within each, there is effectively a portal triad, with branches of the hepatic artery, portal vein and bile duct.

This is the preferred anatomical classification system because it divides the liver into eight independent segments, rather than relying on the traditional morphological description based on the external appearance of the liver.

The main dividing anatomical structures are:

- the hepatic veins – these divide the liver into four segments

- a line through right and left main portal veins – this divides the four segments into eight.

The eight segments (*Fig. 14.4*) are as follows:

1   the posteriorly located caudate lobe

2+3   the superior and inferior lateral segments of the left lobe

4a+4b   the medial segment of the left lobe

5+6   the inferior segments of the right lobe

7+8   the superior segments of the right lobe.

14.1.4 Echogenicity

The liver is described according to its surrounding organs as far as echogenicity is concerned.

A useful reminder here is PLiSK, in order of most echogenic to least:

- **P**ancreas

- **L**iver

- **S**pleen

- **K**idney.

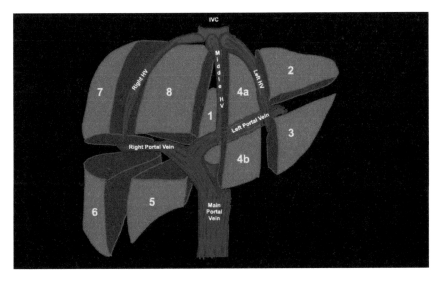

Figure 14.4. The Couinaud segments and associated anatomical relations. HV – hepatic vein.

14.2 Biliary tree ultrasound

Biliary disease is a common cause of acute abdominal pain. Bedside ultrasonography is a sensitive imaging modality for the detection of gallstones and acute cholecystitis. Once the clinician gains good familiarity with general anatomy and sonoanatomy, ultrasonography can be easily mastered and is quick to perform.

Here we will discuss the basic anatomy of the biliary tree, indications for biliary ultrasound, the appearances of common pathologies on ultrasound, and pitfalls of which clinicians should remain cognisant.

There are various key anatomical structures that need to be identified (see *Fig. 14.5* for an overview):

- gallbladder

- hepatic artery

- hepatic portal vein

- common bile duct.

14.2.1 Benefits of biliary ultrasound

Ultrasound of the biliary tree is eminently possible at the patient's bed. Used at the point of care, it is possible to narrow down the differential diagnoses for acute abdominal pain. Amongst skilled users, sensitivity and specificity are high:

- for diagnosing cholelithiasis – 89.8% sensitive and 88.0% specific

- for diagnosing cholecystitis – 87% sensitive and 82% specific.

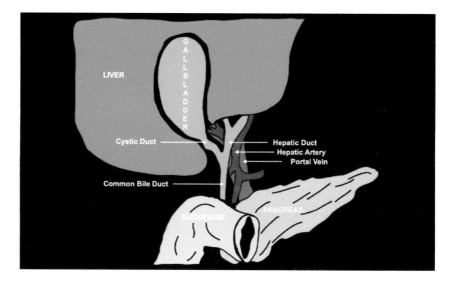

Figure 14.5. Anatomy relevant to biliary ultrasound.

14.2.2 Indications for biliary ultrasound

There are several indications for both hepatic and biliary ultrasound including:

- right upper quadrant pain
- abdominal pain with fever
- history of nausea and flatulent dyspepsia
- jaundice
- vomiting
- infection screen in critical illness.

14.2.3 Performing biliary ultrasound

There are six main things we look for when performing this POCUS modality:

- gallstones
- gallbladder wall thickening
- an enlarged gallbladder
- pericholecystic fluid
- common bile duct (CBD) distension
- detection of sonographic Murphy's sign.

Probe choice

The curvilinear probe is the most used in biliary ultrasound. However, some portable ultrasound devices do not offer a standalone curvilinear probe. In such cases the phased array probe provides a good substitute.

Scanning techniques

Ideally, the gallbladder should be scanned in longitudinal and transverse orientations. There are three commonly used techniques (shown in *Fig. 14.6*).

1. **Traditional sub-xiphoid sweep**

Patient position:
- supine / left lateral decubitus.

Probe placement:
- place the probe in a cephalad/caudad orientation, marker to the patient's head, around 2cm below the xiphoid process.

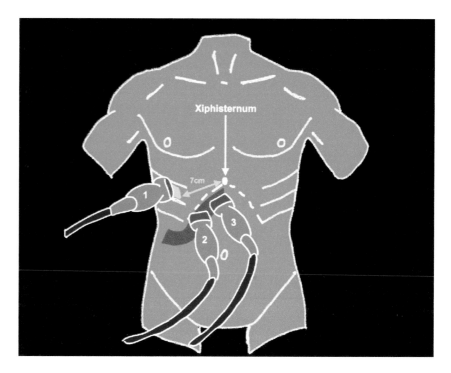

Figure 14.6. Probe positions for biliary ultrasound. (1) X-7 position. (2) Common bile duct position. (3) Traditional sub-xiphoid position.

Movement and optimization:

- sweep the probe along the subcostal margin from left to right until the desired anatomical structures are visualized.

- you may also need to tilt the probe left to right as you do so.

TOP TIPS

Traditional sub-xiphoid sweep

- If bowel gas is in the way, ask the patient to 'puff out their belly' or inhale deeply, holding their breath temporarily at the end.
- Failing the above, try turning the patient into left lateral decubitus position.
- Look for sonographic Murphy's sign:
  - pain when the patient inhales and the gallbladder contacts the probe (equivalent to the traditional examination sign, where the examining hand contacts the gallbladder as the liver moves down on inhalation).

2. X–7

Patient position:
- supine/left lateral decubitus.

Probe placement:
- place the probe in a cephalad/caudad orientation at a point approximately 7cm to the right of the xiphoid process; rotate slightly anticlockwise so the marker is at the 11 o'clock position and the probe lies in the rib space.

Movement and optimization:
- optimize your intercostal window with gentle tilts and lateral movements of the probe

- continue moving laterally across from the xiphoid process if you cannot find the gallbladder.

TOP TIPS

X–7

- Fan the probe back and forth through the liver at each point as you move laterally until you catch the gallbladder (usually black in appearance).

- Once you catch a view of the gallbladder, dip the tail of the probe, aiming for the patient's right shoulder, to ensure you are viewing as wide a section of the gallbladder as possible, in its long-axis.

- If you are still struggling to find the gallbladder, locate the main lobar fissure within the body of the liver (echogenic white structure). Follow this to find the portal triad. The lobar fissure links the portal triad to the gallbladder, appearing as an 'exclamation mark' sign (*Fig. 14.7*).

- Now you have identified the gallbladder, look for the portal triad, which should sit adjacent to it. This consists of:
  - the portal vein
  - the common bile duct
  - the hepatic artery.

- The portal triad has an eponymous sonographic description – the 'Mickey Mouse sign' (*Fig. 14.8*). This is so named because the ears are formed by the hepatic duct and the hepatic artery, whilst the head is formed by the portal vein.

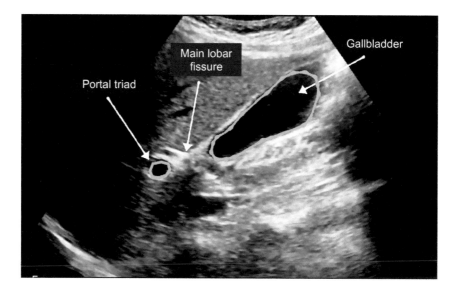

Figure 14.7. Main lobar fissure connecting the portal triad to the gallbladder.

Relevant sono-anatomy

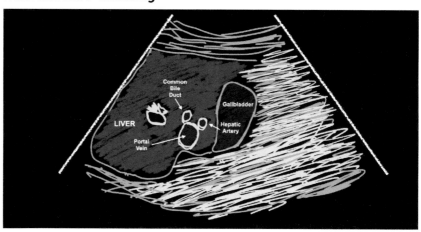

Figure 14.8. The portal triad: the hepatic artery, hepatic portal vein and the common bile duct.

3. Common bile duct view

The common bile duct is often notoriously hard to find. This section focuses on how to locate this structure more exclusively.

Patient position:
- supine/left lateral decubitus.

Probe placement:
- place the probe in a transverse orientation, with the marker to the patient's right at a point approximately 2cm below the xiphoid process.

Movement and optimization:

- locate the abdominal aorta in the centre of the image – this is a pulsatile structure, sitting on top of the vertebral body (this has an echogenic crest with a posterior acoustic shadow)

- locate the superior mesenteric artery (SMA) – this is an anechoic (black) structure with an echogenic (white) collar, sitting on top of the abdominal aorta

- locate the porto-splenic confluence:

  o look for the portal vein – this is a comma-shaped anechoic structure at 11 o'clock to the SMA
  o look for the splenic vein – this is a flattened anechoic structure at 2 o'clock to the SMA (*Fig. 14.9*).

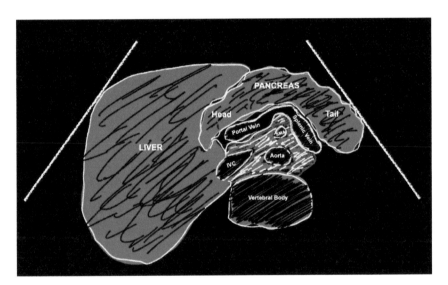

Figure 14.9. Relevant sonoanatomy for location of the common bile duct. IVC – inferior vena cava; SMA – superior mesenteric artery.

- Locate the porta hepatis – rotate the probe clockwise to the 11 o'clock position. This elongates the portal vein and traces it to where it enters the liver at the porta hepatis.

- Locate the common bile duct:

  o with gentle movements of the probe, the common bile duct can be visualized sitting on top of the porta hepatis (in parallel)
  o it is seen as a tubular structure with echogenic walls (*Fig. 14.10*).

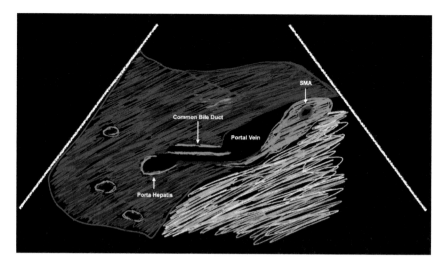

Figure 14.10. The common bile duct viewed after the 11 o'clock tilt from the transverse probe position. SMA – superior mesenteric artery.

TOP TIPS

Common bile duct view

- Another key structure to help locate the common bile duct is the porta hepatis. If you struggle to find it, re-orientate back to the abdominal aorta/SMA and trace the portal vein again.

- Use small tilts and rotations of the probe around the 11 o'clock position to see the common bile duct; it often pops in and out of view.
  - Getting the patient to slowly inspire and hold their breath can minimize this distracting movement.

- Once you find it, zoom onto it.

- Confirm it is the common bile duct by placing colour Doppler over it; there should be no flow (*Figs 14.11* and *14.12*).

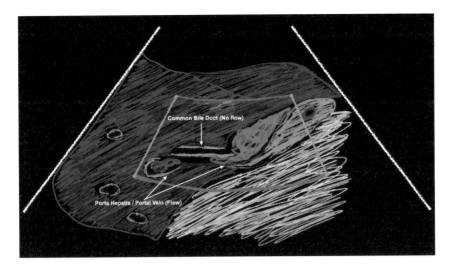

Figure 14.11. Colour flow Doppler demonstrating no flow in the common bile duct (longitudinal orientation), and flow in the surrounding venous structures.

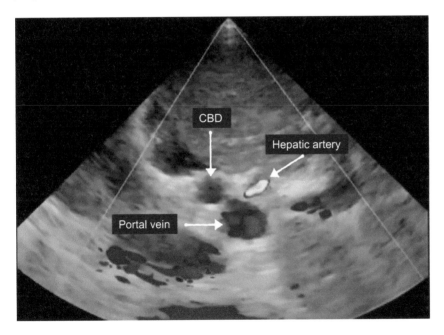

Figure 14.12. Colour flow Doppler demonstrating no flow in the common bile duct (transverse 'Mickey Mouse' orientation), and flow in the surrounding venous structures.

14.2.4 General evaluation and pathology

We will now discuss some of the most common biliary pathologies identifiable on ultrasound.

Gallstones

These are usually hyperechoic. They demonstrate acoustic shadowing behind them because they absorb the sound (hyperechoic white structure with a hypoechoic black run-off shadow). Always attempt to scan the entire gallbladder, because missing the neck will also miss any impacted stones therein. Stones may also lodge in the common bile duct (*Figs 14.13* and *14.14*).

TOP TIP

Gallstones

Altering the patient's position while scanning can demonstrate mobile stones versus impacted ones, because loose stones will tend to fall to dependent areas under gravity.

Gallbladder sludge may be a precursor to gallstones and is sometimes associated with disease. Sludge appears as a dependent fluid with mixed echogenicity within the gallbladder.

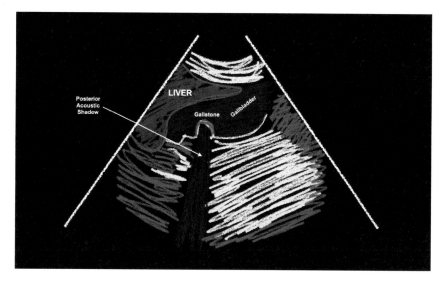

Figure 14.13. Mobile gallstone near the neck of the gallbladder; note the hyperechoic, well-circumscribed cholesterol shell and posterior acoustic shadow.

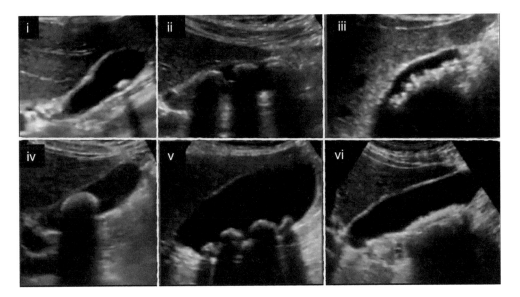

Figure 14.14. Various gallstone appearances. (i) Simple mobile solitary stone and posterior acoustic shadow. (ii) Multiple large stones within a contracted gallbladder; similar acoustic shadows. (iii) Multiple polymorphic gallstones. (iv) Large cholesterol stone and multiple small stones impacted in the neck. (v) Multiple stones, demonstrating dependent collection with the effect of patient movement and gravity. (vi) Multiple small stones collecting posteriorly.

Gallbladder wall thickening

Cholecystitis and cholangiocarcinoma can present as a thickened gallbladder wall. Normal wall thickness should be 3mm or less. Short- and long-axis measurements should be made wherever possible, focusing on the anterior wall of the gallbladder. The posterior wall may appear artificially thickened because of acoustic enhancement or an artefact from bowel gas.

Congestive heart failure, fluid overload, cirrhosis with ascites, hypoalbuminaemia, human immunodeficiency virus, pancreatitis, renal failure or a fully contracted postprandial gallbladder can also present with wall thickening.

It is important to try to see the entire gallbladder, paying particular attention not to miss the neck, to ensure no stones are missed (see *Figs 14.15* and *14.16*).

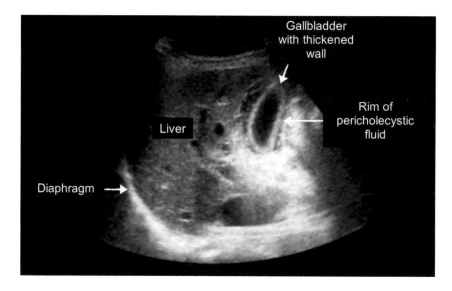

Figure 14.15. Acute cholecystitis.

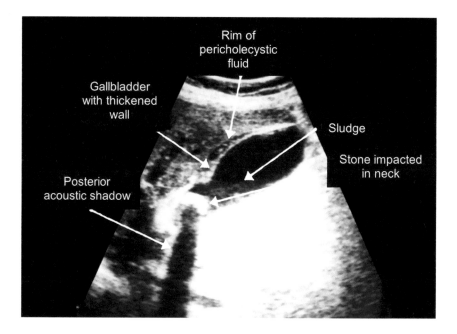

Figure 14.16. Impacted gallbladder neck gallstone causing cholecystitis.

Pericholecystic fluid

Similar in appearance to pericardial fluid, pericholecystic fluid appears during cholecystitis as an anechoic stripe of fluid collecting along the dependent surface of the gallbladder. A good place to look is the space between the gallbladder and liver.

Common bile duct distension

The common bile duct should measure less than 6mm from inner wall to inner wall. Its size increases by approximately 1mm per decade in age. Note: if a patient has had a cholecystectomy, it naturally dilates to up to 1cm (this is a normal phenomenon; see *Fig. 14.17*).

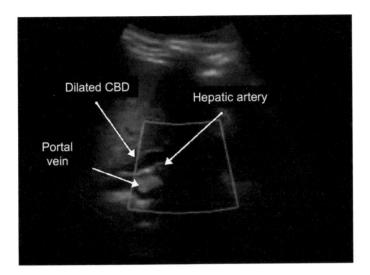

Dilated CBD

Hepatic artery

Portal vein

Figure 14.17. Dilated common bile duct (CBD) (normal variant), in a patient post cholecystectomy.

Sonographic Murphy's sign

This is positive if the point of maximal tenderness in the right upper quadrant is identified while scanning and obtaining a good subcostal view of the gallbladder. *Note: not applicable to the X-7 probe position because the ribs will act as protection.*

14.2.5 Common pitfalls and other signs

Contracted gallbladder

A contracted gallbladder may be difficult to visualize. Walls can look thickened but, on close inspection and zoomed-in, if three distinct layers are seen, this is normal (see *Fig. 14.18*).

Misidentification for other structures

The duodenum, hepatic cysts or renal cysts can look like the gallbladder.

Wall–Echo–Shadow sign (WES sign)

This phenomenon occurs when a gallbladder is filled with stones or is contracted onto a stone(s). You thus cannot see the walls of the gallbladder behind them because there are multiple interferences to the passage of the sound waves through. So, we see the front **WALL**, the **ECHO**genicity of the stone(s), and then the acoustic **SHADOW** created by the stones, hence the **WES** sign. Thus, the anterior gallbladder wall is visualized, followed by the hyperechoic stone(s), and then the shadow of the stone(s) (see *Fig. 14.19*).

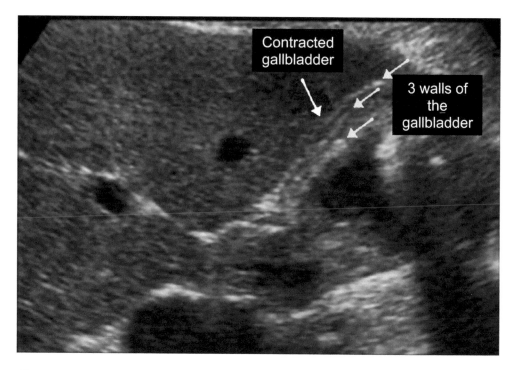

Figure 14.18. Postprandial gallbladder, contracted down but demonstrating the normal '3 layer' appearance.

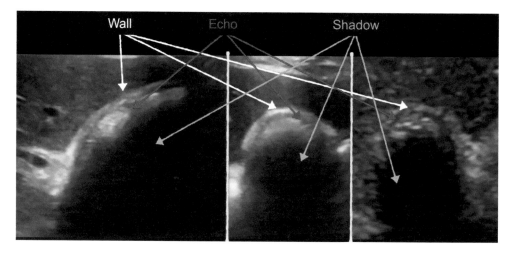

Figure 14.19. The Wall–Echo–Shadow sign.

Gallbladder polyps

Differentiating between gallstones and gallbladder polyps (*Fig. 14.20*) can be challenging. *Table 14.1* shows some tricks the sonographer can use to do this.

Table 14.1. How to differentiate between gallstones and gallbladder polyps on ultrasound.

Gallstone	Gallbladder polyp
Positioned within the gallbladder lumen	Adherent to the gallbladder wall
Usually mobile on repositioning the patient (unless impacted)	Immobile on repositioning the patient
Posterior acoustic shadowing	No posterior acoustic shadowing

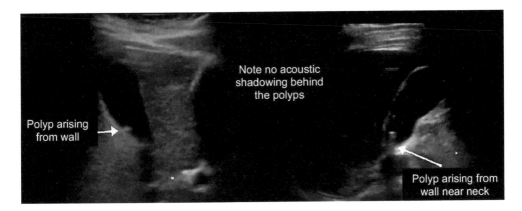

Figure 14.20. Gallbladder polyps.

14.3 Summary

Hepatic and biliary tract ultrasound can be performed rapidly and effectively at the bedside. In correctly trained hands it allows for the rapid, non-invasive identification of a wide range of pathologies and may prove invaluable in patients for whom transfer for other imaging modalities is not possible or safe.

CHAPTER 15

ULTRASOUND ASSESSMENT OF THE RENAL TRACT AND BLADDER

Maryam Khosravi

POCUS assessment of the renal tract and bladder in critical care should be used as a tool to augment clinical thinking and differential diagnosis. As a clinician using POCUS, it is important to first consider the symptoms, signs and circumstances that warrant further investigation with ultrasound, so that the differential diagnosis is formulated before placing the probe on the patient (*Table 15.1*). In this way, POCUS can prevent delays in diagnosis and treatment of conditions that can easily be identified such as urinary retention or hydronephrosis.

With more research, POCUS may also prove useful for the monitoring and management of fluid balance or renal injury, through the measurement of blood flow and calculating the resistive indices within the kidney. Patients with pre-existing renal disease can benefit from POCUS in critical care by allowing assessment of their renal replacement access modalities (e.g. vascular POCUS to detect thrombosis) and possibly their renal transplant.

Table 15.1. Clinical indications for further investigation with POCUS

Clinical symptoms and signs	What are the differential diagnoses for which ultrasound can be helpful?
Abdominal, flank, lower back or groin pain	Pyelonephritis (fat stranding, abscess or nidus for infection, e.g. stone) Hydronephrosis Stone, cyst, tumour, trauma
Trauma	Sub-capsular collection (Page kidney) Rupture and bleeding – abdominal free fluid
Renal impairment	AKI/CKD (small kidneys in CKD and loss of corticomedullary differentiation) Hydronephrosis

Clinical symptoms and signs	What are the differential diagnoses for which ultrasound can be helpful?
Oliguria or anuria	Obstruction/hydronephrosis Retention AKI/CKD
Haematuria	AKI/CKD Stones Cysts Tumour
Dysuria	Stones Obstruction/hydronephrosis Retention

AKI – acute kidney injury; CKD – chronic kidney disease

15.1 Performing the scan

In this section we will discuss the basic steps involved in performing a sonographic assessment of the renal tract and bladder.

15.1.1 Which probe to use?

A curvilinear probe with lower frequency ultrasound allows the deeper penetration required to assess the kidney and bladder. It is also possible to use the phased array probe if a curvilinear probe is not available.

15.1.2 Where to place the probe?

The kidneys are retroperitoneal organs located on either side of the vertebral column (T12–L3). The right kidney is slightly more posterior than the left kidney because the liver is larger than the spleen. With the patient lying supine, the objective is to scan each kidney in long-axis and transverse-axis.

On each side, the probe is first placed in the midaxillary line with the indicator facing cephalad. In this position the kidney can be viewed longitudinally by fanning the probe anterio-posteriorly (*Fig. 15.1*). A 10–20° oblique tilt on the probe may help obtain views between rib shadows.

To obtain transverse views, the probe marker is turned 90° on each side. Fanning the probe cephalo-caudally obtains views from the superior through to the inferior pole.

To assess the bladder, sagittal and transverse views should be obtained at the pubic symphysis by placing the probe over the pelvis with the indicator facing the head and scanning downwards towards the pubic symphysis. The bladder is a dark anechoic fluid-filled sack with posterior enhancement (*Fig. 15.1*). The normal ureters are often difficult to visualize, but ureteral jets may be seen in the bladder with colour flow Doppler (CFD) at the trigone of the bladder.

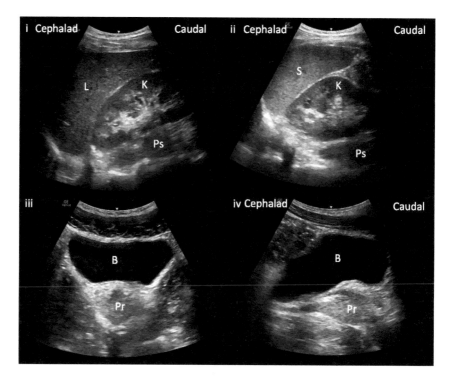

Figure 15.1. (i) Longitudinal view of normal right kidney. (ii) Longitudinal view of normal left kidney. (iii) Transverse view of bladder. (iv) Sagittal view of bladder. Images courtesy of Dr D. Mistry. B – bladder; K – kidney; L – liver; Pr – prostate; Ps – psoas; S – spleen

15.2 Sonoanatomy

Normal kidney size correlates with a person's total body area, approximating to normal pole to pole lengths of 10–12cm in the longitudinal axis, and 5–6cm depth in the transverse axis. The anatomy of the kidney correlates on ultrasound as demonstrated in *Figure 15.2*.

15.3 Scanning objectives

Focused questions should always guide the POCUS scanning protocol.

15.3.1 Are the kidneys of normal size and echogenicity?

With the patient lying supine, the right kidney is easy to find using the liver as an anatomical guide. Placing the probe marker cephalad and in the midaxillary line, the kidney is seen first in its long-axis, with the cortex closest to the probe.

The border of the kidney should be visualized by fanning the probe. The border should be smooth and surrounded by thin bright fascia and perinephric fat; it moves downwards with respiration. The parenchyma of the right kidney can be compared to that of the liver, and normally the renal parenchyma

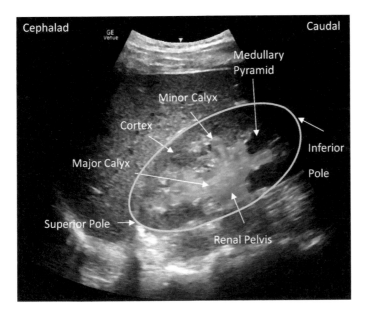

Figure 15.2. Sonographic anatomy of the kidney.

should be isoechoic to the liver parenchyma or darker. The left kidney should be hypoechoic (darker) to the spleen. It usually sits more superior than the right. The fat of the renal sinus and renal pelvis is normally hyperechoic. In renal pathology, the renal parenchyma can be brighter or there may be loss of corticomedullary differentiation.

The longest aspect of the kidney should be viewed and measuring this pole to pole will give a good indication of kidney size. Chronic renal disease is associated with decreased kidney size.

15.3.2 Is there hydronephrosis?

In the hands of an experienced practitioner, POCUS has excellent sensitivity and specificity for the detection of hydronephrosis. Radiological evidence of hydronephrosis is usually graded normal, mild, moderate or severe (*Figs 15.3* and *15.4*).

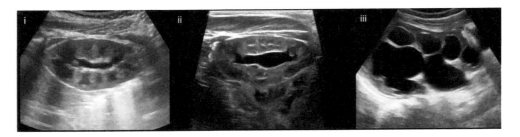

Figure 15.3. (i) Mild hydronephrosis. (ii) Moderate hydronephrosis. (iii) Severe hydronephrosis. Images courtesy of Dr J. Wilkinson.

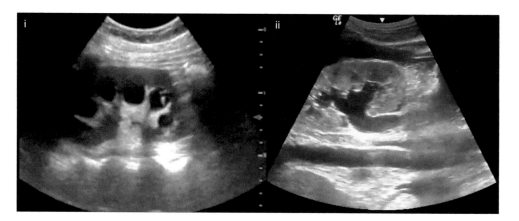

Figure 15.4. (i) Severe hydronephrosis. (ii) Hydronephrosis with hydroureter. Images courtesy of Dr J. Wilkinson.

In mild hydronephrosis the renal pelvis will appear dilated. As the hydronephrosis progresses the renal calyces become involved, to the point where the calyceal dilation is so severe that the cortex appears thinned. It is important to be aware that anatomical variants such an extra-renal pelvis or prominent renal vasculature can also mimic hydronephrosis.

15.3.3 Is there a mass?

It is important to be cognisant of the fact that variations of normal kidney anatomy exist, some of which can be developmental rather than pathological, so they should prompt further radiological investigation. Masses in the kidney can be found coincidentally on POCUS but should also be followed up. Masses can represent renal malignancies such as renal cell cancer, or benign tumours such as angiomyolipomas (which may or may not be related to systemic disease such as tuberous sclerosis).

15.3.4 Is there a cyst?

The prevalence of simple kidney cysts in healthy individuals is approximately 10% and this increases with age. Simple cysts are smooth, thin-walled, anechoic structures within the renal parenchyma (*Fig. 15.5*). If the shape of the cyst is irregular or there are septations, internal elements, or increased echogenicity, then a complex cyst, abscess or malignancy should be considered and investigated further.

Multiple cysts in the kidneys raise the possibility of polycystic kidney disease and these cysts can be susceptible to infection, rupture or haemorrhage. Patients with end-stage renal disease can acquire multiple renal cysts, which may be at higher risk of malignant conversion.

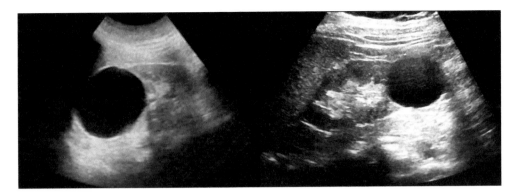

Figure 15.5. Two examples of renal cysts. Images courtesy of Dr J. Wilkinson.

15.3.5 Is there a stone?

Stones can be present at any point in the genitourinary tract from within the renal parenchyma to the bladder. Stones can be single or multiple, of varying sizes and composition. On ultrasound they can be identified by direct visualization as hyperechoic structures with an acoustic shadow, most easily seen within the renal parenchyma. Stones can also be indirectly suspected, for example, if they have caused ureteric obstruction and hydronephrosis. However, smaller stones (usually less than 5mm in size) can still cause renal colic without hydronephrosis, so an absence of hydronephrosis does not rule out small ureteric stones.

15.3.6 Is there normal blood flow?

Measurement of renal haemodynamics is of increasing interest as its value for guidance in resuscitation (venous excess ultrasound – VExUS) is researched. As a POCUS practitioner, the most important question to address is whether there is arterial and venous flow on renal Doppler (scaled at 10–25cm/sec), and whether any vascular malformations are suspected (e.g. post renal biopsy or post renal transplant).

The renal resistive index (RRI) can be calculated by measuring the peak systolic velocity (PSV) and end-diastolic velocity (EDV) of a renal artery.

$$RRI = (PSV - EDV) / PSV$$

The normal range of RRI is 0.50–0.70. Elevated RRI can indicate worse prognosis in renal pathology and renal transplant. This is most useful for monitoring in the acute post-transplant setting.

Venous Doppler tracings in the kidney should be continuous and monophasic. Congestion is indicated if these Doppler flows become discontinuous with biphasic or monophasic flow in systole and/or diastole (described further in *Chapter 24* on fluid assessment).

15.3.7 Is the bladder adequately filled and thin-walled?

Assessment of the bladder can only be made if it is adequately filled, which may not be possible in catheterized patients, but remains a useful tool when oliguria occurs in the catheterized patient. The volume of the bladder can be calculated by:

$$Volume = length \times width \times depth \times 0.52$$

In transverse views, Doppler (scaled at 10–25cm/sec) can be used to detect the ureteral jets on the posterior wall of the bladder. Because urine is sporadically re-released into the bladder, ureteral jets can be difficult to detect, but the complete absence of a ureteral jet can corroborate a differential diagnosis of a stone (preventing urine flow within the ureter or at the uretero-vesical junction). The 'twinkling artefact' can also be sought for stones at the uretero-vesical junction [1].

15.4 Summary

The use of POCUS to assess the renal tract and bladder can prove invaluable in the care of critically unwell patients presenting with suspected urological pathology. However, it should be viewed as one part of the clinical assessment and not as its replacement.

15.5 Reference

1. Ripollés T, Martinez-Perez MJ, Vizutete J, *et al.* (2013) Sonographic diagnosis of symptomatic ureteral calculi: usefulness of the twinkling artifact. *Abdom. Imaging,* **38**:863.

CHAPTER 16

ULTRASOUND-GUIDED ABDOMINAL PARACENTESIS

Charlotte Hateley & Arun Sivananthan

Abdominal paracentesis is a vital procedure that is used to treat the clinical complications of ascites and establish the underlying aetiology. POCUS minimizes complications associated with the collection of ascitic fluid [1]. POCUS also allows the user to find the largest volume of ascites drain, avoid small pockets or loculated ascites, and prevent unnecessary procedures when minimal or no ascites is visualized.

This chapter will focus on the indications for therapeutic abdominal paracentesis, the common complications that occur, how POCUS can reduce these risks, and will then describe how to perform ultrasound-guided abdominal therapeutic paracentesis.

16.1 Advantages and disadvantages

The overall clinical diagnostic accuracy when assessing for ascites on physical examination appears to be low, with one study suggesting only 58% of patients with ascites were identified. Further studies have shown that to identify shifting dullness at least 1L of peritoneal fluid must accumulate [2]. However, when using ultrasound, the user can detect as little as 100ml of fluid which can then be targeted for diagnostic purposes [1]. The characteristics of intraperitoneal fluid can determine whether further investigations or procedures would then be required. For patients with cirrhosis it has also been shown that in-hospital mortality is significantly higher in those patients who do not undergo paracentesis compared to those that do (9% vs. 6%) [1–3].

While the traditional landmark technique is still widely used for abdominal paracentesis, POCUS has been shown to reduce the incidence of complications and therefore benefits short-term outcomes [4]. First, it allows the technician to visualize in real-time the vital organs (the liver, spleen and bowel) to avoid injury and perforation; this is particularly important in this patient group due to the higher incidence of hepatosplenomegaly (*Fig. 16.1*). Secondly, one of the most common complications associated with paracentesis is bleeding (1%) and therefore by utilizing colour flow Doppler (CFD), abdominal wall varices or small vessels can be avoided [2, 5].

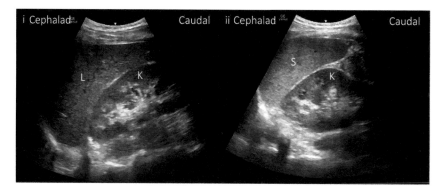

Figure 16.1. (i) Ultrasound image demonstrating the liver and kidney. (ii) Ultrasound image demonstrating the spleen and kidney.
K – kidney; L – liver; S – spleen.

The main disadvantage of using ultrasound guidance for abdominal paracentesis is the training required to ensure that the user is proficient in the technique. However, evidence shows that it is relatively easy to acquire these skills and perform the technique to the standard required [4, 6].

16.2 Aetiology of ascites

The most common cause of ascites is cirrhosis (81%), followed by malignancy (10%), heart failure (3%), tuberculosis (2%), haemodialysis (1%), pancreatic disease (1%) and other causes (2%). Approximately 5% of patients have mixed ascites, i.e. fluid due to more than one cause [7, 8]. The incidence of hospital attendance due to ascites has climbed over the last 5 years as cirrhosis becomes more prevalent [2]. Patients with cirrhosis and ascites have a poor prognosis, with a 40% chance of mortality at 1 year and 50% by 2 years [7]. These patients are also at a higher risk of developing complications of ascites including hyponatraemia, hepatorenal syndrome and spontaneous bacterial peritonitis.

16.3 Indications

All patients with grade 2 or 3 ascites should have ascitic paracentesis to identify the underlying aetiology [7]. Ascitic paracentesis is also required to diagnose spontaneous bacterial peritonitis, while therapeutic paracentesis (drain insertion) can be used to relieve abdominal pressure or respiratory compromise.

16.4 Contraindications

The main contraindication to therapeutic ascitic paracentesis is a surgical abdomen. Relative contraindications include:

- coagulopathy (INR >2)
- thrombocytopenia (platelet count <50 × 10³/µL)
- disseminated intravascular coagulation
- abdominal wall cellulitis
- pregnancy
- urinary bladder distension
- intra-abdominal adhesions
- massive ileus [9].

16.5 Complications

Severe and life-threatening complications of abdominal paracentesis are rare, with the most common complications being peritoneal leakage of fluid following the procedure (5%) and bleeding (1%). The risk of infection is around 0.63% [2].

Removing fluid too fast can lead to circulatory collapse and exacerbate renal failure or hepatorenal syndrome. These can be minimized through controlled removal of fluid, use of human albumin solution and a limit on total volume removed. The patient's renal function should be assessed pre-procedure to ensure it is safe to proceed.

Rarer complications include bladder or bowel perforation, abdominal wall haematoma, mesenteric haematoma, and epigastric artery aneurysm.

16.6 Performing the procedure

16.6.1 Equipment

- Sterile dressing pack:
  - sterile gloves
  - chlorhexidine 2%.
- Analgesia: 10ml of 1% or 2% lidocaine, orange 25G needle, green 21G needle, 10ml syringe.
- 20ml syringe with green 21G needle.
- Specimen containers.
- Blood culture bottles.

- Dressing.

- Drain.

- Human albumin solution (20%).

16.6.2 Laboratory tests

Initially, for diagnostic purposes, 10–20ml of ascitic fluid should be withdrawn. A neutrophil count and culture of ascitic fluid (by inoculation into blood culture bottles) should be performed to exclude spontaneous bacterial peritonitis (SBP). A Gram stain and neutrophil count >250 cells/cm^3 suggests a diagnosis of SBP. Up to 60% of patients will have no growth on culture [7].

Further analysis should include:

- amylase

- cytology

- PCR

- culture for mycobacteria

- lactate dehydrogenase

- triglyceride (high in chylous ascites).

Measurement of the serum–ascites albumin gradient (SAAG) can indicate the underlying cause of ascites, with a SAAG >1.1g/dl (or 11g/L) attributed to portal hypertension. It is also important to measure ascitic total protein concentration, because patients with an ascitic protein concentration of less than 15g/L have an increased risk of developing spontaneous bacterial peritonitis and may benefit from antibiotic prophylaxis [7].

16.6.3 Patient position

The most common site for an ascitic paracentesis is approximately 15cm lateral to the umbilicus in the left or right lower abdominal quadrant [8]. The left lower quadrant has been shown to have a thinner wall and deeper pool of fluid [9]. Rolling the patient to the left can allow fluid to collect in this quadrant.

The inferior and superior epigastric arteries run laterally to the umbilicus towards the mid-inguinal point and should be avoided. For optimal positioning, ensure the patient is lying semi-reclined and tilted toward the iliac fossa of choice.

16.6.4 Using the ultrasound probe to identify fluid: dynamic versus static technique

The ultrasound probe can either be used statically to mark a spot or used in real-time to identify accumulated fluid. Dynamic visualization is preferred when there are small pockets of fluid or a difficult non-traditional location has been identified, particularly if the patient moves in between scanning and the procedure taking place.

To identify the most beneficial place to perform a tap or insert a drain, the largest pocket of ascites should be identified using a 2–5MHz curvilinear probe. Place the probe longitudinally on the abdomen in either the left or right iliac fossa and fan through to measure the depth of fluid [9].

The ascites will appear as anechoic and extraperitoneal while the bowel, liver and spleen are hyperechoic (*Fig. 16.2*). The bowel will be free-floating in the fluid and will be peristalsing and the bladder is located in the midline suprapubic window with a hyperechoic dome and anechoic urine [10]. Fanning through the abdomen allows the depth of fluid to be assessed and the most appropriate aspiration position to be identified.

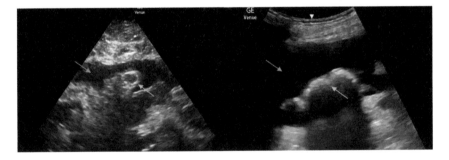

Figure 16.2. Two figures demonstrating ascites (orange arrow) with bowel free-floating within it (blue arrow).

16.6.5 Identifying vessels

Superficial vessels of the abdominal wall vary between individuals, especially lateral branches. Several blood vessels are at risk of injury during paracentesis [11], and a review of 126 cases demonstrated the most likely lacerations to occur were in the superior or inferior epigastric arteries resulting in rectus sheath haematomas [2].

Assessing whether the desired point of insertion is overlying a vessel prior to starting the procedure can reduce the risk of bleeding. This is performed using the linear high frequency transducer and CFD.

16.6.6 Inserting the drain

- On identification of the optimal site of paracentesis, the site and surrounding area should be cleaned with iodine or chlorhexidine solution using a combination of aseptic non-touch technique and drapes to maintain sterility.

- The skin and subcutaneous tissue should then be infiltrated with lidocaine (1%) using an orange (25G) needle parallel to the skin aiming to a raise a bleb.

- A blue (23G) or green needle (21G) should then be inserted using a 'z-track' technique through the bleb perpendicular to the skin to infiltrate deeper. The z-track technique involves pulling the skin down with one hand on insertion of the needle to ensure the skin insertion point and peritoneal insertion point are not in line, helping prevent ascitic leak (*Fig. 16.3*).

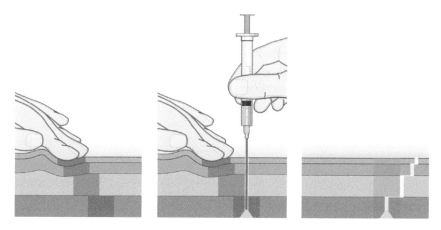

Figure 16.3. The z-track technique. Before insertion of the needle, the free hand gently pulls the skin and subcutaneous tissue to the side and the needle is then advanced as normal. Once the needle is taken out the traction is then removed, leaving a diagonal access tract – the pale line seen in the image on the right. Reproduced from *Anatomy and Physiology: an introduction* (Minett P. and Ginesi L.) with permission from Lantern Publishing.

- The syringe should be aspirated prior to infiltration at each stage of insertion to ensure no intravascular lidocaine is delivered. Aspiration should be intermittent to avoid obstruction of the needle by omentum or bowel.

- Aspiration of fluid indicates successful insertion into the peritoneum and note should be taken of the depth at which this is achieved.

- The paracentesis needle should now be inserted with a syringe attached following the anaesthetic z-track previously established to minimize pain and reduce risk of leakage. For therapeutic paracentesis a larger bore needle is required (ideally 15G).

- Once fluid is aspirated, a diagnostic sample can be taken from the syringe and then the catheter can be advanced, whilst the needle is withdrawn.

- A drainage system should then be attached.

- Patients with cirrhosis should not have drains *in situ* for longer than 6h due to risk of bacterial peritonitis.

- Albumin infusion should be considered in proportion to the amount of fluid drained [12,13].

16.6.7 Managing complications

The most common complication of therapeutic paracentesis is ascites leak after removal of the drain. In the event of a leak, a stoma bag should be placed over the leaking site to quantify and observe the leaking fluid. Most will stop spontaneously but a suture or second ascitic drain can be considered if the leak is continuous. Dressings should be avoided because these can become saturated quickly and inflame the underlying skin. Fluid shift during drainage can result in hypotension and renal dysfunction. This should be managed by appropriate fluid resuscitation. Significant bleeding is rare but may need treatment with blood products and potentially require surgical intervention as it can be fatal.

KEY POINTS

- POCUS in therapeutic abdominal paracentesis reduces complication rate.
- The use of Doppler can help avoid insertion into vessels.
- The z-track technique helps prevent ascites leak (the most common complication).
- Intravenous albumin should be given when draining ascites in cirrhosis.
- Drains for cirrhotic ascites should stay in no longer than 6h.

16.7 Summary

Abdominal paracentesis is a vital technique to identify the underlying aetiology of ascites as well as preventing the complications associated with its accumulation. The use of POCUS either statically or dynamically can reduce the risks of inserting an abdominal drain; most notably bleeding or perforation of surrounding organs.

16.8 References

1. Gaetano JN, Micic D, Aronsohn A, *et al.* (2016) The benefit of paracentesis on hospitalized adults with cirrhosis and ascites. *J Gastroenterol Hepatol*, 31:1025.

2. Cho J, Jensen TP, Reierson K, *et al.* (2019) Recommendations on the Use of Ultrasound Guidance for Adult Abdominal Paracentesis: A Position Statement of the Society of Hospital Medicine. *J Hosp Med*, 14:E7.

3. Orman ES, Hayashi PH, Bataller R, Barritt AS (2014) Paracentesis is associated with reduced mortality in patients hospitalized with cirrhosis and ascites. *Clin Gastroenterol Hepatol*, 12:496.

4. Barsuk JH, Cohen ER, Feinglass J, McGaghie WC, Wayne DB (2013) Clinical outcomes after bedside and interventional radiology paracentesis procedures. *Am J Med*, 126:349.

5. Patel PA, Ernst FR, and Gunnarsson CL (2012) Evaluation of hospital complications and costs associated with using ultrasound guidance during abdominal paracentesis procedures. *J Med Econ*, 15:1.

6. Arora S, Cheung AC, Tarique U, *et al.* (2017) First-year medical students use of ultrasound or physical examination to diagnose hepatomegaly and ascites: a randomized controlled trial. *J Ultrasound*, 20:199.

7. European Association for the Study of the Liver (2010) EASL clinical practice guidelines on the management of ascites, spontaneous bacterial peritonitis, and hepatorenal syndrome in cirrhosis. *J Hepatol*, 53:397.

8. Moore KP, Aithal GP (2006) Guidelines on the management of ascites in cirrhosis. *Gut*, 55:vi1.

9. Sakai H, Sheer TA, Mendler MH, Runyon BA (2005) Choosing the location for non-image guided abdominal paracentesis. *Liver Int*, 25:984.

10. Scheer DM, *et al.* (2012) Ultrasound guided paracentesis. *ACEP Now.*

11. Barsuk JH, Rosen BT, Cohen ER, Feinglass J, Ault MJ (2018) Vascular ultrasonography: a novel method to reduce paracentesis related major bleeding. *J Hosp Med*, 13:30.

12. Arora V, Vijayaraghavan R, Maiwall R, *et al.* (2020) Paracentesis-induced circulatory dysfunction with modest-volume paracentesis is partly ameliorated by albumin infusion in acute-on-chronic liver failure. *Hepatology*, 72:1043.

13. Bernardi M, Caraceni P, Navickis RJ, *et al.* (2012) Albumin infusion in patients undergoing large-volume paracentesis: a meta-analysis of randomized trials. *Hepatology*, 55:1172.

CHAPTER 17

BASIC AORTIC ULTRASOUND

Jonny Wilkinson, Marcus Peck & Ashley Miller

This chapter focuses on the basic sonoanatomy of the aorta and discusses branches, anatomical areas supplied and basic measurements of relevance to POCUS. The main indication for POCUS of the aorta is to rule in an abdominal aortic aneurysm, or to evaluate extension of a Type B aortic dissection.

17.1 Anatomy of the aorta

The abdominal aorta is a retroperitoneal structure that lies anterior to the spine, beginning at the 12th thoracic vertebra or the aortic hiatus of the diaphragm. It ends at around the fourth lumbar vertebra, where it bifurcates into the right and left common iliac arteries.

The abdominal aorta supplies arterial blood to the digestive organs, kidneys, adrenal glands, gonads, abdominal and paraspinal muscles, pelvis, and limbs. It is approximately 10–20cm long in adults, with an external diameter of approximately 2cm in men and slightly narrower in women. It tapers at the bifurcation, where it can measure 1–1.5cm.

17.2 Ultrasound

There are four main things to look for when performing this POCUS modality:

1. Visualization of the entire abdominal aorta, including the main branches.

2. Detection of atheromatous plaques, stenosis, aneurysms, dissections, or other pathology.

3. Measurement of any dilated segments.

4. Assessment of both common iliac arteries at origin.

17.3 Scan preparation

17.3.1 Probe selection

The curvilinear probe is the ultrasound probe of choice, commonly used with the abdominal preset selected.

17.3.2 Patient position

The patient should be supine with the head of the bed flat. It may help to ask the patient to flex their knees to lower abdominal muscle wall tone.

17.3.3 Probe placement

The aorta is classically scanned in two planes requiring the following probe orientations (*Fig. 17.1*):

- transverse
    - the probe marker is to the patient's right
- longitudinal
    - the probe marker is facing cephalad.

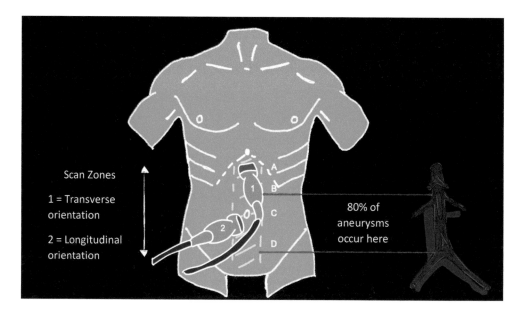

Figure 17.1. Aortic ultrasound probe positioning, scan zone and aneurysm locality.

17.3.4 Movement and optimization

Apply constant, firm pressure with the transducer to displace bowel gas that may otherwise obscure your image. The entire length of the abdominal aorta should be visualized as far as possible.

Start from the xiphoid process and scan down to the umbilicus (bifurcation point). Both transverse and longitudinal planes should be assessed. The identification of key landmark structures can assist in ensuring as much of the abdominal aorta is visualized as possible.

17.3.5 Sonoanatomy and views

Four views are commonly used to scan the abdominal aorta:

1. **High subxiphoid transverse view** (position 'A' using probe 1 in *Fig. 17.1*)

Adjust the depth so that the anterior aspect of the vertebral body is clearly visualized. You will see the aorta and inferior vena cava (IVC) just above the spine (*Fig. 17.2*). This is where the 'seagull' silhouette (the body is the coeliac artery and the hepatic and splenic arteries form right and left wings) can be seen.

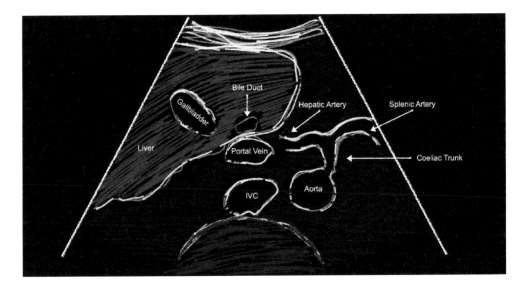

Figure 17.2. High subxiphoid transverse view of the aorta and surrounding structures.

2. **Upper transverse view** (position 'B' using probe 1 in *Fig. 17.1*)

A key landmark in the transverse plane is the vertebral body of the spine (*Fig. 17.3*), which appears as a highly reflective convex structure with dense shadowing posteriorly. The aorta is just anterior to this, slightly left of the midline. Adjust the depth to include the anterior portion of the spine as a point of reference and then move the probe down the abdomen, caudally, to obtain the view.

Origins of the renal arteries are more obvious in this view: the right and the left originate from the lateral wall of the aorta just distal to the superior mesenteric artery (SMA); the right courses under the IVC. Accessory and duplicate renal arteries are common and can often be missed on ultrasound (*Fig. 17.3*).

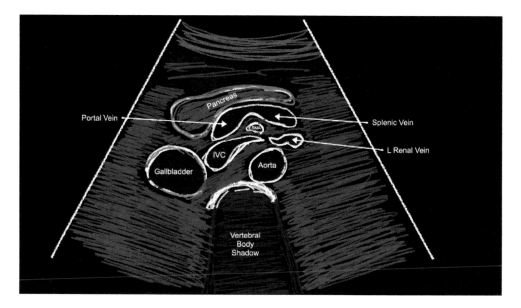

Figure 17.3. Upper transverse view of the aorta and surrounding structures.
IVC – inferior vena cava; SMA – superior mesenteric artery.

3. **Longitudinal view** (positions 'A' to 'C' using probe 2 in *Fig. 17.1*)

The main aortic branches recognizable on ultrasound are the two anterior vessels (*Fig. 17.4*):

● coeliac artery

● superior mesenteric artery.

Next, the renal arteries branch off, 1.5cm or so below the origin of the SMA:

● the right renal artery, as mentioned above, lies posterior to the IVC

● the left renal vein usually lies anterior to the aorta and can be seen passing over the aorta near the origin of the SMA (*Fig. 17.3*).

Other main aortic branches not easily identified on ultrasound include the paired gonadal arteries and the inferior mesenteric artery.

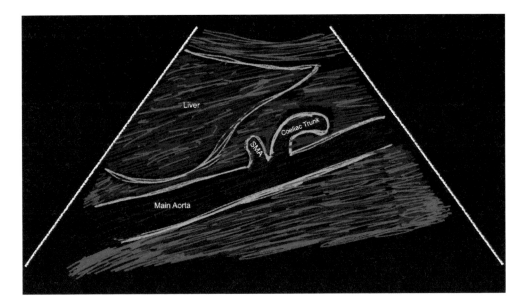

Figure 17.4. Longitudinal aorta view.
SMA – superior mesenteric artery.

4. **Bifurcation view** (position 'D' using probes 1 and 2 in *Fig. 17.1*)

Figure 17.5 shows a longitudinal view of the bifurcation. The transverse view (position 'D' using probe 1 in *Fig. 17.1*), shows the two common iliac arteries: the right common iliac artery and the left common iliac artery, the IVC and the spine posteriorly (*Fig. 17.6*). The maximum normal diameter of the common iliac arteries is approximately 1.4–1.5cm for men and 1.2cm for women.

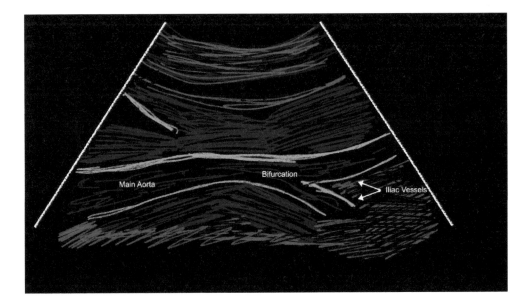

Figure 17.5. Longitudinal view of the aortic bifurcation.

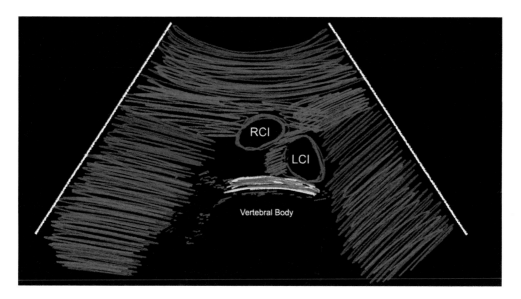

Figure 17.6. Transverse view of the aortic bifurcation. LCI – left common iliac; RCI – right common iliac.

17.4 The renal vessels

17.4.1 Renal arteries

The right and left renal arteries originate just distal to the origin of the SMA and at the level of the left renal vein (LRV), where they travel posteriorly to each kidney. They are harder to image than the LRV, which is why CT angiograms are far more reliable when planning aortic graft surgery or endovascular aneurysm repair.

17.4.2 Renal veins

The LRV is normally easily identified. It must travel further to reach the IVC and is therefore longer than the right. It can be seen anterior to the aorta in the longitudinal view and posterior to the SMA in the transverse view, where it empties into the IVC.

17.5 Measurement tips

- Measurement is more accurate in the longitudinal plane.

- Find the widest point by sweeping the probe across the aorta from one side to the other.

- Antero-posterior diameter measurement should be done in both longitudinal and transverse planes, preferably at the same point with the transducer simply rotated 90°.

- Inner to inner measurement should be undertaken, because this method was found by the Multicentre Aneurysm Screening Study to be the most reproducible method of measuring the aorta [1].

17.6 Common pitfalls

- As mentioned, bowel gas can be your worst enemy. Attempt to displace it by placing gentle downward pressure with the probe.

- Care is needed not to confuse the IVC and the abdominal aorta. Findings that can help you differentiate between the two include:

  - **IVC** – this will normally lie on the patient's right hand side, be non-pulsatile with colour flow Doppler (CFD) and have a low amplitude trace on pulsed wave Doppler (PWD).
  - **aorta** – this will be pulsatile with CFD and have a pulsatile high amplitude trace on PWD.

Sliding the probe laterally and medially (with the probe in a cephalad/caudad orientation) will transition between the two vessels. Rotating to a transverse orientation will allow them each to be seen at the same time. Both manoeuvres will help you identify which vessel is which.

17.7 Abdominal aortic aneurysm

Aneurysms are focal or diffuse swellings within a blood vessel. They may be split into two groups:

- **true aneurysm** – all three layers of the vessel encase the aneurysm

- **false or pseudoaneurysm** – blood escapes through a hole in the innermost vessel lining (the intima) but is contained by either the outer layer (adventitia) or adjacent tissue.

The rupture of an abdominal aortic aneurysm (AAA) is often fatal, with a mortality rate of 85–90%, and it accounts for 2% of all deaths in men aged 65 and over. Around 4% of men aged between 65 and 74 in the UK have an aneurysm and typically manifest no symptoms, thus many aneurysms will progressively expand until they rupture. Risk factors for the development of an aneurysm include:

- smoking

- increasing age

- family history

- hypertension.

17.7.1 Screening and concerns

All men aged 65–75 years who have ever smoked should be screened routinely with the following commonly used as reference values:

- **1.5–2cm** – normal

- **<3cm** – normal and discharged

- **3–4cm** – annual scan

- **4–5cm** – scan every 3 months

- **>5.5cm** – referral to vascular surgeon

- **>7cm** – critical rupture risk.

If the abdominal aorta is fully visualized, emergency ultrasound is 100% sensitive and 98% specific for AAA detection. An AAA should be considered a differential diagnosis in the setting of:

- abdominal, flank or back pain

- hypotension

- pulsatile mass

- abdominal bruit

- presentation of syncope or signs of retroperitoneal haemorrhage.

17.7.2 Subtypes

The main aneurysm subtypes are saccular and fusiform (*Fig. 17.7*).

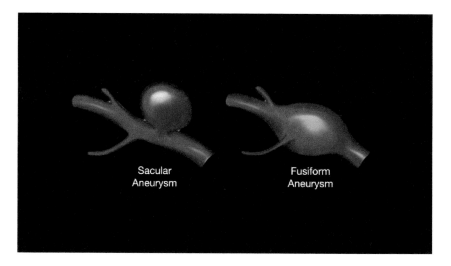

Figure 17.7. Aneurysm subtypes.

17.7.3 Fusiform aneurysms

Fusiform aneurysms (*Figs 17.8* and *17.9*) are the most common AAAs seen and are characterized by uniform dilation across the diameter of the vessel with tapering at each end (making it spindle-shaped).

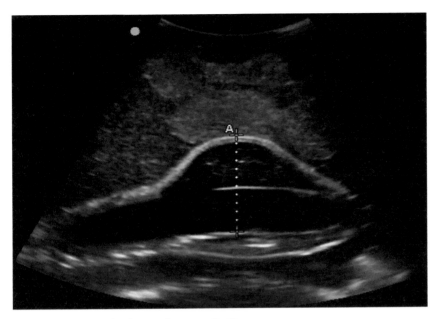

Figure 17.8. Longitudinal scan of a 4.4cm fusiform aneurysm.

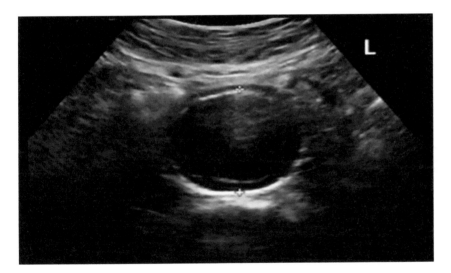

Figure 17.9. Transverse scan of a 5.5cm fusiform aneurysm.

17.7.4 False or pseudoaneurysms

These are rare and may occur after trauma, or as leaks after a graft repair. They consist of round or oval protuberances from the artery and blood can be seen circulating into the protuberance in systole and out in diastole.

17.7.5 Infected aneurysms

These are termed mycotic aneurysms, and are usually saccular in shape and expand rapidly. Surgery is associated with a higher mortality and morbidity rate compared to other aneurysms.

17.8 Aortic emergencies and measurement

17.8.1 Dissection

Dissection occurs when there is disruption of the intimal lining of the vessel, resulting in blood filling the sub-intimal space. Typically, dissections occur in the thoracic region and extend into the abdomen; only 5% occur primarily in the abdominal aorta.

Typical appearances on ultrasound are that of a flap or thin membrane, fluttering in the vessel lumen. CFD can be used to ascertain whether there is flow outside of the intima of the vessel. This is usually preceded by existing weakness or defect in the wall. This causes the intimal lining to detach from the artery wall.

The causes include:

- idiopathic

- Marfan syndrome

- pregnancy

- trauma

- hypertension.

17.8.2 Thrombus

With increasing size, peripheral flow rates in aneurysms drop leading to thrombus formation (*Fig. 17.10*). Thrombus usually forms anteriorly or laterally but can sometimes be circumferential; many embolize.

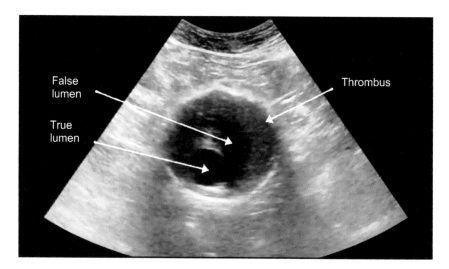

Figure 17.10. Transverse view of a 6cm aneurysm demonstrating true vessel lumen in centre (pulsatile flow on Doppler), a false lumen surrounding it (little to no flow on Doppler) and the presence of a peripheral thrombus.

17.8.3 Rupture

The risk of rupture increases as the aneurysm's diameter increases. The larger the aneurysm, the greater the degree of expansion per year (6cm+ tend to expand potentially 7–8mm per annum). Sonographic signs of rupture include:

- aneurysmal features

- para-aortic fluid collection

- free intraperitoneal fluid

- retroperitoneal haematoma.

17.9 Summary

Visualization of the aorta is relatively simple with ultrasound (if there is no bowel gas in the way). Knowledge of its sonoanatomy, and how to obtain these images, will allow you to rule in emergency and life-threatening pathology.

17.10 Reference

1. Ashton HA, Buxton MJ, Day NE, *et al.* (2002) The Multicentre Aneurysm Screening Study (MASS) into the effect of abdominal aortic aneurysm screening on mortality in men: a randomised controlled trial. *Lancet*, 360:1531.

CHAPTER 18

DEEP VEIN THROMBOSIS SCANNING IN CRITICAL CARE

Rosie Baruah, David Hall & Colum O'Hare

Critical illness is a hyperinflammatory state. When combined with prolonged immobility and indwelling central lines, critical illness predisposes patients to development of venous thromboembolism (VTE). Deep vein thrombosis (DVT) may lead to development of life-threatening pulmonary thromboembolism. The use of POCUS for bedside diagnosis of DVT was particularly beneficial during the SARS CoV-2 pandemic given the high incidence of VTE seen in this patient group.

In this chapter we will outline the anatomy of the deep venous system of the lower limb and describe the use of POCUS to diagnose the presence of DVT at the bedside.

18.1 Anatomy of the deep venous system of the lower limb

The ultrasound examination for DVT involves identifying and examining the common femoral vein (CFV) and greater saphenous vein (GSV) in the groin. The superficial femoral vein (SFV) is then followed down throughout its length and the scan concludes by identifying and examining the popliteal vein and the three crural veins distal to it in the calf (*Fig. 18.1*).

The external iliac vein becomes the CFV as it traverses the inguinal ligament. The GSV comes off proximal to the CFV's division into the SFV and deep femoral vein. Despite its name, the SFV is a part of the deep venous system. Thrombosis within the GSV may propagate into the deep venous system and so it is included in the ultrasound examination for DVT, and assessment of at least the 5cm proximal to the confluence of the GSV and CFV should also form part of the DVT examination (*Fig. 18.2*).

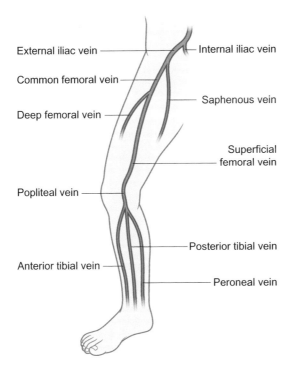

Figure 18.1. Anatomy of the deep venous system of the lower leg.

The SFV travels medially and inferiorly in the thigh, entering the adductor canal in the lower third of the thigh. The vein passes posterior to the knee as it exits the adductor canal, where it becomes the popliteal vein, lying superficial to the popliteal artery. The popliteal vein trifurcates at the inferior margin of the popliteal fossa into the anterior tibial vein (lateral) and the tibioperoneal trunk (medial). The tibioperoneal trunk further divides into the peroneal vein (lateral) and the posterior tibial vein (medial).

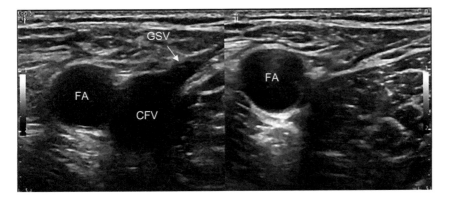

Figure 18.2. (i) Transverse view of the right common femoral vein at its confluence with the great saphenous vein. (ii) Compression applied with the probe showing complete compression of the common femoral vein and great saphenous vein. CFV – common femoral vein; FA – femoral artery; GSV – great saphenous vein.

18.2 Scanning technique

18.2.1 Indications for examination

Indications for a DVT scan include:

- unilateral lower limb swelling, tenderness, or erythema

- clinical suspicion of pulmonary embolism

- as part of a scanning protocol, e.g. BLUE protocol.

18.2.2 Choice of probe and settings

The deep veins of the lower limb should be imaged with a high frequency probe such as the linear array probe. This has a frequency range of approximately 5–13MHz, depending on manufacturer. In the very obese or oedematous patient a lower frequency probe may need to be used to allow adequate penetration. The correct mode for scanning should be selected on the machine – newer machines will have a specific mode for imaging of lower limb veins, otherwise the venous or vascular scanning mode should be chosen.

The depth chosen will depend on the body habitus of the patient, but the aim should be to keep the deep veins in the middle/lower third of the image as you move down the thigh. This will mean a single high frequency linear probe can be used for the full examination in most patients. Gain should be set so the contents of the veins appear black. Ensuring the focal point is adjusted to correlate with the region on the screen where the vessel is being imaged will help optimize the image.

The probe is held in the transverse orientation throughout the scan protocol when visualizing the vein in its transverse axis, and rotated 90° for visualization in longitudinal axis.

18.3 Lower limb

18.3.1 Patient positioning

It is well worth taking some time to position the patient optimally before starting the scan. Tilting the bed 30° head-up will promote filling of the lower leg veins. The patient should be supine with the leg externally rotated and bent at the knee, with a pillow placed under it for support ('Frog's leg' position). By positioning the patient in this manner, it should be possible to complete the whole scan without repositioning the lower limb. In an awake patient who can position themselves, it may be possible to start the scan in the upper thigh with the leg straight, then ask the patient to externally rotate at the hip to examine the mid-thigh and ask the patient to turn on their side with their leg slightly flexed at the knee to examine the popliteal fossa and upper calf.

18.3.2 Scanning protocol

Multiple scanning protocols are in clinical use worldwide, recommending 2-point, 3-point or whole-leg scanning. The UK FUSIC training module in DVT scanning recommends compression of the deep veins at 2cm intervals and interrogation of veins using colour flow Doppler (CFD) and pulsed wave Doppler (PWD), with assessment of compressibility, respiratory variation, and augmentation of flow with calf compression. This is the technique described in this chapter.

18.3.3 Compression scanning

The examination starts by visualizing the CFV at its confluence with the GSV, just inferior to the inguinal ligament. It is important to visualize the GSV, although it is not part of the deep venous system of the lower limb, because a clot within it may propagate into the CFV. At least 5cm of the GSV should be visualized and assessed for compressibility. The vessels should be compressed by the operator pressing down with the transducer until the lumina of the CFV and GSV are *completely* obliterated, with apposition of the walls of the vein. It is crucial to fully compress the vein throughout the examination – if the vein cannot be fully compressed this is highly suspicious for presence of DVT. If sufficient pressure is used it is usual to see a degree of compression of the femoral artery. Compression can be painful for the patient and, if possible, this should be explained to the patient before starting the examination.

The probe is then moved caudally and the vein compressed at 2cm intervals as described above. The vein may be difficult to visualize as it passes through the canal of adductor magnus in the medial aspect of the lower thigh; pressure applied towards the probe with the non-scanning hand can help to visualize the vein more easily. To image the popliteal vessels, the probe should be placed in the popliteal fossa approximately 2cm above the crease of the knee, being careful not to use excessive pressure because this may obliterate the lumen of the popliteal vein. Continue to move inferiorly, compressing every 2cm, until the trifurcation of the popliteal vessels is seen.

18.3.4 Colour flow Doppler imaging

CFD can be used to identify the SFV. This can be useful in the obese or oedematous patient when the vein may be difficult to compress. In the groin the femoral vein has a continuous 'hum', in contrast to the femoral artery which will demonstrate pulsatile flow when interrogated by CFD (*Fig. 18.3*). In the absence of DVT distal to the point of scanning, augmentation of the CFD will be seen when the calf is compressed. There is a theoretical risk of dislodging a DVT with vigorous squeezing of the calf. In the presence of non-occlusive DVT, some residual colour flow signal will be seen in the vessel lumen.

Figure 18.3. (i) Normal colour flow Doppler at the confluence of the common femoral vein and the great saphenous vein. (ii) Transverse view of the common femoral vein with application of pulsed wave Doppler showing normal respiratory variation. (iii) Transverse view of the common femoral vein with application of pulsed wave Doppler and augmentation of flow by squeezing of the calf.

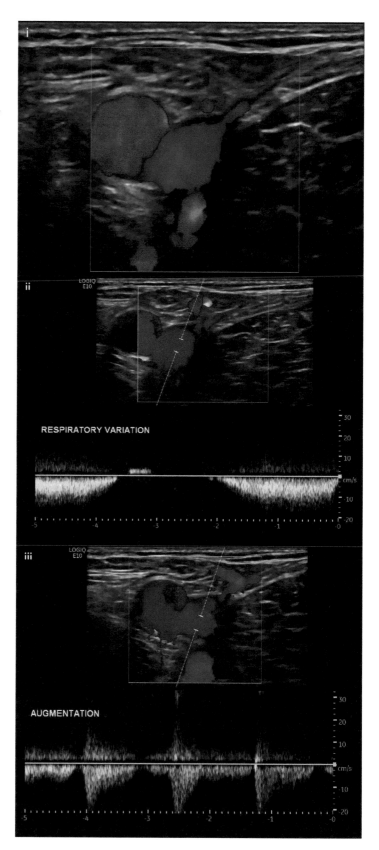

18.3.5 Pulsed wave Doppler

PWD can be used to assess patency of the deep venous system within the lower limb. The femoral vein should be visualized in transverse or longitudinal axis and the sample volume placed within the lumen of the vessel. In the absence of DVT proximal to the point of scanning, undulating respirophasic changes in flow will be seen below the baseline. Flow may be seen both above and below the baseline in the ventilated patient. A monophasic flow pattern is suspicious of venous obstruction proximal to the point of interrogation. Distal augmentation of venous return by compression of the calf will show a sharp 'spike' in anterograde flow in the presence of patent veins distal to the point of interrogation (*Fig. 18.3*). Blunted or no change in flow pattern with distal compression could indicate venous obstruction distal to the point of interrogation.

18.4 Appearance of a clot within the deep veins of the lower limb

The appearance of a clot within the deep venous system will depend on the age of the clot. An acute clot may appear somewhat mobile within the vessel lumen and be hypo- or isoechoic in appearance. Turning up the gain will allow better visualization of an acute clot. It is not uncommon for the vein to appear distended and in the groin the CFV may appear larger than the femoral artery. An acute clot may be somewhat compressible, but it will not be possible to fully oppose the walls of the vein with compression. A chronic clot will not appear mobile within the vessel lumen, it will be more hyperechoic than an acute clot and the vein will not be distended or compressible (*Fig. 18.4*).

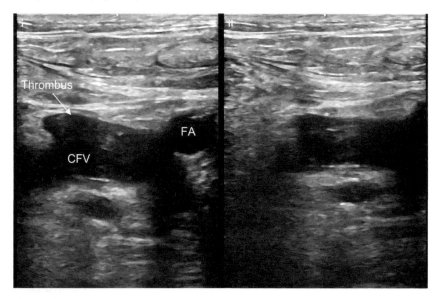

Figure 18.4. (i) Thrombus seen in the common femoral vein. (ii) Inability to fully compress the vein due to presence of thrombus. CFV – common femoral vein; FA – femoral artery.

18.5 Common mimics of DVT

18.5.1 Lymph nodes

Lymph nodes can mimic the appearance of thrombus within a vein, with a hyperechoic core surrounded by a hypoechoic rim. In a longitudinal view, unlike a vein, they will appear ovoid (*Fig. 18.5*).

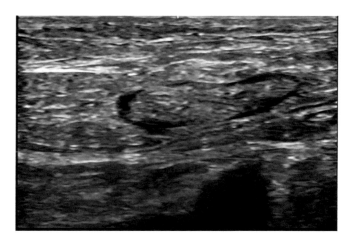

Figure 18.5. Transverse view of a lymph node in the groin.

18.5.2 Superficial veins – superficial thrombophlebitis

It is possible to visualize clots within the superficial veins of the lower limb. Thrombi within the superficial veins are not associated with increased risk of pulmonary embolism and therefore do not need treatment. The exception to this are clots within the GSV within 2–4cm of its confluence with the femoral vein; clots here can propagate into the deep venous system and therefore should be treated as a DVT. To avoid confusing superficial with deep venous thrombus, it is important to have a sound knowledge of the sonoanatomy of the deep venous system.

18.5.3 Thrombosed pseudoaneuryms

Pseudoaneurysms may be seen as a complication of arterial cannulation. A pseudoaneurysm of the femoral artery resembles a rounded structure with a neck connecting to the parent vessel and may be seen adjacent or superficial to the CFV. It may be distinguished from DVT within the CFV by application of CFD which will demonstrate the classic 'ying yang' pattern.

TIPS AND TRICKS

- To avoid unnecessary interruption of the scan it is helpful to apply a strip of ultrasound gel from the top of the thigh infero-medially along the sites of compression before starting scanning.
- It may be challenging to visualize the SFV the further down the leg you go – turning on CFD and positioning the box over where you think the vein is will help confirm you are looking at the correct structure.
- When assessing venous flow with augmentation, having an assistant in place ready to squeeze the patient's calf will allow you to keep the probe steady and focus on image acquisition and interpretation.

18.6 Summary

DVT is common in the critically ill patient and can lead to life-threatening pulmonary thromboembolism. POCUS is an effective way to rule out DVT at the bedside, using a combination of 2D, colour and spectral Doppler ultrasound. There are common mimics of DVT and it is important to be aware of the ultrasound appearance of these.

CHAPTER 19

19

ULTRASOUND-GUIDED VENOUS ACCESS

Zdenek Bares

Venous cannulation is a crucial skill, especially in the acute setting, and its mastery greatly improves patient care. Ultrasound is used widely in intensive care units and emergency departments (and increasingly everywhere else in the hospital) to enhance diagnostic capabilities. It also has a vital role in procedural guidance, changing everyday practice through improved procedural accuracy, first pass success rate and safety, whilst simultaneously shortening the learning time required significantly.

There are many factors that can make cannulation of large veins more challenging, including shock, intravascular volume depletion, body habitus, pressures of the time-critical procedure in an acute situation, and prior cannulation. Before the advent of ultrasound, cannulation of large central veins was a blind procedure guided by surface landmarks and palpation of the underlying structures. Anatomical variation means such an approach is not fully reliable and may inadvertently lead to increased injury of surrounding structures and a lower success rate. Ultrasound use has improved safety, first pass and overall success rate, reduced complications and flattened the learning curve. Long-term complications such as catheter infections have also decreased since the introduction of ultrasound, although other factors may have influenced this (increased use of sterile dressings, bioconnectors, venous catheter care bundles, etc.). The incorporation of ultrasound into central venous cannulation can also help to diagnose vascular pathology (such as thrombosis) with possible implications for further care [1,2].

This chapter will discuss indications and basic considerations for central venous catheter (CVC) insertion, the technique needed to identify the optimal central vessel to cannulate (and which veins may be better left alone due to anatomy, size or pathology), key locations for insertion, and the cannulation technique itself. Peripherally inserted central catheters (PICC), peripheral cannulas and their insertion will also be mentioned.

19.1 Indications for central venous catheter

There are several indications for CVC insertion including:

- Intravenous (IV) access when peripheral access is difficult to obtain or maintain.

- Infusion of irritant substances (such as high concentrations of electrolytes, vasoconstricting drugs, total parenteral nutrition).

- Prolonged IV drug therapy (typically for more than a week).

- Central venous pressure monitoring.

- Advanced haemodynamic monitoring (pulse index contour continuous cardiac output (PICCO) monitors, pulmonary artery catheters, central venous oxygenation).

- Others: haemodialysis, cardiac pacing.

It is important to mention that peripheral IV access has some advantages over central IV access, in particular, fewer short-term complications, less pain on insertion, and better flow due to their short length. Indication for central venous cannulation should thus be clear. It is important for clinicians to challenge decisions (or protocols) to introduce central catheters if there is no proper indication.

19.2 Choosing the best place for cannulation

Before getting prepared in a sterile fashion, you should always spend some time scanning the target vessels to find the one best suited for cannulation. RaCeVA (rapid central vein assessment) is a systematic approach to central veins and should not take more than 2 minutes to perform once it becomes familiar [3]. It follows seven steps performed bilaterally. Scanning and assessment of the femoral veins can also be added for a full assessment of the large calibre veins potentially amenable to cannulation. The linear probe is used for both assessment and further on for ultrasound navigation.

Some criteria to consider when choosing a vein for cannulation include:

- The internal diameter of the vein.

- The depth of the vein from the skin surface.

- Any respiratory variation seen in its diameter.

- Whether it is compressed by adjacent arterial pulsations.

- Its proximity to surrounding structures such as the lung, arteries or nerves.

- The position the catheter will sit in with regard to ongoing care (e.g. maintenance of femoral CVCs can be challenging in prone patients).

Applying a systematic approach to central veins allows clinicians to identify the vein most suited for cannulation and to avoid attempts that are unlikely to be successful, or where complications are more probable [3,4].

19.2.1 Vein versus artery

It may not always be easy to distinguish veins from arteries. Knowledge of anatomy with expected position, collapsibility of veins (in comparison to arteries) and pulsatility of arteries are all very useful, but arteries may become collapsible in intravascularly deplete patients, veins look pulsatile in tricuspid regurgitation and will be difficult to compress when there is thrombosis. When there is *any* doubt, it is vital to check flow through arteries with colour and/or pulsed wave Doppler. It may be necessary to tilt the probe when doing this to ensure proper alignment with flow. Cannulation should not be attempted before you have a very clear idea of which vessels are which.

19.2.2 Vein size

A very important aspect to mention is the size of the vein (or more precisely its internal diameter). This can be measured using the caliper function and should be compared with the diameter of the catheter/catheters that you want to insert. The catheter-to-vessel ratio should be kept at a maximum of 33–45% to minimise risk of thrombosis. Catheter circumference (in Fr) can be found on the package of a given central catheter and can be roughly converted to the diameter in mm using 1 Fr = 0.33mm.

Note that the common circumference of vascular catheters for dialysis is 15.5Fr, which is approximately 5.1mm. To maintain good flow in the given vein, it should therefore have a diameter of at least 11.3mm. If there is no identifiable vein with a safe diameter, a catheter with a smaller circumference should be used.

19.2.3 The RaCeVA protocol

The RaCeVA protocol starts by scanning at the level of laryngeal prominence on the right side and moves caudally down and then laterally to evaluate the supraclavicular level. The probe is then moved to the infraclavicular region and finally to the axilla (*Fig. 19.1*). The last step is a quick lung ultrasound assessment. This is then repeated on the contralateral side and the optimal vein for cannulation is chosen. It is important to note that medical and surgical history (especially history of previous cannulations) also play an important role in determining the optimal vein.

The lung assessment can identify lung pathology and confirm the pre-cannulation state, which is then compared to lung ultrasound post insertion.

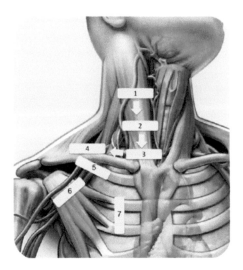

Figure 19.1. The RaCeVA approach with ultrasound positions highlighted. Reproduced from Spencer TR & Pittiruti M (2019) *J. Vasc. Access*, 20:239 with permission from Sage Publishing.

The operator's experience and preference shouldn't play a significant role in vessel choice, although this is often not the case in clinical settings. Use of the RaCeVA protocol may help clinicians select vessels in a more patient-based manner.

Once the optimal vein is identified, ultrasound 'knobology' comes into play to optimize the image. Depth should allow visualization of the whole target vessel and gain is adjusted to provide the best contrast between the interior of the vein and surrounding structures. A marker can be used to speed up further ultrasound navigation.

19.3 General technique of ultrasound-guided central venous cannulation

Ergonomics is of the utmost importance when attempting any procedure. When it comes to central venous cannulation, it is crucial to find a comfortable position in which the area of interest, the direction of cannulation and the screen are in one line. This allows simultaneous control over both the ultrasound image and the cannula used and prevents turning and unnatural positioning. Once the correct vein is identified and the ultrasound image optimized, standard preparation for central venous cannulation follows (the full technique is not described here).

The patient's position should be optimized before draping. This involves a gentle Trendelenburg position for all upper body veins. When cannulating the internal jugular vein, turning the head towards the contralateral side to cannulation may optimize the view, but excessive turning distorts the anatomy and is not recommended.

Sterile precautions should be used throughout and only when the patient is fully draped, with a fenestrated drape over the cannulation site, is it appropriate to begin. The probe is covered in a dedicated sterile cover and an ultrasound image of the target vein is found. Various techniques can be used to approach the cannulation including (*Fig. 19.2*):

- short-axis out-of-plane approach

- short-axis in-plane approach

- long-axis in-plane approach.

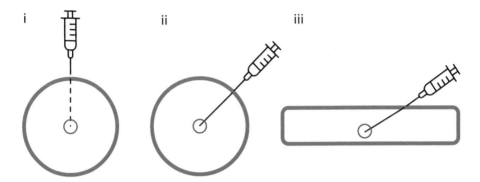

Figure 19.2. Examples of different ultrasound cannulation approaches. (i) short-axis out-of-plane, (ii) short-axis in-plane, and (iii) long-axis in-plane approach. Adapted from Spencer TR & Pittiruti M (2019) *J. Vasc. Access*, 20:239 with permission from Sage Publishing.

Short/long-axis refer to how the vein is visualized:

- a vein in short-axis appears as a circular compressible structure with a hypoechogenic interior

- a vein in long-axis appears as a compressible stripe-like structure with a hypoechogenic interior.

In-plane/out-of-plane approaches refer to whether the needle is visible as a dot (out-of-plane) or its whole length is visible (in-plane).

19.3.1 Short-axis out-of-plane approach

This is probably the most commonly used approach. It is used to cannulate the internal jugular, femoral, axillary and subclavian veins. An elementary maths refresher can be helpful when determining how far away from the probe the needle should be introduced and at what depth the vein will be encountered by the needle. As a simple rule, if we approach the vein at an angle of 45°, the needle should be introduced at the same distance from the probe as the depth of the interior of the vein. The depth from the skin at which the vein is encountered by the needle will then be roughly 1.4 times the depth of the vein interior on ultrasound (*Fig. 19.3*).

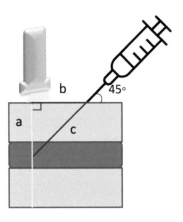

Figure 19.3. Here a right-angled triangle is imagined using the ultrasound beam, skin and needle with angles a,c and b,c both equal to 45°. Pythagorean theory then tells us that if a = b then c ≈ 1.4 × a.

When the needle enters the skin, it is not visible on ultrasound, it must first enter the ultrasound plane where it appears as a hyperechogenic dot. The probe then needs to be gently moved further from the needle so that the dot disappears. The needle is then advanced further until the dot appears again. This is repeated until the needle enters the vein (*Fig. 19.4*). This technique provides direct visualization of the needle, but there are also indirect signs that the needle tip is in close proximity, such as movement of tissues, tenting of the vein or (undesirably) tenting of the artery (*Fig. 19.5*).

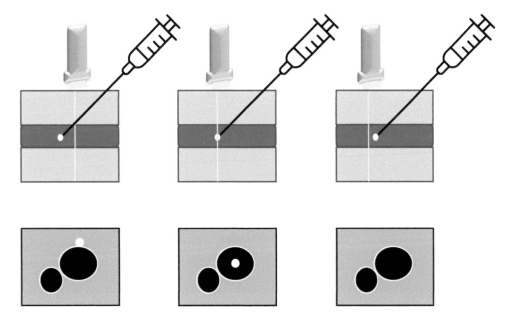

Figure 19.4. Illustration of how sliding the probe from the shaft of the needle (left) to the tip (middle), and beyond this (right) can alter the appearance of the needle with regard to the vein.

Although cannulation may be successful based solely on indirect signs, without visualization of the needle tip, it is an inferior and less safe technique.

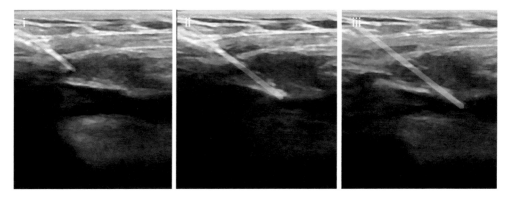

Figure 19.5. Ultrasound-guided insertion of a central venous catheter in the longitudinal plane. From left to right (i) needle visible away from vessel, (ii) needle visible tenting the vessel, and (iii) needle visible within the vessel.

19.3.2 Long-axis in-plane approach

This is technically more challenging but allows for much better control of the position of the needle and its angle. It is necessary to make sure the visualized longitudinal structure is a vein; the best way to do this is by finding a vein in a good short-axis view and then rotating the probe slowly to 90°. As the rotation is being done, the circular vein slowly stretches until it becomes a longitudinal structure in the long-axis view. The needle is then introduced so that it can be tracked all the way to the vein. This allows optimal alignment with the vein and good control of the needle (*Fig. 19.5*). It is, however, more technically demanding to keep the ultrasound probe in exactly the correct plane and then maintain the needle within it as it is advanced towards the vein.

19.3.3 Short-axis in-plane approach

This is the least commonly used approach but can prove very helpful when attempting to cannulate technically difficult veins (e.g. caused by the patient's body habitus, intravascular depletion, challenging anatomy). This approach can prove particularly useful for cannulation of the internal jugular vein and is described below (*Fig. 19.6*).

19.3.4 Cannulation

Before the cannulation is started, the skin should be cleaned with chlorhexidine and local anaesthetic infiltrated. This is carried out under ultrasound guidance and will cover the skin but also the expected track of the larger needle for cannulation. Some local anaesthetic should also be infiltrated into the surrounding skin if sutures will be used to secure the catheter.

Once the patient is draped, the skin cleaned and local anaesthetic injected, cannulation can start. The needle with connected syringe is slowly introduced

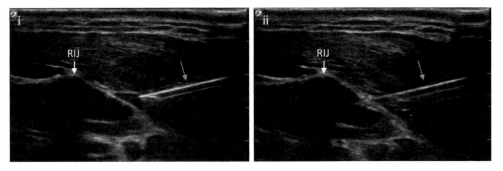

Figure 19.6. Images of short-axis in-plane internal jugular vein cannulation. (i) Needle (orange arrow) just lateral to the internal jugular vein. (ii) Needle (orange arrow) seen to puncture the internal jugular vein. RIJ – right internal jugular vein.

– the trick here is being aware of its position both on the screen and in the patient. The piston of the syringe is gently pulled back during advancement of the needle. This is technically challenging and can therefore be limited to when the needle is near the vein. The operator should always be aware of the needle position in relation to the structures on the screen, ideally visualizing the needle itself.

Once flashback of blood is seen inside the syringe, the probe, held in the left hand, is gently dropped onto the sterile drapes. The right hand passes the needle over to the now free left hand, the syringe is removed and the guidewire is introduced (it is recommended that the wire is ready on the drape close to the right hand, so no turn is required). The correct position of the guidewire in the target vein should then be confirmed with ultrasound and followed as far centrally as possible. A dilator is then threaded over the guidewire, with a small cut made adjacent to the wire where it meets the skin. Once the dilator is removed, a central catheter is then introduced using the Seldinger technique over the wire and its position is again checked by ultrasound. It is vital the guidewire is seen to be removed. Following this, all catheter ports should be checked for patency and lung ultrasound performed to rule out a pneumothorax (not required in femoral catheters).

Note that POCUS can also help confirm correct line position for certain insertion sites including the subclavian and internal jugular. Fluid can be flushed through the catheter whilst echocardiography is being performed and, if correctly placed, spontaneous contrast will be seen in the right atrium.

19.4 Specific locations

19.4.1 Internal jugular vein

Positives of using the internal jugular vein (IJV) include:

- it is compressible, so excessive bleeding can be avoided in the event of an unsuccessful puncture

- it can normally be visualized throughout its course

- it is close to skin.

Negatives of using the IJV include:

- it is often collapsible making cannulation more challenging

- the carotid artery is in proximity

- there is a potential risk of iatrogenic pneumothorax.

Sonoanatomy

The IJV is lateral to the carotid artery with the vagus nerve lying medial to it between the two vessels (*Fig. 19.7*). The sternocleidomastoid muscle lies over most of the course of the IJV.

The probe is usually put perpendicularly in short-axis at the level of the laryngeal prominence and is then moved up and down along the IJV to find the optimal spot. Turning the patient's head may improve the relation between artery and vein; ideally the vein lies to the side of the artery and close enough to the skin.

Technique

As previously mentioned, the short-axis out-of-plane approach is used more commonly and is easy to perform. The danger lies in relying on indirect signs and inadvertently damaging underlying structures, especially the subclavian vein, subclavian artery and pleura. The key to avoiding this is visualization of the tip of the needle; the probe can be tilted towards the needle to decrease the distance travelled until the needle tip reaches the ultrasound plane. The long-axis in-plane approach is a good option if the operator is comfortable performing it.

The short-axis in-plane approach or its modification, the oblique-axis in-plane approach, represents an underused and particularly useful technique

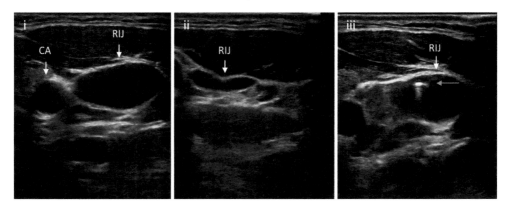

Figure 19.7. (i) Right internal jugular vein and carotid artery. (ii) Tenting of right internal jugular vein during line insertion. (iii) Guidewire (orange arrow) visualized in the lumen of the internal jugular vein. CA – carotid artery; RIJ – right internal jugular vein.

in this location. While these are not recommended for the introduction of vascular dialysis catheters (these need to be optimally aligned), they can be very useful in other situations. The upside is perfect control of the track of the needle and clear visualization of the vein, which makes cannulation of even very collapsible small veins possible. Despite approaching the vein from its side, the guidewire will still normally go in the correct direction. To avoid any problems with guidewire direction, the approach can be modified with gentle rotation of the probe towards the long-axis to achieve an oblique-axis view; the needle is then more aligned with the vein.

19.4.2 Innominate vein

Positives of this approach include:

- the innominate vein is less collapsible than the IJV and may therefore be used in intravascularly deplete patients

- it is usually well visualized.

Negatives include an increased risk of pneumothorax.

Sonoanatomy

The vein can be found at the confluence of IJV and subclavian vein when tracking the IJV distally. It should be approached in the long- or oblique-axis in-plane. The needle must be visualized at all times because there is a risk of pneumothorax.

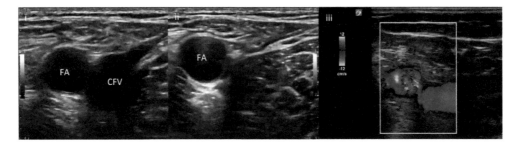

Figure 19.8. (i) Transverse view of the right common femoral vein at confluence with the great saphenous vein. (ii) Compression applied with probe showing complete compression of the common femoral vein and great saphenous vein. (iii) Colour flow Doppler applied to help differentiation between the femoral artery and common femoral vein. CFV – common femoral vein; FA – femoral artery.

19.4.3 Femoral vein

Positives of femoral vein cannulation include:

- the femoral vein is compressible so excessive bleeding can be avoided in the event of an unsuccessful puncture

- it is normally relatively well visualized in the groin

- it is often better tolerated than lines placed in the neck

- the calibre of the vessel means it is good for vascular dialysis catheter insertion

- there is no risk of pneumothorax.

Negatives of the femoral approach include:

- a potentially increased risk of line infection

- insertion can be challenging in obese patients

- it may not be a reliable access source in abdominal bleeding

- it can be difficult to maintain in the prone patient.

The femoral vein is medial to the femoral nerve and artery *(Fig. 19.8)*. To optimize visualization the patient should have their ipsilateral leg abducted and externally rotated. If attempted in obese patients, their abdominal apron can completely cover the required area. In such cases it may be possible to use an assistant to hold the apron or it can be taped to the side of the bed. Both short-axis out-of-plane and long-axis in-plane approaches are possible.

19.5 Peripherally inserted central catheter

Unlike CVCs, peripherally inserted central catheters (PICCs) can be used long-term whilst offering similar advantages (e.g. blood sampling, multiple infusions, irritant infusions, etc.) and a lower risk of line infection [5]. It is worth noting that the ability to deliver very rapid infusions is limited due to their length and diameter (as per the Hagen–Poiseuille law). The use of PICCs is gaining in popularity and they are certainly worth learning about.

Almost the exact same technique (Seldinger) is used to insert PICCs and CVCs, and the insertion sets look strikingly similar, differing only by the size of the set and the longer length of the PICC catheter *(Fig. 19.9)*. It is important to have an idea of what length of catheter is needed; this can be estimated by measuring from the expected site of insertion along the normal course of the target veins towards the superior vena cava and right atrial junction.

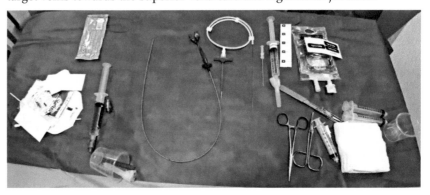

Figure 19.9. Peripherally inserted central catheter (PICC) kit.

PICCs are usually inserted into one of the large peripheral veins of the arm, mostly at its inner aspect. Although insertion is possible without ultrasound navigation, it is virtually never done, with ultrasound playing a crucial role. Identification of the main vessels is performed using ultrasound and the most convenient vessel is chosen based on position, size, proximity to arteries, and vascular pathology. As with a CVC, it is important to choose an appropriately sized vein in order to keep sufficient flow and minimize risk of thrombosis.

Once the optimal length of PICC is determined and an appropriately sized and safely positioned vessel identified, the ultrasound-guided insertion can proceed. Insertion may be complicated by misplacement, because catheters introduced via veins in the arm are more likely to go the wrong way. The most common misplacement is the ipsilateral IJV and contralateral subclavian vein. It is useful to scan the IJV with ultrasound during the final part of insertion to identify any poor positioning. If repeated attempts end up in the wrong place, alterations to patient position may be helpful, e.g. stretching or abducting the arm or stretching and rotating the neck.

19.6 Midline insertion

A midline is basically a long peripheral line (8–12 cm) that does not terminate in a central vein, but can remain *in situ* for longer than peripheral cannulas and may be used out of hospital. Rapid fluid infusion is less efficient than with standard peripheral lines.

Again, ultrasound is invaluable in identifying the optimal vein for insertion and is used for navigation. The insertion technique commonly involves venous cannulation with a large cannula and consequently threading a wire through it. After confirming good position, the cannula is removed and a midline is inserted over the wire and the wire removed.

19.7 Peripheral cannulas

One of the most common procedures in hospital is the insertion of peripheral cannulas. Although mostly very straightforward, it can be challenging in some patients. Ultrasound can be of great help, but it is usually possible to identify a peripheral vein amenable to cannulation without it [6]. Only if no good vein is identified despite warm water immersion of the limb (if possible), good quality tourniquet application, pumping and gravity, should ultrasound then be considered.

The forearm, cubital and arm veins in general are the most useful and the whole circumference of the arm may need to be scanned. That being said, there are typical locations for the main veins of the limbs (although there is of course anatomical variety) as shown in *Figure 19.10*. Because the veins cannulated with ultrasound navigation are usually deeper, it is advisable to use longer cannulas (at least 4–5cm). The lifespan of peripheral cannulas is improved when at least two-thirds of the cannula is placed intravenously.

The confluence of two veins is a useful site for cannulation because the position is more fixed. Peripheral veins are generally more fragile and tend to escape the needle, roll or pop, so utmost care and precision must be used to succesfully cannulate.

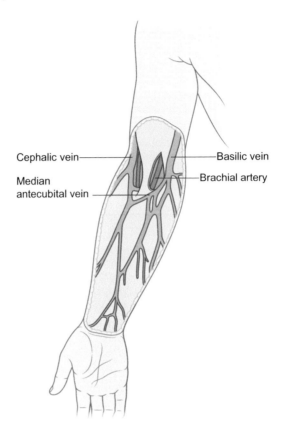

Cephalic vein

Median antecubital vein

Basilic vein

Brachial artery

Figure 19.10. Arm vasculature. The basilic vein, brachial artery, cephalic vein, and median antecubital vein are shown. The superficial and deep brachial veins flank the brachial artery but are not shown here.

19.8 Summary

Ultrasound is an invaluable tool to aid venous cannulation, be it for central access, haemofiltration, PICC, or peripheral line insertion. Time should be taken to identify the optimal vessel for cannulation in order to increase the chance of success and reduce complications.

19.9 References

1. McGee DC, Gould MK (2003) Preventing complications of central venous catheterization. *N Engl J Med,* 348:1123.

2. Troianos CA, Hartman GS, Glas KE, *et al.* (2012) Special articles: guidelines for performing ultrasound guided vascular cannulation: recommendations of the American Society of Echocardiography and the Society of Cardiovascular Anesthesiologists. *Anesth Analg,* 114:46.

3. Spencer TR, Pittiruti M (2019) Rapid Central Vein Assessment (RaCeVA): a systematic, standardized approach for ultrasound assessment before central venous catheterization. *J Vasc Access*, 20:239.

4. Pittiruti M, Malerba M, Carriero C, Tazza L, Gui D (2000) Which is the easiest and safest technique for central venous access? A retrospective survey of more than 5,400 cases. *J Vasc Access*, 1:100.

5. Lamperti M, Bodenham AR, Pittiruti M, *et al.* (2012) International evidence-based recommendations on ultrasound-guided vascular access. *Intensive Care Med*, 38:1105.

6. Costantino TG, Parikh AK, Satz WA, Fojtik JP (2005) Ultrasonography-guided peripheral intravenous access versus traditional approaches in patients with difficult intravenous access. *Ann Emerg Med*, 46:456.

CHAPTER 20

TRANSCRANIAL DOPPLER AND OPTIC NERVE SHEATH DIAMETER

Manni Waraich

Transcranial colour-coded duplex (TCCD) ultrasonography allows direct non-invasive imaging of intracranial vascular structures and brain parenchyma. It has several advantages over traditional transcranial Doppler (TCD) sonography through identification of the cerebral vessels in relation to anatomical landmarks as well as allowing, by angle correction, more accurate insonation of the vessels. The main obstacle to TCCD is ultrasound penetration of the skull. The use of the low frequency cardiac phased array probe reduces the attenuation of the ultrasound wave caused by bone. There are acoustic windows representing specific points of the skull where the bone is thin enough to allow penetration of the ultrasound waves. Despite this, in approximately 10–20% of the population, it is not possible to find an adequate acoustic window.

20.1 Anatomy

There are four commonly used acoustic windows (*Fig. 20.1*):

- submandibular – allows insonation of the extracranial carotid arteries

- transtemporal – allows insonation of the anterior, middle, and posterior cerebral arteries

- transorbital – used to insonate the ophthalmic artery as well as the cavernous portion of the internal carotid artery

- suboccipital – allows insonation of the vertebral and basilar arteries.

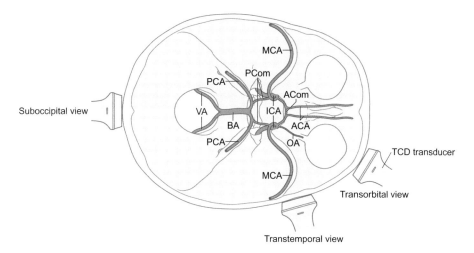

Figure 20.1. The acoustic windows used in transcranial colour-coded duplex ultrasonography. ACA – anterior cerebral artery; ACom – anterior communicating artery; BA – basilar artery; ICA – internal carotid artery; MCA – middle cerebral artery; OA – ophthalmic artery; PCA – posterior cerebral artery; PCom – posterior communicating artery; VA – vertebral artery.

20.2 Technique

The most commonly used acoustic window is the transtemporal window. In this window identification of some anatomical landmarks allows for correct TCCD technique. The ultrasound transducer is placed in the orbitomeatal line, over the temporal area just above the zygomatic arch and in front of the tragus of the ear, with the index marker anteriorly. In this mesencephalic plane, visualization of the contralateral skull is usually found at a depth of 12–15cm and appears as a curved bright line. The next landmarks to identify are a hypoechoic butterfly structure which are the cerebral peduncles (marked 'P' in *Fig. 20.2*) surrounded by the hyperechoic basal cisterns (marked by an asterisk in *Fig. 20.2*). Angulating the probe cephalad by 10° brings the view to the diencephalic plane where two central hyperechoic lines, corresponding to the third ventricle, are seen with the hypoechoic thalami each side (*Fig. 20.3*). Further cephalad angulation of the probe to the ventricular plane allows visualization of the frontal horns of the lateral ventricle. The mesencephalic and diencephalic planes are used for vascular diagnosis because the circle of Willis is found here.

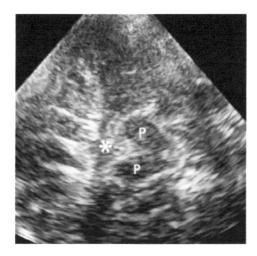

Figure 20.2. Transtemporal window mesencephalic plane. P = cerebral peduncle, asterisk = basal cisterns.

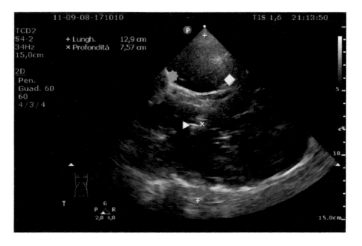

Figure 20.3. Transtemporal window diencephalic plane. White arrowhead = third ventricle, yellow diamond = petrous bone; orange star = sphenoid wing.

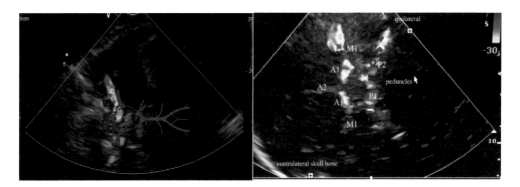

Figure 20.4. Transtemporal window demonstrating the circle of Willis.

In the mesencephalic plane, the area immediately lateral to the peduncles can then be interrogated with colour and pulsed wave Doppler to demonstrate the vessels as well as attaining measurements (*Fig. 20.4*) [1,2].

20.3 TCCD characteristics and calculations

A typical TCCD waveform has a systolic peak and a diastolic stepdown (*Fig. 20.5*). The shape of the waveform is important to note because changes in systolic and diastolic morphology indicate pathology. Once the waveform has been recorded, calculated values for peak systolic (PSV), end-diastolic (EDV) and time-averaged mean flow velocities (TAMV) are obtained. From these measurements, two derived measurements are calculated:

- the pulsatility index (PI) = (PSV − EDV)/TAMV; normal value 0.6–1.2

- the resistivity index (RI) = (PSV − EDV)/PSV

These give an indication of the resistance to blood flow. Remember that the brain maintains a low resistance circulation to allow preferential blood flow to it at all times. Changes in the PI correspond to changes in cerebral haemodynamics, so a rise in PI could indicate a drop in cerebral perfusion pressure, hypocapnia or distal resistance, whereas a decrease in PI could be due to an arteriovenous malformation. The PI value needs to be interpreted together with the clinical picture.

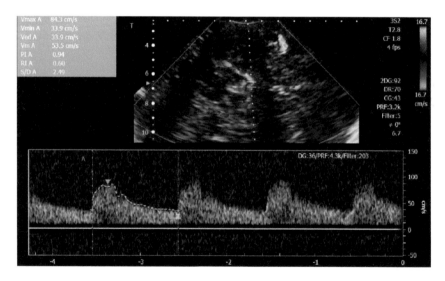

Figure 20.5. A typical transcranial colour duplex waveform with a pulsatility index (PI) of 0.9.

Knowledge of the depth of insonation, direction of blood flow relative to the transducer probe and the mean velocity of the flow allows correct identification of the vessel (*Table 20.1*).

Table 20.1. Reference characteristics and velocities for vessels

Artery	Window	Depth (mm)	Direction of flow (relative to transducer)	Peak systolic velocity (cm/sec)	End-diastolic velocity (cm/sec)	Time averaged mean flow velocity (cm/sec)
MCA	Transtemporal	45–65	Towards	90–110	35–55	55–80
ACA	Transtemporal	60–65	Away	80–90	30–40	50–60
PCA	Transtemporal	60–75	P1 towards; P2 away	66–81	26–33	42–53
BA	Suboccipital	90–120	Away	54–74	23–34	35–50
VA	Suboccipital	65–85	Away	52–66	22–31	33–44
OA	Transorbital	45–60	Towards	–	–	20–30

ACA – anterior cerebral artery; BA – basilar artery; MCA – middle cerebral artery; OA – ophthalmic artery; PCA – posterior cerebral artery; VA – vertebral artery.

20.4 Clinical applications of TCCD

20.4.1 Detection of vasospasm in aneurysmal subarachnoid haemorrhage

Eighty percent of aneurysmal subarachnoid haemorrhages (aSAHs) occur in the anterior circulation, and the transtemporal acoustic window allows adequate visualization of the middle and anterior cerebral arteries. Mean velocities between 120 and 200cm/sec indicate vasospasm in those vessels. To differentiate these high velocities from a hyperdynamic vascular state such as sepsis, the Lindegaard ratio is calculated by using the middle cerebral artery (MCA) or anterior cerebral artery (ACA) velocity as numerator and, through the submandibular window, insonation of the ipsilateral extracranial carotid artery velocity as the denominator. A Lindegaard ratio greater than 3 indicates mild spasm, a ratio between 3 and 6 indicates moderate spasm and a ratio above 6 indicates severe vasospasm. It must be noted that the velocities measured depend again on other physiological parameters such as changes in blood pressure and carbon dioxide, so the clinical neurological picture should be taken into consideration when interpreting these velocities [3].

20.4.2 Acute ischaemic stroke

In large vessel occlusion, ischaemic findings on plain computed tomography of the head may take hours to be evident. If there is clinical suspicion, then TCCD of the MCA of both cerebral hemispheres may confirm the absence of flow in the occluded large vessel, as well as looking at flow in collateral vessels. Through the collateral circulation, the cerebral circulation will attempt to maintain constant cerebral perfusion. In MCA occlusion, flow is commonly diverted from the distal internal carotid artery (ICA) to the ACA, so on TCCD there would be higher velocity flow in the ipsilateral ACA when compared to the velocity flow in the contralateral ACA [4].

Serial TCCD can also be used to monitor recanalization post endovascular or thrombolytic intervention in stroke. Nedelmann and colleagues developed a TCCD-based grading system called the Consensus on Grading Intracranial Flow Obstruction (COGIF) score which is similar in principle to the radiographic Thrombolysis In Cerebral Infarction (TICI) grading system [5].

Another potential use of TCCD in the hyperacute stroke ward setting would be in those patients with malignant MCA syndrome. Malignant MCA syndrome is a term used to describe the deterioration of GCS score and neurological symptoms following an MCA infarction, which is attributed to the space-occupying vasogenic oedema caused by the infarcted area, potentially leading to midline shift and raised intracranial pressure. Prognostic factors for developing a malignant infarction are 50% or more of the MCA territory being affected and early signs of midline shift on CT head imaging. Early decompressive hemicraniectomy is the treatment option. To calculate midline shift, the transtemporal acoustic window in the diencephalic plane is used to identify the third ventricle. Bilateral measurements (in millimetres) are taken from the start of the ultrasound beam at the top of the screen to the centre of the third ventricle (between the hyperechoic lines). The difference between the two measurements divided by two gives the midline shift, i.e.

Midline shift = (right side – left side)/2

A midline shift >2.5mm on TCCD is considered significant and has been shown to have good correlation with CT imaging. Of note, in the post decompressive craniectomy patient, this method of measuring midline shift is inaccurate.

Lastly, in post-operative carotid endarterectomy patients, reperfusion can lead to a clinical syndrome called cerebral hyperperfusion syndrome (CHS) which presents as a triad of ipsilateral headache, seizure and focal neurological symptoms occurring in the absence of cerebral ischaemia. It is accompanied by post-operative hypertension in almost all patients. If left untreated the hyperperfusion causes cerebral oedema and midline shift. In CHS, hyperperfusion is defined as a greater than 100% increase in MCA velocity. Baseline measurement of MCA velocity before induction of anaesthesia is a quick non-invasive assessment and allows continued measurement, because CHS can appear immediately post-operatively or up to a month later. Given the signs of CHS are similar to stroke, the MCA velocity is a useful diagnostic differential in this clinical scenario.

20.4.3 Cerebral circulatory arrest

Increasing intracranial pressure (ICP) causes decreasing cerebral perfusion pressure (CPP) until critical closing pressure is reached. Critical closing pressure is the arterial pressure below which cerebral blood flow (CBF) approaches zero. The step-wise changes in CBF can be observed via transtemporal TCCD of the MCA flow in an emergency setting (*Fig. 20.6*).

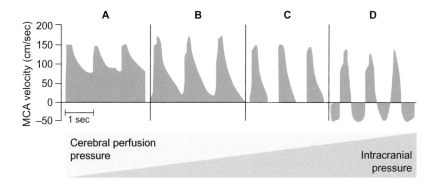

Figure 20.6. Step-wise changes in middle cerebral artery waveform shape as intracranial pressure increases.

With increasing ICP, the diastolic step-down of the waveform is lost (B). The end-diastolic velocity becomes zero when the ICP reaches the diastolic blood pressure value (C). When ICP is above diastolic blood pressure, the brain will only receive blood in systole. At this stage CPP is still higher than ICP so there is forward flow. This is seen as the complete loss of the diastolic step-down and the appearance of systolic peaks only. With a continued rise in ICP, the systolic peak duration is shortened and diastolic back or reverse flow is seen to give an oscillating systolic forward flow and diastolic backward flow (D). As the ICP continues to rise, the diastolic reverse flow disappears so there are only isolated smaller amplitude systolic spikes and eventually no forward systolic flow is seen when the critical closing pressure is reached.

To confirm cerebral circulatory arrest, all anterior and posterior circulation vessels bilaterally should be insonated, with extracranial circulation assessed through ICA insonation submandibularly to demonstrate physiological forward flow bilaterally. At least two studies should be undertaken 30 minutes apart to confirm circulatory cerebral arrest. It must be remembered that TCCD in this scenario is evaluating cerebral circulatory arrest rather than brainstem function and so should be used with caution as an ancillary test for diagnosing death by neurological criteria [4].

20.5 Optic nerve sheath diameter and raised intracranial pressure

The optic nerve sheath is continuous with the dura mater and its contents are thus continuous with the subarachnoid space where cerebral spinal fluid (CSF) circulates from the posterior to anterior part. The anterior retrobulbar part of the peri-optic subarachnoid space is surrounded by fat and thus is more distensible than the posterior part. Providing there is no obstruction to CSF flow, a rise in CSF pressures is transmitted along the optic nerve sheath.

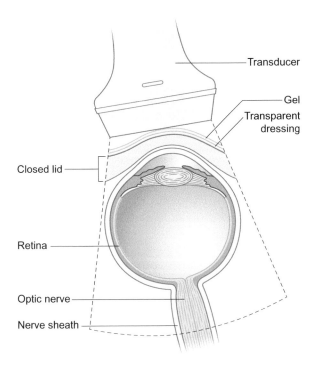

Figure 20.7. Anatomy of the optic nerve sheath.

A high frequency (7.5MHz) probe is used with the ophthalmic setting selected according to the ALARA (as low as reasonably achievable) principle. Protecting the closed eye with a transparent dressing and a generous amount of gel, the probe is gently placed on the upper eyelid. Steadying the operating hand on either the bridge of the patient's nose or maxilla, in addition to the gel, will avoid transmitting undue pressure to the globe. The anechoic globe is seen with the optic nerve sheath behind it (*Fig. 20.7*). Optimization of the image by rocking the probe from medial to lateral allows full appreciation of the course of the optic nerve and reduces refraction artefacts related to insonation through the lens. The optic nerve sheath diameter is measured 3mm from the back of the globe and across between the external borders of the hyperechogenic area surrounding the optic nerve (*Fig. 20.8*). The 3mm

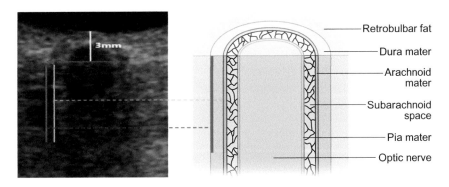

Figure 20.8. Optic ultrasound anatomy.

marker from the back of the globe is where the optic nerve sheath is most distensible. Measuring the optic nerve sheath diameter in both the transverse and the sagittal planes in both eyes and averaging the measurement allows for a more accurate assessment.

The normal optic nerve sheath diameter in the adult population ranges between 5.6 and 5.9mm depending on gender and ethnicity. An optic nerve sheath diameter above 6mm would indicate an ICP greater than 20mmHg. Meta-analysis has suggested that optic nerve sheath diameter above 6mm has a sensitivity of 100% and specificity of 95% for raised ICP when compared to CT scan [6].

There are a few pitfalls with optic nerve sheath diameter measurements. Insonation through the lens is the most common. Shadow artefacts from the lamina cribrosa, which is a mesh-like structure through which the optic nerve fibres pass through the sclera, can mimic the optic nerve root. To avoid this artefact, the central retinal artery can be used as a guide. It is seen entering the centre of the optic nerve sheath at the level of the vitreoretinal junction and will remain central in the optic nerve tract. However, with raised ICP, the central retinal artery may be compressed and therefore not be visible on insonation.

As a simple, non-invasive tool, optic nerve sheath diameter can be used in various settings (prehospital, operating theatres, labour ward) and clinical scenarios (traumatic brain injury, pre-eclampsia, meningitis, high altitude mountain sickness, idiopathic intracranial hypertension, acute liver failure, post laparoscopic cerebral oedema and ventriculoperitoneal shunt obstruction) where invasive ICP monitoring is not available or contraindicated [6]. There is one particular scenario where it should be used with caution. It is known that in aSAH there is an initial sudden rise in ICP on aneurysm rupture. Observational studies have shown that the recoil of the optic nerve sheath post rupture is slow and that an optic nerve sheath diameter value higher than 6mm should be verified with invasive ICP monitoring through external ventricular drains, ICP bolts and continuous brain tissue oxygen (PbtO$_2$) monitors.

Orbital ultrasound can also be used to diagnose papilloedema when two sonographic findings are present. The optic nerve sheath diameter must be greater than 6mm and optic disc elevation must be greater than 0.6mm. Studies have suggested that optic disc elevation on ultrasound is 82% sensitive and 76% specific for papilloedema. The added benefit of using ultrasound to diagnose papilloedema is that it does not need pupillary dilatation.

20.6 Summary

Neuro POCUS is a useful non-invasive tool that can help guide clinical assessment and decision making in a variety of scenarios. Through the transtemporal acoustic window, the circle of Willis and the ventricular system can be visualized. Optic nerve sheath diameter provides a simple way to ascertain whether there is evidence of raised ICP. Combining clinical history, examination and POCUS findings allows the bedside clinician to institute swift measures to reduce secondary cerebral ischaemia.

20.7 References

1. Robba C, Goffi A, Geeraerts T, *et al.* (2019) Brain ultrasonography: methodology, basic and advanced principles and clinical applications. A narrative review. *Intensive Care Med*, 45:913.

2. Lau VI, Arntfield RT (2017) Point-of-care transcranial Doppler by intensivists. *Crit Ultrasound J*, 9:21.

3. Robba C, Taccone FS (2019) How I use transcranial Doppler. *Crit Care*, 23:420.

4. Blanco P, Abdo-Cuza A (2018) Transcranial Doppler ultrasound in neurocritical care. *J Ultrasound*, 21:1.

5. Nedelmann M, Stolz E, Gerriets T, *et al.* (2009) TCCS Consensus Group. Consensus recommendations for transcranial color-coded duplex sonography for the assessment of intracranial arteries in clinical trials on acute stroke. *Stroke*, 40:3238.

6. Robba C, Sarwal A, Sharma D (2021) Brain echography in perioperative medicine: beyond neurocritical care. *J Neurosurg Anesthesiol*, 33:3.

CHAPTER 21

ULTRASOUND-GUIDED SPINAL PROCEDURES

John Dick & Kay Mak

Central neuraxial blocks (CNBs), which include spinals, epidurals, and combined spinal–epidurals (CSEs), are used widely in anaesthesia to provide highly effective analgesia for a variety of indications. Performance of these blocks has traditionally relied on the palpation of bony anatomical landmarks and identification of endpoints such as loss of resistance or presence of cerebral spinal fluid (CSF). Needle angulation and its trajectory, along with estimation of the depth of the spinal space, relies on the operator's tactile perception and previous experience. In a patient with no obvious spinal deformities, it is often difficult to predict or anticipate technical difficulties or needle placement until skin puncture has been made. As a result, multiple puncturing attempts may be required, resulting in patient discomfort and dissatisfaction.

In this chapter, we discuss how the use of spinal ultrasonography has emerged as a superior technique compared with the surface landmark approach and describe its use as an adjunct to improve the success rate of performing CNBs.

21.1 Problems associated with the surface landmark technique

Several potential shortcomings are associated with the traditional surface landmark approach. First, the surface landmark which is typically used is Tuffier's (intercristal) line – an imaginary horizontal line connecting the top of the iliac crests – to identify the L3/4 intervertebral space. However, this landmark has been shown to be highly variable between patients and can lead to incorrect identification of the spinal level, resulting in placement of the needle in a space higher than intended, potentially causing significant harm [1]. Secondly, bony landmarks may not always be palpable, especially in patients with high BMI, back oedema, abnormal spinal anatomy or previous back surgery. Both potential drawbacks can be overcome with the use of ultrasound imaging.

21.2 Advantages of spinal sonography

The use of spinal ultrasonography was first reported in 1971 and has since developed into a reliable technique for identifying the spinal interspace level and locating the midline of the spine, the angulation and exact point of needle insertion, and the depth to the spinal space [2]. The operator is therefore able to anticipate patients in whom CNB may be technically challenging, and to have the relevant equipment available, such as a longer needle. Real-time guided CNBs with visualization of the injectate into the spinal space have previously been demonstrated, although this technique remains experimental at present and so is not discussed further in this chapter [3].

Performing a pre-procedural scan of the back has been shown to increase the success rate of CNBs and significantly reduces the number of puncture attempts, thus increasing patient comfort and satisfaction [4,5]. Although more time is required for successful location of the space with ultrasound, the overall procedure time remains relatively unchanged [6]. The safety profile is also increased, with fewer reports of dural puncture and 'severe' headaches when used with epidural performance [7]. Additionally, it can serve as an invaluable teaching tool to aid understanding of the relevant spinal anatomy, especially in those with scoliosis, and prediction of spinal space depth.

The use of ultrasound itself confers many inherent advantages. It is portable, simple to use, and non-invasive, and can be performed as a point-of-care test by the bedside to visualize real-time images. Furthermore, its safety profile in pregnant women makes it extremely useful in the obstetric population, where neuraxial blocks are often performed. We use the technique routinely for both emergency and elective blocks in theatre and the labour room and would argue that this adds little delay because image acquisition can be performed within seconds once adequate experience has been gained.

21.3 Gross anatomy of the lumbar spine

The lumbar spine comprises five bony vertebrae (L1–L5). Each vertebra consists of an anterior vertebral body and a posterior vertebral arch and, together, they form an enclosed ring – the vertebral canal. From the vertebral arch arise several bony prominences: a single spinous process which is centred posteriorly; two transverse processes which extend laterally; two laminae which connect the transverse and spinous processes; two pedicles which connect the transverse processes and the vertebral body; and the four articular processes (two superior and two inferior), which form the joints between the vertebrae (*Fig. 21.1*). The space between the spinous processes (interspinous space) and the one between the laminae (interlaminar space) allows for the penetration of the ultrasound beam and visualization of the contents within the spinal canal.

Multiple ligaments can be found throughout the vertebral column. The thicker supraspinous and thinner infraspinous ligaments connect the spinous processes of each adjacent vertebrae. There are also anterior and posterior longitudinal ligaments, which are attached along the length of the anterior and posterior walls of the vertebral canal, respectively. The ligamentum flavum, a thick and dense layer of connective tissue, connects the laminae of each adjacent vertebrae.

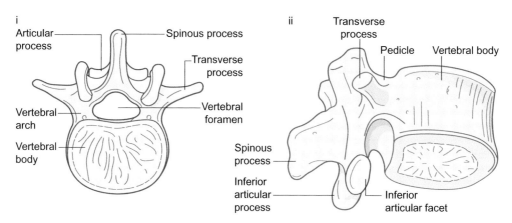

Figure 21.1. Diagram showing (i) the superior and (ii) lateral and inferior view of the lumbar spine. Reproduced from *Anatomy and Physiology in Healthcare* (Marshall P. *et al.*) with permission from Scion Publishing.

21.4 Preparation for procedure

The patient is placed in a sitting or lateral decubitus position and asked to adopt a reverse lordosis position which opens the interspinous spaces. A low frequency 2–5MHz curvilinear probe is used to provide deeper penetration and a wide field of view. A 10cm depth setting is used initially. The simplified technique involves just two scanning angles: para-sagittal oblique (interlaminar) and axial midline (transverse).

21.5 Para-sagittal oblique (interlaminar) view

The probe is placed a few centimetres lateral to the spinous processes (with the pointer placed cephalad) in the lower back, over the transverse processes. The sacrum, which has a characteristic flat shape and gives a continuous bright signal due to maximal reflection of the sound waves, is identified. From here, the probe is adjusted cephalad or caudally in the sagittal plane and tilted medially to visualize the vertebral bodies and laminae in an oblique view. The space between the sacrum and the L5 lamina is the L5/S1 interlaminar space, and the desired space can be obtained by counting upwards. A characteristic sawtooth pattern shown in *Figure 21.2* can be seen, with the 'teeth' corresponding to the laminae and the radiolucent areas in between representing the contents of the vertebral canal. The structures that should be visible are the ligamentum flavum, posterior dura, anterior dura,

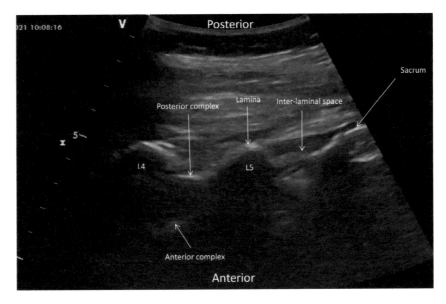

Figure 21.2. Paramedian sagittal oblique sonographic view of the lumbar spine.

and posterior longitudinal ligament. The depth should be adjusted at this point to maximize the image size and optimize the image.

The epidural space is located between the ligamentum flavum and the posterior dura, both of which appear as hyperechoic structures. Collectively, this is known as the posterior complex. The anterior complex, on the other hand, is made up of the anterior dura, posterior longitudinal ligament, and the posterior border of the vertebral body, as shown in *Figure 21.3*. Both the posterior and anterior complexes are often seen as a single linear hyperechoic structure, with the clear delineation of the two structures generally not distinguishable.

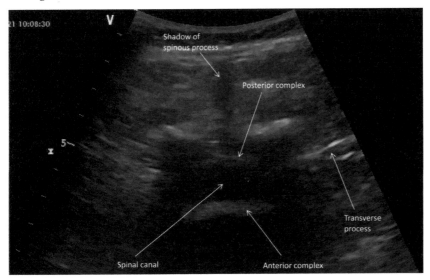

Figure 21.3. Transverse sonographic view of the lumbar spine. The transducer probe is positioned such that the ultrasound beam passes through the interspinous space.

21.6 Axial midline (transverse) view

Once the L5 vertebral body is identified, the probe is slid superiorly to identify L4 and positioned in a horizontal orientation for the axial view, with the centre of the probe placed over the midline (*Fig. 21.3*). The spinous processes will appear as tall, hypoechoic peaked shadows on the ultrasound. The next step is to identify the interspinous space. This is done by sliding the probe superiorly or inferiorly combined with angling, until the beam passes through the interspinous space to the vertebral body. Angling of the probe upwards is usually required to account for the angulation of the spinous processes. The parallel hyperechoic lines of the posterior and anterior complexes should then be visualized in the interspinous view. This view would also correspond to the optimal needle trajectory. Occasionally, if it is not possible to obtain a good image of the anterior complex, the space should be avoided. Conversely, if the ultrasound wave passes through to the back of the vertebral body with clear visualization of the anterior complex, then it usually confers a simple needle trajectory.

Estimation of the spinal space depth is generally best achieved by identifying the posterior complex in the axial midline view, because this represents the reflections from the ligamentum flavum and posterior dura. The image can be 'frozen' on the ultrasound machine with the spinous process in the true midline. The calliper or 'measure' function can then be used to measure the distance from the line to the skin (*Fig. 21.4*). This function is particularly useful in estimating the depth of the epidural space and in avoiding accidental dural punctures.

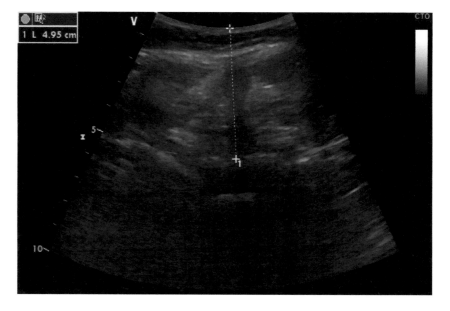

Figure 21.4. The distance from the skin to the posterior complex can be used as an estimate of the spinal space depth; in this example it is 4.95cm.

21.7 Marking the 'spot'

This is the technique used by us to mark the spot for needle insertion once the optimal interspinous space has been identified. With the ultrasound probe held in the midline view and the optimal view obtained (ensuring that the probe is in the midline), the space can be marked by carefully peeling off the ultrasound probe and making a mark by indenting the skin with a needle hub. This creates a temporary circular mark on the skin and the ultrasound probe can be safely stowed before injecting a few millilitres of local anaesthetic into the centre of the mark. This will ensure that the spot is both numb and clearly visible as a tiny bleed point by the time the operator has prepared and is ready to perform the block (*Fig. 21.5*).

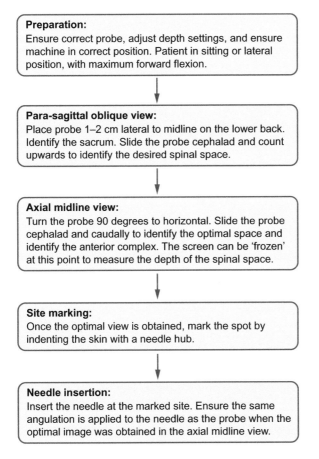

Preparation:
Ensure correct probe, adjust depth settings, and ensure machine in correct position. Patient in sitting or lateral position, with maximum forward flexion.

Para-sagittal oblique view:
Place probe 1–2 cm lateral to midline on the lower back. Identify the sacrum. Slide the probe cephalad and count upwards to identify the desired spinal space.

Axial midline view:
Turn the probe 90 degrees to horizontal. Slide the probe cephalad and caudally to identify the optimal space and identify the anterior complex. The screen can be 'frozen' at this point to measure the depth of the spinal space.

Site marking:
Once the optimal view is obtained, mark the spot by indenting the skin with a needle hub.

Needle insertion:
Insert the needle at the marked site. Ensure the same angulation is applied to the needle as the probe when the optimal image was obtained in the axial midline view.

Figure 21.5. Suggested approach in performing pre-procedural spinal sonography scanning.

TIPS

- It may not be possible to obtain optimal images in morbidly obese patients, but ultrasound can still be useful for identifying the midline from the shadow cast by the spinous process (which is often impalpable).
- For category 1 caesarean sections, a skilled anaesthetic sonographer can quickly identify the 'spot' with the patient in the lateral or sitting position whilst a second anaesthetist prepares for a rapid spinal.
- A plastic model of the lumbosacral complex can aid understanding of ultrasound penetration and the images generated using different probe angles.

21.8 Summary

The use of spinal sonography as a pre-procedural tool for performing CNBs is fast becoming a helpful adjunct and alternative to the surface landmark approach, particularly in those with impalpable anatomy. In pregnant women, it has been shown to increase the success rate and improve patient comfort and satisfaction. A clear understanding of the relevant anatomy and ultrasound probe technique is of paramount importance for optimizing visualization of the desired structures and guidance of needle placement.

21.9 References

1. Snider KT, Kribs JW, Snider EJ, *et al.* (2008) Reliability of Tuffier's line as an anatomic landmark. *Spine,* 33(6):E161.

2. Bogin IN, Stulin ID (1971) Application of the method of 2-dimensional echospondylography for determining landmarks in lumbar punctures. *Zh Nevropatol Psikhiatr Im S S Korsakova,* 71:1810.

3. Grau T, Leipold RW, Fatehi S, Motsch J (2004) Real-time ultrasonic observation of combined spinal-epidural anaesthesia. *Eur J Anaesth,* 21:25.

4. Grau T, Leipold RW, Conradi R, Martin E, Motsch J (2002) Efficacy of ultrasound imaging in obstetric epidural anesthesia. *J Clin Anesth,* 14:169.

5. Tao B, Liu K, Ding M, *et al.* (2021) Ultrasound increases the success rate of spinal needle placement through the epidural needle during combined spinal-epidural anaesthesia: a randomised controlled study. *Eur J Anaesth,* 38:251.

6. Creaney M, Mullane D, Casby C, Tan T (2016) Ultrasound to identify the lumbar space in women with impalpable bony landmarks presenting for elective caesarean delivery under spinal anaesthesia: a randomised trial. *Int J Obstet Anesth,* 28:12.

7. Grau T, Leipold RW, Conradi R, Martin E, Motsch J (2001) Ultrasound imaging facilitates localization of the epidural space during combined spinal and epidural anesthesia. *Reg Anesth Pain Med,* 26:64.

CHAPTER 22

ULTRASOUND TO CONFIRM AIRWAY PLACEMENT AND GUIDE PERCUTANEOUS DILATATIONAL TRACHEOSTOMY

Adrian Wong

The use of ultrasound in acute and critical care continues to evolve, enhancing bedside care. Airway assessment and its subsequent management is often the first step in any structured, systematic approach to the acutely unwell patient.

The National Audit Project 4 carried out by the Royal College of Anaesthetists in the UK reported on the incidence of intubation failure [1]. Key findings include an incidence of:

- 1 in 2000 in the elective setting

- 1 in 300 during rapid sequence intubation in the obstetric setting

- 1 in 50–100 in the emergency department (ED), intensive care unit (ICU) and pre-hospital settings [2].

Crucially, they found a significant increase in morbidity and mortality associated with airway management in the ICU environment compared to that in the operating theatre.

The difficult airway can be, to some extent, inherently unpredictable. In particular, it is influenced by situational factors, including the clinical context and operator skill [2]. In the ICU setting, with its mixture of situational, environmental and patient-related factors, airway management can be particularly challenging.

When comprehensive anaesthetic/airway history taking is limited in time critical situations, ultrasound can play a valuable role in the assessment and subsequent planning of airway strategies in both the non-emergency and emergency setting. This is especially true in patients who are traditionally considered to be at higher risk, such as those with a significantly raised BMI.

In addition to assessing the airway, other clinical applications of airway ultrasound include confirmation of endotracheal tube (ETT) position, guidance of percutaneous tracheostomy and cricothyroidotomy. Less well-described uses of ultrasound include the detection of subglottic stenosis, post-extubation stridor and prediction of ETT size [3]. Other potential uses include real-time assessment of a patient's swallow.

The purpose of this chapter is to review the ultrasonographic anatomy of the upper airway and provide an overview on the use of ultrasound in the management of endotracheal intubations and front-of-neck access in the critically ill patient.

22.1 Sonoanatomy of the airway

A linear array or curvilinear probe can be used to identify most of the structures of the upper airway, which are superficial [3]. Visualization of deeper structures is limited by air – a poor medium for ultrasound transmission.

The larynx is mainly composed of various muscles built around a cartilaginous framework comprising the cricoid cartilage, thyroid cartilage and tracheal rings. Ultrasound enables identification of important upper airway sonoanatomy including the thyroid cartilage, epiglottis, cricoid cartilage, cricothyroid membrane, tracheal rings and oesophagus (*Figs 22.1 and 22.2*).

Bony structures, e.g. mandible, hyoid bone and sternum, appear hyperechoic (bright) on ultrasound with a hypoechoic (dark) acoustic shadow posteriorly. Cartilaginous structures, e.g. thyroid and cricoid cartilages, appear homogeneously hypoechoic. Muscle and connective tissue have a heterogeneously hypoechoic and striated appearance.

The cricoid cartilage is seen as a bump in the longitudinal plane and an oval structure in transverse. The cricothyroid membrane is seen on sagittal and parasagittal views as a hyperechoic band linking the hypoechoic thyroid and cricoid cartilages.

The epiglottis appears as a hypoechoic curvilinear structure in transverse and parasagittal views through the thyrohyoid membrane. In the transverse plane, it is identified by cephalad or caudad angulation of the linear transducer. It is visible as a discrete mobile structure inferior to the base of the tongue during tongue protrusion and swallowing.

Tracheal cartilage rings appear as a 'string of beads' in the longitudinal plane (*Fig. 22.2*), and as inverted 'U'-shaped structures in transverse. A linear hyperechoic line posterior to the trachea (in both transverse and longitudinal planes) is the result of reverberation artefacts at the air–mucosa interface.

Both transverse and sagittal views can be used to visualize the hyoid bone. In the transverse plane, it appears as a superficial hyperechoic inverted U-shaped linear structure with posterior acoustic shadowing. The vocal cords form an isosceles triangle, with a central tracheal shadow.

The oesophagus is best seen with a transverse approach, posterolateral to the trachea at the level of the suprasternal notch. Identification is confirmed in the presence of peristaltic motion upon swallowing.

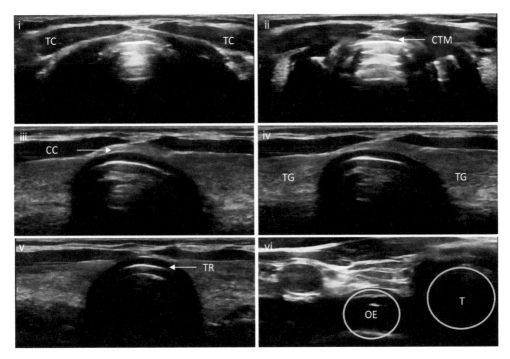

Figure 22.1. Ultrasound of the airway. (i) Thyroid cartilage, (ii) cricothyroid membrane, (iii) cricothyroid cartilage, (iv) thyroid gland, (v) tracheal rings, (vi) laterally displaced probe showing oesophagus and trachea. CC – cricoid cartilage; CTM – cricothyroid membrane; OE – oesophagus; T – trachea; TC – thyroid cartilage; TG – thyroid gland; TR – tracheal rings.

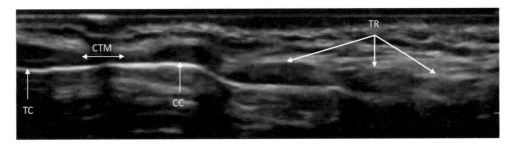

Figure 22.2. Lateral view of the airway on ultrasound. CC – cricoid cartilage; CTM – cricothyroid membrane; TC – thyroid cartilage; TR – tracheal rings.

22.2 Ultrasound in airway assessment and predicting airway difficulty

Traditionally, the assessment of a potentially difficult airway relies on a combination of history taking with clinical examination. Individual predictors of a difficult airway, e.g. mouth opening, Mallampati grading, etc. have poor sensitivity, specificity and positive predictive value [4]. Their use is limited in scenarios where the patient is unconscious or unable to cooperate. To improve the performance of prediction scores, composite multiparametric airway scoring systems have been proposed; the MACOCHA score is most commonly used, comprising seven items:

- Mallampati score III or IV

- obstructive sleep apnoea syndrome

- limited cervical spine mobility

- limited mouth opening

- severe hypoxia

- coma

- non-anaesthetist operator.

It has sensitivity and specificity of 73% and 89%, respectively [5].

Beyond the identification of various neck and airway structures, ultrasound also enables length/distance and volume measurements, a non-exhaustive list of which includes skin–epiglottis distance, hyomental distance ratio and tongue thickness [6–8]. The caveat is that most of the studies using these measurements in the prediction of difficult airway involve small sample sizes; other than demonstrating feasibility of such measurements, they often lack dependable sensitivity and specificity. Indeed, even though ultrasound assessment can be performed in both elective and emergency situations, most international airway guidelines have not yet recommended the use of ultrasound as part of routine airway assessment.

In obese patients, ultrasound measurement of pre-tracheal soft tissue can help predict a difficult airway. Depth measurements from skin to the anterior aspect of the trachea are taken at three levels: the vocal cords, thyroid isthmus, and suprasternal notch. At each level, the measurements are made centrally overlying the trachea as well as two further measurements either side of the midline, then an average value is calculated [9].

22.3 Confirming endotracheal tube position

Clinical examination for confirmation of ETT placement has its limitations, with auscultation and chest rise observation failing to detect up to 55% of endobronchial intubations [10]. Capnography is considered the standard of care for ETT placement confirmation; however, ultrasound can be invaluable in the presence of cardiorespiratory arrest, bronchoconstriction or conditions that prevent accurate capnography or end-tidal carbon dioxide measurement.

Correct placement of the ETT is confirmed by the presence of two hyperechoic lines – the 'double tract' sign in the trachea (*Fig. 22.3*) [11]. Conversely, oesophageal intubation can be identified by the Tracheal Rapid Ultrasound Exam (TRUE). This static transtracheal approach uses a convex transducer in the suprasternal notch window, and has an overall accuracy of 98% (98.9% sensitive; 94.1% specific) in emergency intubations [12]. A cadaver study showed that novice sonographers can accurately identify a saline-inflated ETT cuff at the level of the suprasternal notch [13].

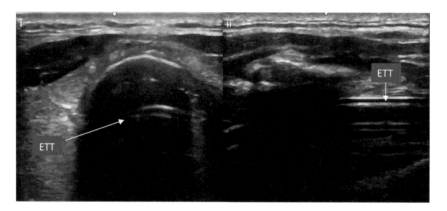

Figure 22.3. Examples of the 'double tract' sign, confirming placement of the endotracheal tube within the trachea in (i) a transverse, and (ii) a longitudinal view of the trachea. ETT – endotracheal tube.

22.4 Ultrasound in intubations and predicting endotracheal tube size

There is growing academic interest in the use of ultrasound in the estimation of airway size and hence appropriate ETT size.

Ultrasound as a tool for assessing the subglottic airway has been validated against MRI and CT [14,15]. It has several practical advantages over these radiological techniques – ultrasound requires minimal training, is quick to perform at the bedside and does not require complete immobilization or sedation.

The subglottic transverse diameter measured on ultrasound correlates well with the outer ETT diameter, giving accurate predictions of ETT size (both cuffed and uncuffed) [16]. Ultrasound is superior to age-based and height-based formulae in estimating ETT size; formulae prediction is 35% and 60% accurate for cuffed and uncuffed ETT size, respectively, compared to over 98% and 96%, respectively, using ultrasound prediction [16].

It should be noted that age-dependent calcification of the laryngeal cartilages begins during the third decade of life; the resultant acoustic shadowing presents an important limitation to laryngeal ultrasound in older patients.

22.5 Ultrasound in emergency front-of-neck access

Cricothyroidotomy is potentially lifesaving in 'cannot intubate, cannot ventilate' situations; however, the cricothyroid membrane is not always easily identified using the landmark techniques.

Ultrasound improves the speed and accuracy with which the cricothyroid membrane can be located. The feasibility of real-time ultrasound-guided bougie-assisted cricothyroidotomy has been demonstrated; in one study, identification of the cricothyroid membrane required a median time of under 4 seconds and cricothyroidotomy was completed in under 30 seconds with a high success rate [17]. Importantly, there is no steep learning curve for this technique [18].

A randomized trial comparing digital palpation with ultrasound by non-experienced ultrasound operators in cadavers found the incidence of airway injury to be three times lower in the ultrasound-guided group, even in the presence of distorted neck anatomy. However, it did increase the time to completion of procedure (196 vs 110 seconds) [19].

22.6 Ultrasound in percutaneous dilatational tracheostomy

A systematic analysis of percutaneous dilatational tracheostomy (PDT) related deaths found a mortality rate of 1 per 600 procedures, with one-third of deaths occurring during PDT; the major causes of death were haemorrhage (38%) and airway complications (29.6%) [20].

The most common complication of PDT is haemorrhage related to vascular anatomical variants. Accurate identification of anterior neck structures can significantly reduce the risk of haemorrhage, as well as other complications including thyroid isthmus damage, tracheal stenosis and erosion into high mediastinal vessels.

Pre-procedural ultrasound improves the safety of PDT by identifying high-risk patients with vascular or tracheal anatomical variants. One study found a change in the management decision from PDT to open surgical tracheostomy in 25% of patients [21]. A separate study found that ultrasound assessment led to a change in PDT puncture location in 25% of cases [22].

In cases where PDT is not contraindicated, ultrasound provides an excellent overview of the anatomical landmarks for PDT and allows estimation of appropriate tracheostomy tube size and length [23].

22.6.1 Performing PDT

1. The pre-tracheal area is examined to identify the tracheal midline, approximate level of tracheal cartilages, anterior jugular veins (with their diameter and location), thyroid isthmus, vulnerable thyroid vessels and any other aberrant vessels.

2. Tracheal puncture should be between the first and fifth tracheal rings in a location without intervening structures, as mentioned above. Transverse plane imaging first allows identification of the tracheal midline.

3. Rotation of the probe 90° gives a longitudinal view of the cricoid cartilage and tracheal rings. Scanning in-plane permits visualization of the needle during its introduction and advancement. A change in resistance indicates tracheal entry, and air or fluid can be aspirated into an attached syringe which is then disconnected.

4. The guide wire is passed down the needle; its position can be confirmed using a transverse or oblique transverse view prior to dilatation.

Real-time ultrasound guidance has been shown to increase the rate of first-pass puncture (TARGET), increase the success rate of midline puncture, and reduce the number of needle punctures compared to a landmark technique [24,25]. It also accurately predicted tracheal ring space insertion in 90% of patients [25]. There was no statistically significant difference in procedural complications [24,25].

Real-time in-plane ultrasound guidance for tracheal puncture and wire insertion has been shown to be feasible in cadaver models [26]. The TRACHUS randomized controlled trial compared the incidence of procedural failure and major complications for ultrasound-guided PDT versus bronchoscopy-guided PDT in critically ill patients; ultrasound-guided PDT was found to be non-inferior to bronchoscopy-guided PDT [27].

With regard to the learning curve for real-time ultrasound-guided PDT, a minimum of 50 procedures is necessary to perform this technique with an acceptable complication rate and procedure time [28].

22.7 Other uses of ultrasound in airway management

22.7.1 Detecting complications

Endotracheal intubation can be associated with a range of local complications. The most common laryngeal injuries include laryngeal oedema and vocal cord dysfunction, both of which can cause stridor and extubation failure, resulting in prolonged mechanical ventilation and length of stay. These injuries can be identified with ultrasound.

22.7.2 Laryngeal oedema

Changes in width of the air column at the level of the vocal cords before and after deflation of an ETT cuff have been used to predict/pre-empt stridor. However, the sample sizes involved are small and the study of this technique is still at an early stage [29].

22.7.3 Vocal cord dysfunction

The diagnosis of vocal cord dysfunction is often made via nasopharyngoscopy, which is invasive and contraindicated in the presence of craniofacial injury and coagulopathy. Glottic oedema can also prevent adequate examination. In comparison, ultrasound is non-invasive and not precluded by the aforementioned conditions.

22.8 Summary

While airway management and intervention have traditionally relied on landmark techniques and clinical assessment, the combination of high-resolution imaging and real-time visualization makes ultrasound an ideal non-invasive tool for airway assessment.

An airway scoring system using ultrasound measurements (e.g. skin-to-epiglottis distance or pre-tracheal soft tissue depth), along with the clinical predictors, can help identify potentially difficult intubations. Upper airway ultrasound is also invaluable in the care of critically ill patients, especially for airway management because of its portability, non-invasiveness, cost-effectiveness and reproducibility. The evidence for the use of ultrasound has been very encouraging thus far; with continuing research and learning it is anticipated that upper airway ultrasound will play an important role in the future standard of care for airway assessment, monitoring and imaging.

22.9 References

1. Cook T, MacDougall-Davis SR (2012) Complications and failure of airway management. *Br J Anaesth*, 109(Suppl 1):i68.

2. Nickson C (2020) Airway assessment. www.litfl.com [accessed 8 March 2022].

3. Kundra P, Mishra SK, Ramesh A (2011) Ultrasound of the airway. *Indian J Anaesth*, 55:456.

4. Daggupati H, Maurya I, Singh RD, Ravishankar M (2020) Development of a scoring system for predicting difficult intubation using ultrasonography. *Indian J Anaesth*, 64:187.

5. De Jong A, Molinari N, Terzi N, *et al.* (2013) Early identification of patients at risk for difficult intubation in the intensive care unit: development and validation of the MACOCHA score in a multicenter cohort study. *Am J Respir Crit Care Med*, 187:832.

6. Parameswari A, Govind M, Vakamudi M (2017) Correlation between preoperative ultrasonographic airway assessment and laryngoscopic view in adult patients: a prospective study. *J Anaesthesiol Clin Pharmacol*, 33:353.

7. Petrisor C, Szabo R, Constantinescu C, *et al.* (2018) Ultrasound-based assessment of hyomental distances in neutral, ramped and maximum hyperextended positions, and derived ratios, for the prediction of difficult airway in the obese population: a pilot diagnostic accuracy study. *Anaesthesiol Intensive Ther*, 50:110.

8. Yao W, Wang B (2017) Can tongue thickness measured by ultrasonography predict difficult tracheal intubation? *Br J Anaesth*, 118:601.

9. Ezri T, Gewurtz G, Sessler DI, *et al.* (2003) Prediction of difficult laryngoscopy in obese patients by ultrasound quantification of anterior neck soft tissue. *Anaesthesia*, 58:1111.

10. Sitzwohl C, Langheinrich A, Schober A, *et al.* (2010) Endobronchial intubation detected by insertion depth of endotracheal tube, bilateral auscultation or observation of chest movements: randomised trial. *BMJ*, 341:c5943.

11. Osman A, Sum KM (2016) Role of upper airway ultrasound in airway management. *J Intensive Care*, 4:52.

12. Chou HC, Tseng WP, Wang CH, *et al.* (2011) Tracheal rapid ultrasound exam (T.R.U.E.) for confirming endotracheal tube placement during emergency intubation. *Resuscitation*, 82:1279.

13. Uya A, Spear D, Patel K, Okada P, Sheeran P, McCreight A (2012) Can novice sonographers accurately locate an endotracheal tube with a saline-filled cuff in a cadaver model? A pilot study. *Acad Emerg Med*, 19:361.

14. Lakhal K, Delplace X, Cottier JP, *et al.* (2007) The feasibility of ultrasound to assess subglottic diameter. *Anesth Analg*, 104:611.

15. Sustic A, Miletic D, Protic A, Ivancic A, Cicvaric T (2008) Can ultrasound be useful for predicting the size of a left double-lumen bronchial tube? Tracheal width as measured by ultrasonography versus computed tomography. *J Clin Anesth*, 20:247.

16. Shibasaki M, Nakajima Y, Ishii S, Shimizu F, Shime N, Sessler DI (2010) Prediction of pediatric endotracheal tube size by ultrasonography. *Anesthesiology*, 113:819.

17. Curtis K, Ahern M, Dawson M, Mallin M (2012) Ultrasound-guided, Bougie-assisted cricothyroidotomy: a description of a novel technique in cadaveric models. *Acad Emerg Med*, 19:876.

18. Nicholls SE, Sweeney TW, Ferre RM, Strout TD (2008) Bedside sonography by emergency physicians for the rapid identification of landmarks relevant to cricothyrotomy. *Am J Emerg Med*, 26:852.

19. Siddiqui N, Arzola C, Friedman Z, Guerina L, You-Ten KE (2015) Ultrasound improves cricothyrotomy success in cadavers with poorly defined neck anatomy: a randomized control trial. *Anesthesiology*, 123:1033.

20. Simon M, Metschke M, Braune S, *et al.* (2013) Death after percutaneous dilatational tracheostomy: a systematic review and analysis of risk factors. *Crit Care*, 17:R258.

21. Even-Tov E, Koifman I, Rozentsvaig V, *et al.* (2017) Pre-procedural ultrasonography for tracheostomy in critically ill patients: a prospective study. *Isr Med Assoc J*, 19:337.

22. Kollig E, Heydenreich U, Roetman B, Hopf F, Muhr G (2000) Ultrasound and bronchoscopic controlled percutaneous tracheostomy on trauma ICU. *Injury*, 31:663.

23. Rajajee V, Fletcher JJ, Rochlen LR, Jacobs TL (2011) Real-time ultrasound-guided percutaneous dilatational tracheostomy: a feasibility study. *Crit Care*, 15:R67.

24. Rudas M, Seppelt I, Herkes R, Hislop R, Rajbhandari D, Weisbrodt L (2014) Traditional landmark versus ultrasound guided tracheal puncture during percutaneous dilatational tracheostomy in adult intensive care patients: a randomised controlled trial. *Crit Care*, 18:514.

25. Dinh VA, Farshidpanah S, Lu S, *et al.* (2014) Real-time sonographically guided percutaneous dilatational tracheostomy using a long-axis approach compared to the landmark technique. *J Ultrasound Med*, 33:1407.

26. Kleine-Brueggeney M, Greif R, Ross S, *et al.* (2011) Ultrasound-guided percutaneous tracheal puncture: a computer-tomographic controlled study in cadavers. *Br J Anaesth*, 106:738.

27. Gobatto AL, Besen BA, Tierno PF, *et al.* (2016) Ultrasound-guided percutaneous dilational tracheostomy versus bronchoscopy-guided percutaneous dilational tracheostomy in critically ill patients (TRACHUS): a randomized noninferiority controlled trial. *Intensive Care Med*, 42:342.

28. Petiot S, Guinot P-G, Diouf M, *et al.* (2017) Learning curve for real-time ultrasound-guided percutaneous tracheostomy. *Anaesth Crit Care Pain Med*, 36:279.

29. Ding LW, Wang HC, Wu HD, Chang CJ, Yang PC (2006) Laryngeal ultrasound: a useful method in predicting post-extubation stridor. A pilot study. *Eur Respir J*, 27:384.

CHAPTER 23

POCUS IN THE ASSESSMENT OF SHOCK

Ashraf Roshdy

The use of POCUS is rapidly expanding and its ability to contribute to a haemodynamic assessment is likely an important reason for this [1,2]. In 2014, the European Society of Intensive Care Medicine (ESICM) recommended echocardiography as a first line tool in the assessment of shock [3]. Whilst echocardiography remains the main modality, ultrasound of other organs can serve as an important adjuvant. In this chapter we highlight the unmatched potential of POCUS as a haemodynamic monitoring tool.

23.1 The shock state

Shock is a state of acute circulatory failure associated with significant morbidity and mortality. Treatment of the cause remains the cornerstone of management. However, the haemodynamic consequences can last significant time, risking hypoperfusion and multi-organ failure. In such cases, well-guided haemodynamic support is fundamental as a bridge to recovery until the cause is reversed.

Aetiologically, shock is divided into obstructive, distributive, hypovolaemic and cardiogenic. Whatever the type, three main physiological variables interplay to cause haemodynamic instability: fluid status, cardiac pump function, and vascular tone. The haemodynamic profile differs from patient to patient. Moreover, targeting one variable can affect the other two. As such, clinicians look to obtain real-time accurate and detailed haemodynamic data to guide tailored management, especially in complex and refractory cases.

23.2 The role of POCUS

No bedside tool is better than echocardiography at directly visualizing and assessing the heart. In fact, it serves a diagnostic as well as a haemodynamic role. In some circumstances it can be used as a stand-alone tool (e.g. resource limited and pre-hospital/emergency settings) where other haemodynamic monitors are not available. Alongside cardiac studies, ultrasound of other organs can also help to identify the underlying cause of shock (e.g. pneumonia in septic shock, tension pneumothorax, intra-abdominal collection) and to assess fluid tolerability.

23.3 Haemodynamic assessment with POCUS

POCUS is usually performed and interpreted by the treating physician. It should be applied early and integrated into the initial resuscitation. It can be utilized through three main approaches:

1. focused echocardiographic screening study

2. advanced comprehensive echocardiography

3. adjunct ultrasound exam of other relevant organs.

Different protocols exist with no clear boundaries between the three components. They can be performed in any order or integrated together into one study. This usually depends on the clinical case, the operator's skills and the available device.

23.4 Focused echocardiography

Facing a haemodynamically unstable patient, the treating clinician can perform a rapid screening study during the initial resuscitation. It usually takes only a few minutes and aims to:

- spot any obvious contributing cardiac pathology

- identify the need for an urgent comprehensive study, specialist referral and/or intervention.

An initial echocardiographic screening can yield useful information in less time than the application and calibration of most haemodynamic monitors [4]. Non-cardiologists can achieve the required competencies after a short training period (including simulation) and there are many simple, relatively cheap, and small devices available (e.g. hand-held ultrasound probes). A focused study should follow a goal-directed approach to answer a range of important clinical questions, such as:

1. Is there a significant pericardial effusion/tamponade?

2. Is there significant LV systolic dysfunction?

3. Is there acute cor pulmonale?

4. Is the patient fluid responsive?

If the operator is skilled in lung ultrasound, it can also answer a fifth question:

5. Is there evidence of a pneumothorax?

If a pneumothorax is present and the patient is haemodynamically unstable, this will require an urgent decompression (see *Chapters 11–13* for more detail on thoracic ultrasound).

Scenarios that need immediate management include:

- pericardiocentesis in cardiac tamponade
- thrombolysis for pulmonary embolism
- adaption of mechanical ventilator settings in acute cor pulmonale
- cardiology referral in acute myocardial infarction
- inotropes in cardiogenic shock
- decompression of a tension pneumothorax.

A focused study relies mainly on 2D imaging, although Doppler imaging can sometimes be useful. While not a continuous real-time monitor, serial studies can overcome this limitation, assessing response to treatment, and guiding further management.

23.5 Comprehensive echocardiography

A comprehensive study may be part of the initial assessment or follow a focused one (if any alarming pathology is flagged). It is also indicated if a haemodynamic monitor shows low cardiac output (CO) or signs of hypoperfusion (e.g. rising lactate) despite adequate filling and/or blood pressure. Some haemodynamic monitors can flag the need for such an examination (e.g. global ejection fraction and cardiac function index in PICCO). Comprehensive echocardiography should be performed by adequately trained and certified staff. In addition to its gold standard role as a cardiac diagnostic tool, echocardiography is useful in the assessment of preload and afterload.

The modality of choice is usually transthoracic echocardiography (TTE), but transoesophageal echocardiography (TOE) may also be used. While it mimics a formal full echocardiographic study, there is a need for special emphasis on haemodynamic indices, and usually serial exams. Nevertheless, subsequent studies can be more focused. The operator is usually a member of the treating team and, while they should be skilled in conducting the study, it is vital that they are also able to interpret the scan, integrate the findings with data from other haemodynamic monitors and formulate a management plan [5].

Broadly speaking comprehensive echocardiography has two main roles:

1. **diagnostic** – detect any structural cardiac pathology contributing to the shock

2. **haemodynamic** – guide haemodynamic management.

23.5.1 Diagnostic role

Any significant structural cardiac pathology (whether acute or chronic) can affect the haemodynamic management. It may sometimes be difficult to differentiate acute from chronic and an incidental diagnosis of a chronic cardiac pathology is not exceptional. *Table 23.1* shows some examples of echocardiographic findings and proposed management.

Table 23.1: Echocardiographic findings and impact on haemodynamic management

POCUS finding	Window/way to assess	Interpretation		Management	Further useful tests
		Acute	Chronic		
Left ventricle					
Impaired left ventricular systolic function	Eye-balling LV ejection fraction	Cardiogenic shock Septic cardiomyopathy Viral myocarditis	Chronic left ventricular dysfunction	Pharmacological – inotropes Mechanical support (e.g. IABP) Treatment of the cause (e.g. PCI)	Troponin ECG Coronary angiography
Regional wall motion abnormality	Eye-balling (17-segment assessment)	Acute MI Conduction defect (e.g. LBBB) Takotsubo cardiomyopathy	Previous MI Conduction defect (e.g. LBBB)	Urgent referral to intervention cardiology Medical ACS treatment	Troponin ECG
Ventricular septal defect	Colour Doppler CW Doppler	Mostly new MI if acute	Less probable (e.g. congenital heart disease)	Urgent referral to cardiology	TOE
LVOT obstruction	SAM of the anterior mitral leaflet CW Doppler Colour Doppler	Acquired LVOT obstruction Takotsubo cardiomyopathy	Chronic HOCM	Fluid (keep the LV filled) Beta-blockade	Serial echocardiography
Apical ballooning syndrome (takotsubo cardiomyopathy)	2D imaging (apical ballooning and hypercontractile base) Atypical forms exist and can involve the right ventricle	Stress cardiomyopathy	-	Exclusion of ACS	Troponin ECG Coronary angiography
Mural thrombus	2D imaging	Underlying MI or dilated cardiomyopathy Risk of arterial embolization		Anticoagulation	TOE
Valves					
Mitral regurgitation	Colour Doppler PISA	If acute think of acute ischaemia (+/− ruptured chordae) Infective endocarditis	Chronic MR	Vasopressors by way of increasing SVR may aggravate MR Cautious fluid resuscitation as risk of pulmonary oedema	Work-up for ACS and infective endocarditis
Mitral stenosis (chronic)	PW Doppler	−	Almost always chronic	Stroke volume depends on diastolic time Avoid tachycardia (BB) Usually associated with AF Cautious fluid resuscitation as risk of pulmonary oedema	−

Acute aortic regurgitation	CW Doppler	Infective endocarditis Aortic dissection	Chronic AR	High SVR may aggravate regurgitation Low DBP does not reflect low SVR	Work-up for ACS and infective endocarditis Aortic imaging (CT, TOE)
Aortic stenosis (chronic)	CW Doppler (Continuity equation)	–	Almost always chronic	Fixed cardiac output May respond to inotropes (pseudo-AS) Be aware of low flow low gradient states especially in shock patients Frequently associated with LVH and LV diastolic dysfunction	TOE
Tricuspid regurgitation	Colour Doppler CW doppler	Acute cor pulmonale	Pulmonary hypertension Dilated RV and TV annulus	Increased RAP High CVP and venous congestion	–
Vegetations	2D imaging	Infective endocarditis Risk of embolization	Can be subacute	Antimicrobials Cardiothoracic surgical referral	Blood culture TOE Serial echo
Right heart					
Dilated right ventricle with paradoxical septum	2D imaging Eye-balling	Acute cor pulmonale: (PE, ARDS)	Chronic pulmonary hypertension	Reduce RV afterload Thrombolysis/ thrombectomy/ anticoagulation	CTPA
Patent foramen ovale	Colour Doppler (SC view and TOE)	Chronic, but may become patent in context of an acute increase in pulmonary arterial pressure		Hypoxia Paradoxical embolization	TOE
Intra-cardiac thrombi	2D imaging Eye-balling	–	–	Risk of PE	–
McConnell's sign 60/60 sign	2D imaging CW of tricuspid valve PW of pulmonary valve	Differentiate acute PE from chronic pulmonary hypertension		Thrombolysis Thrombectomy Anticoagulation	CTPA
Others					
IVC	2D imaging M-mode	Fluid responsiveness Can reflect CVP		Fluid administration	Serial echocardiography

ACP: acute cor pulmonale; AF: atrial fibrillation; ARDS: acute respiratory distress syndrome; AV: aortic valve; BB: beta-blocker; CO: cardiac output; CT: computed tomography; CTPA: CT pulmonary angiography; CVP: central venous pressure; CW: continuous wave Doppler; HOCM: hypertrophic obstructive cardiomyopathy; IABP: intra-aortic balloon pump; IVC: inferior vena cava; LBBB: left bundle branch block; LV: left ventricle; LVOT: left ventricular outflow tract; MV: mitral valve; PCI: percutaneous coronary intervention; PE: pulmonary embolism; PFO: patent foramen ovale; PISA: proximal isovelocity surface area; PW: pulsed wave Doppler; RAP: right atrial pressure, RV: right ventricle; RWMA: regional wall motion abnormality; SAM: systolic anterior motion; SC: subcostal; SV: stroke volume; TOE: transoesophageal echocardiography; TV: tricuspid valve; VSD: ventricular septal defect

23.5.2 Haemodynamic role

A stepwise approach is again warranted (see *Figs 23.1–23.3*) [2]. As a general rule, it is important to target adequate haemodynamic parameters (i.e. supply meets demand) not normal values, and thus it is imperative the end-organ response to treatment is assessed.

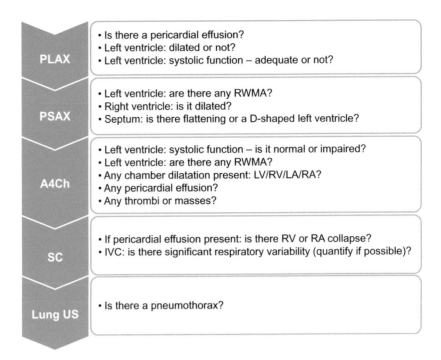

PLAX
- Is there a pericardial effusion?
- Left ventricle: dilated or not?
- Left ventricle: systolic function – adequate or not?

PSAX
- Left ventricle: are there any RWMA?
- Right ventricle: is it dilated?
- Septum: is there flattening or a D-shaped left ventricle?

A4Ch
- Left ventricle: systolic function – is it normal or impaired?
- Left ventricle: are there any RWMA?
- Any chamber dilatation present: LV/RV/LA/RA?
- Any pericardial effusion?
- Any thrombi or masses?

SC
- If pericardial effusion present: is there RV or RA collapse?
- IVC: is there significant respiratory variability (quantify if possible)?

Lung US
- Is there a pneumothorax?

Figure 23.1. Focused POCUS: Initial screening approach in shock state. IVC – inferior vena cava; LA – left atrium; LV – left ventricle; RA – right atrium; RV – right ventricle; RWMA – regional wall motion abnormality.

Step 1

The first step is to exclude **obstructive shock** which is usually amenable to immediate correction (e.g. cardiac tamponade, acute cor pulmonale, tension pneumothorax). Chest ultrasound can help spot if a pneumothorax is contributing to the haemodynamic instability. Whilst rare, acquired left ventricular outflow tract (LVOT) obstruction can be a cause especially in patients with left ventricular hypertrophy or those who are under-filled and on high inotropic support. In many instances, an obstructive contribution to the shock would never have been identified if an echocardiographic study had not been performed, with grave consequences for the patient.

Step 2

The second step is to quantify the **CO/stroke volume (SV)** or their indexed value, which echocardiography can do both accurately and precisely [6]. This second step can help differentiate between two types of shock: high and low cardiac output shock states (warm and cold shock). Hypoperfusion associated with high CO is usually seen in distributive shock. Clinicians should consider vasopressors if the patient has a low blood pressure and a low systemic vascular resistance (SVR). Otherwise, microcirculatory and cellular/mitochondrial dysfunction can be the underlying mechanism.

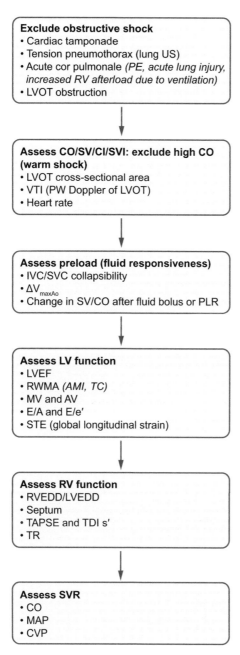

Exclude obstructive shock
- Cardiac tamponade
- Tension pneumothorax (lung US)
- Acute cor pulmonale *(PE, acute lung injury, increased RV afterload due to ventilation)*
- LVOT obstruction

Assess CO/SV/CI/SVI: exclude high CO (warm shock)
- LVOT cross-sectional area
- VTI (PW Doppler of LVOT)
- Heart rate

Assess preload (fluid responsiveness)
- IVC/SVC collapsibility
- ΔV_{maxAo}
- Change in SV/CO after fluid bolus or PLR

Assess LV function
- LVEF
- RWMA *(AMI, TC)*
- MV and AV
- E/A and E/e'
- STE (global longitudinal strain)

Assess RV function
- RVEDD/LVEDD
- Septum
- TAPSE and TDI s'
- TR

Assess SVR
- CO
- MAP
- CVP

Figure 23.2. Comprehensive echocardiograhic stepwise approach to the shocked state. AMI: acute myocardial infarction; AV: aortic valve; CO: cardiac output; CVP: central venous pressure, IVC: inferior vena cava; LV: left ventricle; LVEDA: LV end-diastolic area; LVEF: left ventricular ejection fraction; LVOT: LV outflow tract; MAP: mean arterial pressure; MV: mitral valve; PLR: passive leg raise; RV: right ventricle; RVEDA: RV end-diastolic area; RWMA: regional wall motion abnormality; STE: speckle tracking echocardiography, SV: stroke volume; SVC: superior vena cava; TAPSE: tricuspid annular plane systolic excursion; TC: takotsubo cardiomyopathy; TDI: tissue Doppler imaging; TR: tricuspid regurgitation; US: ultrasound; VTI: velocity–time integral

In most cases, shock is associated with low CO, where CO is the product of the SV and the heart rate. The SV can be calculated through the measurement of the LVOT and the velocity–time integral by pulsed wave Doppler (PWD):

$$SV = LVOT\ VTI \times LVOT\ cross\text{-}sectional\ area$$

$$CO = SV \times HR$$

$$SVR = (MAP - RAP/CO) \times 80$$

where: SV – stroke volume (ml); LVOT – left ventricular outflow tract (cm²); VTI – velocity–time integral (cm); CO – cardiac output (L/min); HR – heart rate (beats/min); SVR – systemic vascular resistance (dynes.sec/cm⁵); MAP – mean arterial pressure (mmHg); RAP – right atrial pressure (mmHg).

Calculating LVOT VTI: TTE is classically used for this. The same approach can be applied to the right ventricular outflow tract (RVOT) (parasternal short-axis view). TOE can also be used (LVOT diameter measurement in the mid-oesophageal long-axis view (LAX) and LVOT PWD in the deep trans-gastric LAX view) [7].

An LVOT VTI of >18cm is considered normal, but this will depend on many factors, most importantly the heart rate (HR) [7,8]. It has shown prognostic value in heart failure patients [9]. As the LVOT size does not dramatically change within short intervals, serial studies can track the change in VTI as a surrogate of the SV. This approach avoids mistakes in measuring LVOT, especially when serial studies are performed by different operators (i.e. inter-observer variability).

Heart rate: bradycardia should be excluded as a contributing factor (e.g. beta blocker or calcium channel blocker toxicity, profound hypothyroidism, and spinal injury/anaesthesia). If the HR is appropriate, the next step would be to investigate the reasons for a low SV, given that SV is determined by the interaction of the preload, afterload and cardiac contractility.

Step 3

The third step is to optimize the preload by assessing *fluid responsiveness* (FR). Only 50% of critically ill patients (beyond the initial resuscitation phase) are fluid responsive (FR+) [10], and so POCUS can improve current practice, given that studies have shown fluid therapy is given unguided in 50% of cases [11].

Respiratory failure is not rare in shocked patients and excessive fluid therapy may be associated with harm. Consequently, it would be wise to assess fluid tolerability in parallel to FR especially when the risk of pulmonary oedema is high (e.g. cardiogenic shock, pre-existing heart disease, septic shock associated with acute respiratory distress syndrome).

FR is defined as a 10–15% increase in SV/CO or a 10% increase in VTI (after giving 500ml fluid) [12]. Of note, the maximum effect of fluid therapy occurs within a few minutes, and thus POCUS should be available to detect any

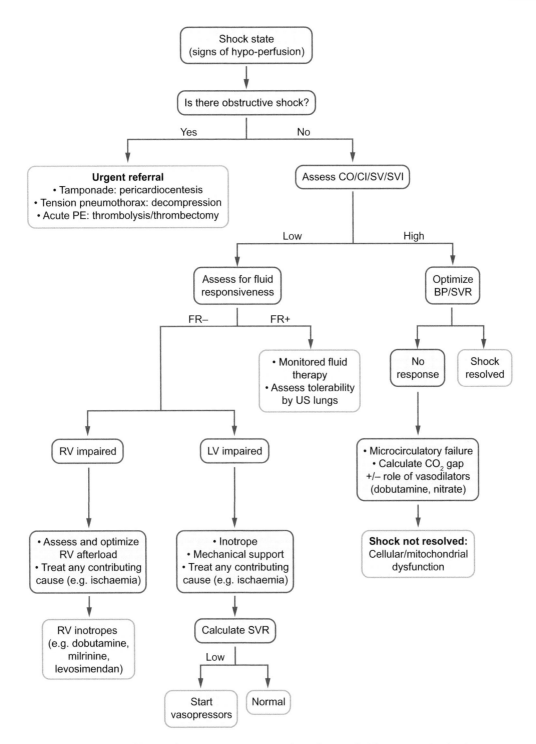

Figure 23.3. Advanced haemodynamic management algorithm guided by POCUS in shock state. BP: blood pressure; FR+: fluid responsive; FR–: non fluid responsive; CI: cardiac index; CO: cardiac output; LV: left ventricle; PE: pulmonary embolism; RV: right ventricle; SV: stroke volume; SVI: stroke volume index; SVR: systemic vascular resistance; US: ultrasound

potential effect within 1–3 minutes [13]. As a general principle, FR requires preserved biventricular function (i.e. cardiac muscle performing on the ascending limb of the Frank–Starling curve). Dynamic parameters outperform static ones (i.e. % change secondary to either a fluid bolus, positive pressure ventilation or a passive leg raise). Examples of static parameters include pulmonary capillary wedge pressure and ventricular end-diastolic volume. Dynamic echocardiographic parameters include:

- inferior vena cava (IVC) collapsibility (assessed using TTE)

- superior vena cava (SVC) collapsibility (assessed using TOE)

- maximal Doppler velocity in LVOT (ΔV_{maxAo}).

Both the IVC (TTE) and SVC (TOE) collapsibility share the same principle: greater venous collapsibility when squeezed by positive pressure ventilation indicates a potential benefit for volume expansion and hence FR. In mechanically ventilated patients, the cut-off value is >12% for the IVC and >36% for the SVC [14]. The evidence for spontaneously breathing patients is less clear (a suggested threshold for the IVC is >42%) [15,16]. FR can also be confirmed by observing a 10–15% increase in SV after a fluid bolus or PLR.

One study showed SVC collapsibility to be the most specific and ΔV_{maxAo} to have the highest sensitivity [14]. However, and in the author's experience, IVC collapsibility is the easiest, especially for novice users (SVC collapsibility, for example, requires a TOE study). It is important to note that a low tidal volume, low lung compliance, high intra-abdominal pressure and an open chest can affect the results and should be taken into consideration when interpreting them.

Fluid therapy should stop when the patient is no longer fluid responsive or the patient can no longer tolerate fluids, especially if they are not mechanically ventilated. Lung ultrasound or assessment of the LV filling pressure can be useful in such cases (see below). Serial measurements of the left ventricular filling pressure (e.g. E/e') is an alternative approach.

Whilst many other monitors can be used to investigate FR, echocardiography carries specific advantages:

- the feasibility of using IVC collapsibility during cardiac arrhythmias [16]

- by directly assessing RV function, echocardiography avoids the pitfalls of a false positive pulse pressure variation [17].

The next step after optimizing the preload is to assess the **LV and RV function** (in any order). Echocardiography is the gold standard tool to assess the heart and can discriminate LV from RV dysfunction.

Step 4
The fourth step is to **assess the left ventricle.**

LV systolic function: traditionally, LV ejection fraction (LVEF) is the parameter most commonly used to assess LV systolic function. However, a good understanding and correct interpretation in the context of shock is necessary [5]:

- LVEF reflects LV systolic function while CO reflects blood supply to other organs.

- A dilated heart with greater end-diastolic volume can pump adequate SV despite a mild to moderately reduced LVEF.

- Preload and afterload are important determinants of the LVEF. As such, its value can be significantly affected in the context of shock resuscitation.

- While LVEF was not clearly associated with poor outcome in severe sepsis, more subtle systolic changes detected by speckle tracking echocardiography showed a correlation (a less negative LV global longitudinal strain was associated with increased mortality) [18]. Speckle tracking echocardiography is a cardiac imaging technique that can detect myocardial strain and help overcome the limitations of LVEF. Its use is showing promise in intensive care, but it requires more resources and a high level of skill and experience and currently remains mainly a research tool.

It is important to differentiate chronic from acute heart failure as acute interventions can be indicated. If no old echocardiographic studies are available, LV dilatation and thin scarred walls may be a marker of chronicity.

If an inotropic treatment (e.g. dobutamine) is initiated, detection of a 20% increase in SV may reasonably be considered to be a positive inotropic response, although it may be more useful to consider end-organ perfusion parameters (e.g. lactate, urine output, central venous oxygen saturation) [19].

LV diastolic function: echocardiography has the unique advantage of measuring LV diastolic function [20]. Filling pressure is the hallmark of diastolic dysfunction in the absence of increased LV end-diastolic volume [21]. The LV filling pressure can be assessed by PWD and tissue Doppler (*E/A* ratio, *E/e'* ratio) and can guide fluid tolerability. In general, patients suffering diastolic dysfunction will tolerate less fluid therapy. An *E/A* ratio >2 and/or average *E/e'* ratio >14 are signs of increased left atrial pressure [21]. Assessment of LV diastolic function is discussed in more depth in *Chapter 7*.

Pulmonary capillary wedge pressure: PCWP is one of the static haemodynamic parameters. PCWP and LV filling pressure can be calculated during an echocardiographic study. This is done by using the PWD trace of the mitral inflow (maximum *E* velocity) and the tissue Doppler imaging (TDI) of the mitral annulus (maximum *e'* velocity) [22]:

$$PCWP = 1.24 \times (E/e') + 1.9$$

$$e' = (e'\ lateral + e'\ septal)/2$$

PCWP reflects the LV filling pressure and while not very useful when initiating fluid therapy, it can help in assessing fluid tolerability.

If the LV is impaired, the operator should look for an underlying cause including:

- acute coronary syndrome: regional wall motion abnormality

- acute myocarditis: global hypokinesia and sometimes a thickened LV wall

- septic cardiomyopathy: global hypokinesia, sometimes associated with a dilated LV; this can also affect diastolic function and the RV

- takotsubo cardiomyopathy: stress and excessive catecholamines can lead to apical ballooning syndrome associated with ECG changes (this may sometimes involve the RV too); classically, echocardiography shows a hypercontractile base, apical ballooning and sometimes LVOT obstruction

- infective endocarditis: vegetations or an aortic root abscess.

Step 5

The fifth step is to **assess the right ventricle.** The RV plays an important role in the haemodynamic profile and optimization of its function is crucial. The thinner muscular wall of the RV and lower elastance makes it very sensitive to any sudden change in afterload. Pulmonary disease (e.g. chronic obstructive pulmonary disease or acute respiratory distress syndrome), deranged blood gases (hypoxia, hypercapnia) or exposure to positive pressure ventilation can significantly increase the pulmonary vascular resistance (PVR) leading to RV pressure overload, dilatation, RV ischaemia and failure. The two ventricles are contained within the pericardium and are hence interdependent. A dilated RV can lead to LV diastolic dysfunction. A reduced RV SV in association with LV diastolic dysfunction will ultimately lead to a reduced CO.

When examining the RV, it is important to consider 3 conditions:

1. acute cor pulmonale

2. RV systolic dysfunction

3. moderate to severe tricuspid regurgitation.

Acute cor pulmonale: defined as:

- RV dilatation: RV and LV end-diastolic area ratio >0.6 (RVEDA/LVEDA >0.6)

and

- paradoxical interventricular septal motion.

In most cases, it is secondary to either a pulmonary embolism or acute respiratory distress syndrome.

- Pulmonary embolism (PE): echocardiography can rule in but not out PE [23]. RV dilatation usually occurs when pulmonary artery obstruction (as evidenced by CT) is more than 40%. An RVEDA/LVEDA ratio >0.6 has the best correlation to pulmonary arterial obstruction [24,25]. The incidence of acute cor pulmonale depends on the location of the PE: 87% in proximal versus 13% in sub-segmental PE [26]. In cases of RV dilatation and dysfunction, the treating clinician should balance the benefits and risks of thrombolysis.

  Acute RV failure leads to low RV SV. The pulmonary artery systolic pressure may not accurately reflect the severity of PE and PA obstruction because the increase of PVR is offset by the reduction in RV SV (flow) [24,27]:

$$Pressure = Flow \times Resistance.$$

  It is also important to differentiate acute PE from chronic pulmonary hypertension (e.g. the McConnell's and 60/60 signs) [28].

- Acute respiratory distress syndrome: acute cor pulmonale occurs in up to 50% of mechanically ventilated patients with severe acute respiratory distress syndrome [29]. Management is by reducing RV afterload (e.g. pulmonary vasodilators, PE treatment, the prone position, tuning of mechanical ventilation settings and avoiding hypoxia and hypercapnia).

RV systolic dysfunction. This can be assessed by measuring:

- tricuspid annular plane systolic excursion (TAPSE): normal ≥17 mm

- RV s': by tissue Doppler imaging, normal is ≥9cm/sec [30].

If RV systolic dysfunction persists after optimizing the RV afterload, inotropic support can be initiated. Assessment of the RV is discussed in more depth in *Chapter 8.*

Tricuspid regurgitation: this can be due to increased RV afterload (pulmonary hypertension) and RV dilatation. It can lead to a high central venous pressure (organ venous congestion) and reduces the gradient for venous return and hence FR.

Step 6
The sixth step is to **calculate the SVR**, to investigate the need to initiate/increase vasopressors. This can be done using the following equation:

$$SVR = (MAP – RAP/CO) \times 80$$

where: MAP – mean arterial pressure; RAP – right atrial pressure.

23.6 Ultrasound of other organs

Combining multi-organ POCUS with echocardiography in the acute setting can save time and direct the clinician towards a more tailored management plan. Examples which may be of particular importance include the following.

- **Lung ultrasound** looking for:

  - pneumothorax: to identify a tension pneumothorax as the cause of haemodynamic instability
  - pulmonary congestion: may be suggestive of cardiogenic shock and less fluid tolerability, especially if not yet intubated
  - pulmonary consolidation: to identify pneumonia as a potential cause of sepsis
  - pleural effusion: to identify an empyema as a potential cause of sepsis.

- **Vascular ultrasound:** to assess for the presence of DVT in cases of pulmonary embolism and acute cor pulmonale.

- **Abdominal ultrasound:** to identify the presence of intra-abdominal fluid or collections in abdominal sepsis, trauma, a ruptured abdominal aortic aneurysm or ectopic pregnancy.

- **Urinary tract ultrasound:** to assess the bladder, look for hydroureter/ obstruction and calculate the renal resistive index.

The extent of the multi-organ ultrasound examination possible will depend on the operator's skills and local protocols. The use of full body ultrasound is integrated into many focused protocols, including the Focused Ultrasound in Intensive Care (FUSIC) modules and Jean-François Lanctôt et al.'s Echo-Guided Life Support [31].

23.7 POCUS-guided haemodynamic interventions

In some cases, POCUS can guide necessary haemodynamic interventions, including:

- mechanical circulatory support

- pericardiocentesis

- thrombolysis in pulmonary embolism

- prosthetic valve thrombolysis monitoring.

23.7.1 Septic shock

Septic shock has arguably the most complex pathophysiology: hypovolaemia (relative or absolute), vasoplegia and myocardial dysfunction (e.g. septic cardiomyopathy) may all interplay. Five different haemodynamic patterns can prevail:

- hyperkinetic

- persistent fluid responsiveness

- well resuscitated

- predominant LV dysfunction

- severe RV failure [32].

On top of the macrovascular derangement, microcirculatory, cellular and mitochondrial dysfunctions can also be present.

23.7.2 Valvular lesions

It is important to assess all four cardiac valves. In most cases, the pathology is chronic. However, it can have a significant impact on haemodynamic data and management (e.g. severe mitral regurgitation/aortic regurgitation may be associated with a hyperkinetic LV but be directing the flow in the wrong direction) (*Table 23.1*).

23.8 Advantages and limitations of POCUS in the assessment of shock

23.8.1 Advantages

A focused study is widely feasible. The setup can be as short as five minutes, outperforming most invasive and non-invasive haemodynamic monitors [4]. POCUS is non-invasive and can be applied in numerous different settings (e.g. pre-hospital, the emergency department, acute medical wards, perioperative or on intensive care units) with negligible side-effects. Apart from guiding shock management, POCUS haemodynamic data can be used to assess volume status, help perioperative optimization, adjust mechanical ventilator settings, and guide mechanical cardiac support.

Many devices are available including ultra-portable hand-held probes. Once the machine has been purchased, the cost of maintenance and training is low, which has allowed increasing use in resource-limited settings where advanced haemodynamic monitors are less accessible. The availability of multiple probes and software means the machines can usually also serve other purposes (e.g. vascular access, assessment of lung disease, abdominal scanning, etc.).

A comprehensive study is more likely to be undertaken in the intensive care unit and takes longer to perform (30–45 minutes), needs a skilled operator and more sophisticated machines. Echocardiography is unique in detecting certain pathologies: cardiac tamponade, LVOT obstruction and diastolic dysfunction. Classically, the approach is TTE, however, a TOE may be necessary and should be part of any advanced CCE certification. TOE can often provide better windows and is less operator-dependent.

A further advantage of echocardiography is its ability to act as both a diagnostic and a monitoring tool. It can diagnose the cause of haemodynamic instability and has an advantage over most other haemodynamic monitors (with the exception of a pulmonary artery catheter) in that it can assess the right and left side of the heart separately.

While acute physicians may be less skilled at echocardiography than cardiologists and sonographers, the most striking benefit remains the immediate integration of the findings into the patient management, because in most cases the operator is the managing physician [5]. This was demonstrated during the Covid-19 pandemic, when POCUS reduced the risk of transport and cross-contamination while providing immediate data for the treating teams.

23.8.2 Limitations

The limits include its non-continuous nature and operator dependency (with huge variability in training across specialties and countries). To overcome its non-continuous nature, POCUS is usually performed in a serial pattern allowing regular review of a patient's response to treatment.

Arguably the most important limit is incorrect interpretation of findings in the context of sub-optimal windows and inexperience, with the risk that less experienced operators may miss a significant pathology (e.g. vegetations, a ventricular septal defect, patent foramen ovale or significant valvular pathology) [5].

23.8.3 Quality measures

The use of structured reporting and vigilant digital storage are useful for training, follow-up, re-interpretation and quality improvement. It is also important to report the conditions under which the POCUS study was performed (e.g. mechanical ventilation, inotropes, sedation, etc.).

If a structural pathology has been identified, it is useful to confirm the findings after discharge from the intensive care unit with a repeat echocardiographic study.

23.9 Summary

POCUS has proved its role as a valuable tool in assessing the shocked patient. This role starts at the initial resuscitation and extends to the follow-up of patients. It is important for POCUS operators to follow a structured approach to ensure it is used to its full potential. Its popularity and value will likely continue to expand as the technology surrounding it advances.

23.10 References

1. Hüttemann E, Schelenz C, Kara F, *et al.* (2004) The use and safety of transesophageal echocardiography in the general ICU – a minireview. *Acta Anaesthesiol Scand*, 48:827.

2. Roshdy A, Francisco N, Rendon A, Gillon S, Walker D (2014) Critical Care Echo Rounds: Haemodynamic instability. *Echo Res Pract*, 1:D1.

3. Cecconi M, De Backer D, Antonelli M, *et al.* (2014) Consensus on circulatory shock and hemodynamic monitoring. Task force of the European Society of Intensive Care Medicine. *Intensive Care Med*, 40:1795.

4. Volpicelli G, Lamorte A, Tullio M, *et al.* (2013) Point-of-care multiorgan ultrasonography for the evaluation of undifferentiated hypotension in the emergency department. *Intensive Care Med*, 39:1290.

5. Roshdy A (2018) Echodynamics: interpretation, limitations, and clinical integration! *J Intensive Care Med*, 33:439.

6. Mercado P, Maizel J, Beyls C, *et al.* (2017) Transthoracic echocardiography: an accurate and precise method for estimating cardiac output in the critically ill patient. *Crit Care*, 21:136.

7. Porter TR, Shillcutt SK, Adams MS, *et al.* (2015) Guidelines for the use of echocardiography as a monitor for therapeutic intervention in adults: a report from the American Society of Echocardiography. *J Am Soc Echocardiogr*, 28:40.

8. Blanco P, Aguiar FM, Blaivas M (2015) Rapid Ultrasound in Shock (RUSH) Velocity–Time Integral. *J Ultrasound Med*, 34:1691.

9. Tan C, Rubenson D, Srivastava A, *et al.* (2017) Left ventricular outflow tract velocity time integral outperforms ejection fraction and Doppler-derived cardiac output for predicting outcomes in a select advanced heart failure cohort. *Cardiovasc Ultrasound*, 15:18.

10. Michard F, Teboul JL (2002) Predicting fluid responsiveness in ICU patients: a critical analysis of the evidence. *Chest*, 121:2000.

11. Cecconi M, Hofer C, Teboul JL, *et al.* (2015) Fluid challenge in intensive care: the FENICE study. A global inception cohort study. *Intensive Care Med*, 41:1529.

12. Monnet X, Rienzo M, Osman D, *et al.* (2006) Passive leg raising predicts fluid responsiveness in the critically ill. *Crit Care Med*, 34:1402.

13. Aya HD, Ster IC, Fletcher N, Grounds RM, Rhodes A, Cecconi M (2016) Pharmacodynamic analysis of a fluid challenge. *Crit Care Med*, 44:880.

14. Vignon P, Repesse X, Begot E, *et al.* (2017) Comparison of echocardiographic indices used to predict fluid responsiveness in ventilated patients. *Am J Respir Crit Care Med*, 195:1022.

15. Corl K, Napoli AM, Gardiner F (2012) Bedside sonographic measurement of the inferior vena cava caval index is a poor predictor of fluid responsiveness in emergency department patients. *Emerg Med Australas*, 24:534.

16. Airapetian N, Maizel J, Alyamani O, *et al.* (2015) Does inferior vena cava respiratory variability predict fluid responsiveness in spontaneously breathing patients? *Crit Care*, 19:400.

17. He HW, Liu DW (2015) The pitfall of pulse pressure variation in the cardiac dysfunction condition. *Crit Care*, 19:242.

18. Sanfilippo F, Corredor C, Fletcher N, *et al.* (2018) Left ventricular systolic function evaluated by strain echocardiography and relationship with mortality in patients with severe sepsis or septic shock: a systematic review and meta-analysis. *Crit Care*, 22:183.

19. Nishimura RA, Grantham JA, Connolly HM, Schaff HV, Higano ST, Holmes DR (2002) Low-output, low-gradient aortic stenosis in patients with depressed left ventricular systolic function: the clinical utility of the dobutamine challenge in the catheterization laboratory. *Circulation*, 106:809.

20. Vieillard-Baron A, Millington SJ, Sanfilippo F, *et al.* (2019) A decade of progress in critical care echocardiography: a narrative review. *Intensive Care Med*, 45:770.

21. Nagueh SF, Smiseth OA, Appleton CP, *et al.* (2016) Recommendations for the evaluation of left ventricular diastolic function by echocardiography. *J Am Soc Echocardiogr*, 29:277.

22. Nagueh SF, Middleton KJ, Kopelen HA, Zoghbi WA, Quiñones MA (1997) Doppler tissue imaging: a noninvasive technique for evaluation of left ventricular relaxation and estimation of filling pressures. *J Am Coll Cardiol*, 30:1527.

23. Fields JM, Davis J, Girson L, *et al.* (2017) Transthoracic echocardiography for diagnosing pulmonary embolism: a systematic review and meta-analysis. *J Am Soc Echocardiogr*, 30:714.

24. Mansencal N, Joseph T, Vieillard-Baron A, *et al.* (2003) Comparison of different echocardiographic indices secondary to right ventricular obstruction in acute pulmonary embolism. *Am J Cardiol*, 92:116.

25. Qanadli SD, El Hajjam M, Vieillard-Baron A, *et al.* (2001) New CT index to quantify arterial obstruction in pulmonary embolism: comparison with angiographic index and echocardiography. *Am J Roentgenol*, 176:1415.

26. Mansencal N, Redheuil A, Joseph T, *et al.* (2004) Use of transthoracic echocardiography combined with venous ultrasonography in patients with pulmonary embolism. *Int J Cardiol*, 96:59.

27. McIntyre KM, Sasahara AA (1977) The ratio of pulmonary arterial pressure to pulmonary vascular obstruction: index of preembolic cardiopulmonary status. *Chest*, 71:692.

28. Kurzyna M, Torbicki A, Pruszczyk P, *et al.* (2002) Disturbed right ventricular ejection pattern as a new Doppler echocardiographic sign of acute pulmonary embolism. *Am J Cardiol*, 90:507.

29. Vieillard-Baron A, Price LC, Matthay MA (2013) Acute cor pulmonale in ARDS. *Intensive Care Med*, 39:1836.

30. Harkness A, Ring L, Augustine D, *et al.* (2020) Normal reference intervals for cardiac dimensions and function for use in echocardiographic practice: a guideline from the British Society of Echocardiography. *Echo Res Pract*, 7:G1.

31. Lanctôt JF, Valois M Beaulieu Y (2011) EGLS: Echo-guided life support. *Crit Ultrasound J*, 3:123.

32. Geri G, Vignon P, Aubry A, *et al.* (2019) Cardiovascular clusters in septic shock combining clinical and echocardiographic parameters: a post hoc analysis. *Intensive Care Med*, 45:657.

CHAPTER 24

POCUS ASSESSMENT OF FLUID STATUS

Olusegun Olusanya & Ashley Miller

24.1 The concept of 'volume status'

The fluid volumes of various body compartments (blood, interstitium, lung) have been a central concept to the management of the critically ill since the early days of Max Harry Weil and the 'Shock Unit' [1]. Successful navigation of shock requires the manipulation of these volumes, either by replenishing plasma and extracellular fluids, removal of oedema, or both.

The phrase 'volume status' is commonly used to refer to intravascular volume, which is estimated to be around 70ml/kg in the adult male [2]. In some cases, this refers to total body water (which is normally around 60% of body weight). The terms 'dehydration' and 'hypovolaemia' are used interchangeably to refer to a state of reduced volume status; however, the two terms are not equivalent. Dehydration is a term commonly used to suggest an absolute deficit in body water; this can be hypertonic (such as is seen with insufficient drinking), or isotonic (as can be seen with diarrhoeal losses). The definition of dehydration is complex and inconsistent, and relying on this term could lead to inappropriate intervention. The term 'hypovolaemia' should be reserved to refer specifically to intravascular volume depletion. While this may be a sequela to isotonic dehydration, the two are not synonymous [2,3]. In this chapter we will delve into these concepts and discuss how ultrasound can be used in the management of volume in the critically ill.

24.2 Total body water and its compartments

As mentioned earlier, in the adult male total body water is about 60% of body weight. This body water is then divided between extracellular and intracellular compartments in a proportion of 1:2. Extracellular fluid is then further divided into interstitial fluid (which is about 80%) and intravascular fluid which comprises the remaining 20% (*Fig. 24.1*) [3].

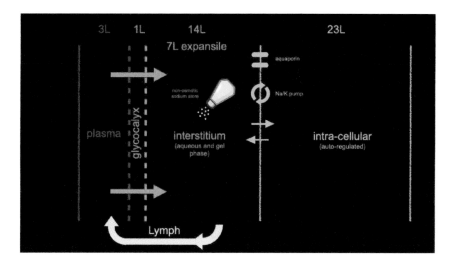

Figure 24.1: Total body water and its constituents.

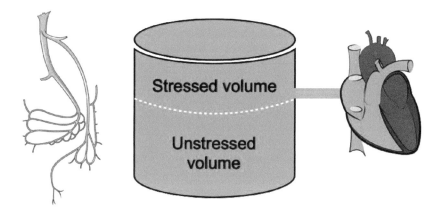

Figure 24.2. Total body water and a Guytonian model of the circulation.

Blood volume is of particular interest, because this is the volume of fluid involved in oxygen delivery. The heart as a pump is designed to circulate this blood volume, and usually circulates the total blood volume around every minute as the cardiac output. Thus, oxygen delivery can be calculated by the equation below:

$$oxygen\ delivery = oxygen\ content \times cardiac\ output$$

Blood volume can further be conceptually divided into two compartments:

- the stressed volume, which is the volume of venous return that actively 'pressurizes' the vessels

- the unstressed volume, which is the blood pooled in the splanchnic veins that can be mobilized during exercise or physiological stress by modulating vascular tone [4].

With the above, one can see how the measurement of absolute 'volume status' becomes challenging. Which component does one measure, total body water, extracellular fluid, plasma volume or stressed volume?

A detailed discussion of this is beyond the scope of this text; for simplicity, for the rest of the chapter we will focus on methods of assessing plasma volume and stressed volume. Various ultrasound modalities can be used including echocardiography (both transthoracic (TTE) and transoesophageal (TOE)), lung ultrasound, and abdominal imaging. A skilled practitioner will combine multiple parameters to give an accurate assessment and guide therapy in the critically unwell patient.

24.3 Static assessments of volume status

If we think of the stressed volume as a 'tank', as demonstrated in *Figure 24.2*, we can estimate how much fluid is present in a distensible tank by measuring the size of the chambers.

Cardiac imaging would fulfil this purpose. Direct heart visualization ('eyeballing') can give an impression of volume status, especially with experienced eyes. A low stressed volume results in relatively empty cardiac chambers, with the left ventricle becoming hyperdynamic and the walls meeting (or 'kissing') in systole. The inferior and superior vena cavae give some reflection of venous return, and collapse when venous return is low. In situations of volume overload, the opposite is seen – the heart chambers and vena cavae become dilated.

These states can be quantified for those with an advanced skillset in echocardiography. Ventricular end-diastolic area can be measured and has been shown to correlate particularly well with low stressed volume states [5]. A measurement of inferior vena cava (IVC) diameter can be performed, with an IVC expiratory diameter of <1cm correlating with a low stressed volume [6]. Echocardiography can be used to measure stroke volume, either via 2D methods (Teicholz, Simpson's method of discs), 3D methods, or Doppler. A hyperdynamic heart with a low stroke volume is strongly suggestive of a low stressed volume state.

Outside the heart, the hepatic portal vein is easily visualized via a transhepatic window. An absolute portal vein velocity of <20cm/sec is suggestive of low preload; however, this must be interpreted in context of the rest of the patient [7].

24.4 Fluid responsiveness

Estimating absolute volumes with ultrasound is remarkably difficult, as one can imagine; fluid is trapped in multiple compartments, not all of which can be visualized. Arguably in the ICU in a shocked patient we are not interested in absolute compartment volumes – what we want to know is whether this shock state can be improved with the administration of volume, so-called 'volume responsiveness' [8].

A patient is termed 'volume responsive' when the administration of a fixed volume of fluid (normally 250–500ml, or 10–20ml/kg) results in an increase in stroke volume of 10–15% (*Figs 24.3* and *24.4*) [9]. To demonstrate this, a cardiac output monitor is required, and the patient needs to be observed during the administration of the fluid bolus, normally performed over 5–30 minutes.

Ultrasonography is well suited to assessing volume responsiveness during a fluid challenge. The gold standard is to directly measure cardiac output before or after the challenge, through a measurement of stroke volume [8,9]. In the critically unwell, left ventricular outflow tract (LVOT) or right ventricular outflow tract (RVOT) Doppler are the most accurate ways of assessing this. To fully assess this, an accurate measurement of the LVOT diameter is required; Simpson's method of discs or 4D stroke volume measurements can also be used in patients with excellent windows.

Several surrogate measures exist for stroke volume. The velocity–time integral (VTI) and/or peak velocities of the LVOT or RVOT would also increase with a fluid challenge and are simpler to measure. In the same vein, peak velocity of ascending or descending aortic flow can be used. In patients with challenging echocardiographic windows, peripheral arteries can be monitored – carotid, brachial, and femoral peak velocities/VTI have been studied for this purpose [10,11].

It is important to recognize that fluid responsiveness exists as part of the normal physiological spectrum [12]; this is discussed further below.

24.5 Dynamic measures of volume status

In patients who are hypovolaemic and mechanically ventilated, heart–lung interactions become exaggerated, leading to a visible variation in left- and right-sided stroke volumes with inspiration and expiration [13]. Such 'stroke volume variation' (SVV) can easily be visualized with ultrasound. This involves interrogating the LVOT or RVOT with pulsed wave Doppler (PWD) on a low sweep speed setting and monitoring the peak velocity (or VTI) in inspiration and expiration. SVV can also be demonstrated using mitral or tricuspid inflows, or outside the heart by interrogating carotid, brachial, or femoral arteries [14].

A passive leg raise allows for an autotransfusion of roughly 300ml of blood from the lower extremities [15]. This autotransfusion is reversed on restoring the patient to their original position, making passive leg raise an extremely attractive option for assessing fluid responsiveness without giving fluid. The changes in stroke volume are easily assessed with ultrasound using the same techniques as above.

A slightly different way of assessing fluid responsiveness with ultrasonography is by assessing the superior and inferior vena cavae [16]. In the mechanically ventilated patient, the SVC will distend with insufflation of the lungs, and collapse in expiration; the IVC performs the opposite. An SVC distensibility index of more than 36%, and an IVC collapsibility index of more than 18% have both been shown to be predictive of fluid responsiveness [16]. As attractive as this assessment may seem, they are sadly limited – the SVC is best assessed via TOE, and both indices are poorly validated in the awake patient [17].

To assess fluid responsiveness using heart–lung interactions, several criteria must be present: the patient must be ventilated at 8ml/kg of ideal body weight or more, must have an intact thorax, no intra-abdominal hypertension, and must be in sinus rhythm. Unfortunately this excludes a significant majority of intensive care patients [18]. If the tidal volumes are lower, they can be transiently increased to allow the detection of fluid responsiveness – a so-called 'tidal volume challenge'. Flow from the ventilator can also be interrupted at end-inspiration (or end-expiration) to exaggerate heart–lung interactions and potentially unmask fluid responsiveness [19].

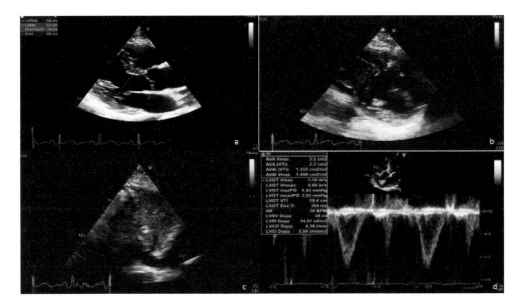

Figure 24.3. Normal circulation. (a) and b) Normal left ventricular cavity size. (c) Normal inferior vena cava size. (d) Normal stroke volume as measured by Doppler; velocity–time integral (VTI) 18.4cm, stroke volume 58ml, cardiac output 4.39L/min.

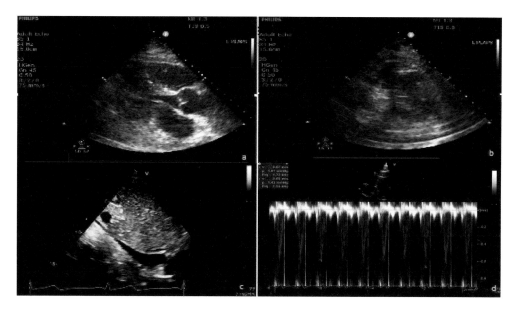

Figure 24.4. High likelihood of fluid response. (a) and b) Show a small collapsed left ventricular cavity in systole. (c) Collapsed inferior vena cava. (d) Significant respiratory left ventricular outflow tract peak velocity variation.

24.6 Fluid tolerance and fluid excess

Due to the limitations of assessments of fluid responsiveness, especially in awake patients, some people prefer the concept of 'fluid tolerance'. Rather than assessing for a potential increase in stroke volume with fluid, a global assessment of whether the patient can safely tolerate fluid loading may be a much more pragmatic and valuable approach [20].

Assessment of fluid tolerance involves assessing for fluid 'stop points' – essentially looking for signs of fluid excess, or near excess. Signs of fluid excess can be divided into right-sided changes, left-sided changes, and other organs (*Fig. 24.5*).

24.6.1 Right-sided changes

Fluid overload results in increased venous pressures which are easily detected on ultrasound, either visually or with PWD. Venous congestion can be seen in the IVC, which will dilate beyond 2cm. The jugular veins and hepatic veins also become dilated, with an altered PWD wave form. The portal vein velocities change, and the portal vein becomes increasingly pulsatile. Veins in encapsulated organs like the spleen, kidneys, and cerebral vessels also change their flow patterns and become pulsatile [21].

The Venous Excess Ultrasound (VExUS) score is a recent semi-quantitative system, which uses the IVC, hepatic veins, portal vein, and renal vein to assess the degree of right-sided volume overload. It has been shown to

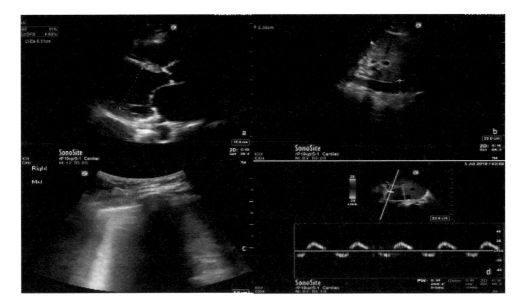

Figure 24.5. Volume overloaded circulation. (a) Significantly dilated left ventricle (6.31cm). (b) Dilated inferior vena cava (2.38cm). (c) B-line lung profile. (d) Pulsatile portal vein with flow reversal in diastole.

correlate with renal outcomes in a study of critically ill patients, with further studies in progress [22].

Performing VExUS can be split into the following main steps.

- **Step 1 – assessment of the IVC:** the IVC longitudinal diameter should be measured as previously described, and if it is <2cm then the exam can be stopped because no significant venous congestion is present. If the IVC diameter is ≥2cm then venous congestion may be present and the examination should be continued.

- **Step 2 – assessment of hepatic vein flow:** here, once one of the three hepatic veins has been identified, PWD is placed over it at its coalescence with the IVC. The PWD findings can then be interpreted as demonstrated in *Figure 24.6*.

- **Step 3 – assessment of portal vein flow:** once identified, PWD should be placed over the portal vein and the findings interpreted as demonstrated in *Figure 24.6*.

- **Step 4 – assessment of intrarenal venous flow:** interlobar renal vessels should be identified, aided by colour flow Doppler, with PWD then placed over the vessel with the best signal. The venous component of the Doppler signal is the more important here and interpreted as per the waveforms demonstrated in *Figure 24.6*.

- **Calculating the VExUS score:** the above findings are then combined, as demonstrated in *Figure 24.6*, to give a VExUS score from Grade 0 (no congestion) through to Grade 3 (severe congestion).

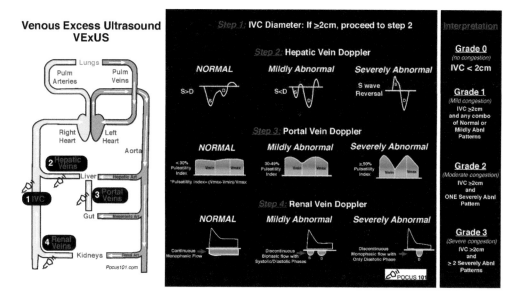

Figure 24.6. Demonstration of how to perform and interpret VExUS. Reproduced with kind permission from www.pocus101.com/vexus-ultrasound-score-fluid-overload-and-venous-congestion-assessment/.

24.6.2 Left-sided changes

Volume overload may result in a raised left atrial pressure, which can be seen as an increase in mitral inflow velocity (an '*E* wave' above 1.2m/sec is suggestive of volume overload), a dilated left atrium, or B-lines on lung ultrasonography [23].

24.6.3 Other organs

Ultrasound can detect subcutaneous oedema, ascites, and organ oedema (e.g. gallbladder wall thickening) which are all signs of volume overload. As a result, ultrasound can be used to direct diuresis, and there is increasing data showing the superiority of an ultrasound-guided approach over traditional markers such as clinical examination or weight-based assessments [24].

24.7 Pitfalls in volume state assessment with ultrasound

These can be classified as errors in image acquisition, errors in image interpretation, and errors in clinical integration (*Fig. 24.7*).

24.7.1 Image acquisition

Errors in stroke volume measurement
Every effort should be made to ensure pinpoint accuracy of measurements, using either Simpson's method or LVOT VTI. Due to the nature of the

calculations, any errors (particularly those of LVOT diameter) will be amplified, resulting in significant over- or underestimates of stroke volume [25].

Errors in measuring changes in stroke volume

Following an intervention such as a passive leg raise or fluid bolus, reassessments of stroke volume to assess fluid responsiveness require the patient and probe to be in almost exactly the same position, and ideally should be performed by the same operator. Changes in any of these can lead to drifts in measurement and inaccuracy [25].

Incorrect Doppler angles

This can affect stroke volume assessment using VTI, and VExUS assessments. Angle correction should be used wherever possible, and colour flow Doppler (CFD) used to ensure that the Doppler cursor is truly aligned with the direction of flow [25].

24.7.2 Image interpretation

Mistaking the inferior vena cava for the aorta

This is particularly relevant in profoundly hypovolaemic patients where the IVC can be difficult to appreciate [26]. Care should be taken to ensure the proper vessel is identified; both by anatomical relationships (the IVC can be identified using its conjunction with the hepatic veins and right atrium) and CFD.

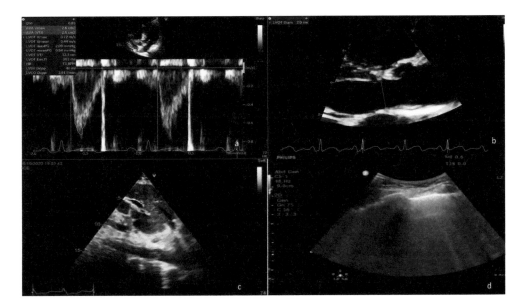

Figure 24.7. Pitfalls in fluid assessment. (a) and b) Importance of accuracy in stroke volume assessment; this demonstrates an accurately placed pulsed wave Doppler in the left ventricular outflow tract (LVOT) (showing a closing click), an accurate trace, and an accurate LVOT diameter measured at the level of the aortic valve cusps. (c) Descending aorta – easily mistaken for the IVC. (d) B-line profile in a Covid-19 patient, that could easily be mistaken for pulmonary oedema.

Mistaking the IVC for hepatic veins

This can be very easily done, as all three hepatic veins connect to the right atrium. This mistake may be avoided by assessing the IVC in both long- and short-axis, thus ensuring the correct vessel is assessed.

Interpreting all B-lines as fluid overload

An 'interstitial syndrome' profile can be generated by several other conditions – infection, viral pneumonitis, and pulmonary fibrosis [27]. Close attention needs to be paid to the patient's history, the appearances of the pleural line, and the presence or absence of effusions to help quantify this. Nonetheless, the presence of B-lines should encourage caution with further fluid administration because it is most likely related to the presence of increased extravascular lung water [28].

24.7.3 Clinical integration

Presuming all 'fluid responsiveness' must be treated with fluid

This is one of the biggest pitfalls. Approximately 50% of normal healthy people are fluid responsive [12]. Many conditions can give false positives for fluid responsiveness (right ventricular failure, constrictive pericarditis, abdominal compartment syndrome). This can lead to unnecessary fluid administration and cause harm. More than this, a state of volume non-responsiveness is *abnormal* – administering large amounts of fluid to reach such a state is likely to result in venous congestion and harm.

Acting on single parameters

A dilated IVC in a hypotensive patient does not eliminate the potential benefit from volume expansion. For instance, this can be a normal finding in some individuals (e.g. athletes) and can be seen in anaphylaxis. Conversely, a small IVC can be seen in some forms of volume overload, particularly some forms of sympathetically mediated acute pulmonary oedema. A holistic approach to the assessment of fluid status is necessary. Use every parameter available to you and treat the patient, not the ultrasound images.

24.8 Summary

Volume status is difficult to define and measure in the critically ill; the phrase normally refers to the 'stressed volume' of blood. Rather than measuring absolute volume status, it is more pragmatic to assess volume responsiveness, tolerance, and signs of overload. Ultrasound is well suited to assess the above three categories of volume. Echocardiography is the mainstay of this, but lung ultrasound and imaging of solid organs can also be used. Just because a patient is volume responsive does not mean they need fluid. When all else fails, put the probe down and be a clinician.

24.9 References

1. Weil MH, Henning RJ (1979) New concepts in the diagnosis and fluid treatment of circulatory shock. Thirteenth annual Becton, Dickinson and Company Oscar Schwidetsky Memorial Lecture. *Anesth Analg*, 16:124.

2. Pain RW (1977) Body fluid compartments. *Anaesth Intensive Care*, 5:284.

3. Lacey J, Corbett J, Forni L, *et al.* (2019) A multidisciplinary consensus on dehydration: definitions, diagnostic methods and clinical implications. *Annals Med*, 51:232.

4. Maas J (2015) Mean systemic filling pressure: its measurement and meaning. *Neth J Crit Care*, 19:6.

5. Slama M, Maizel J (2011) Assessment of fluid requirements: fluid responsiveness. In *Hemodynamic Monitoring Using Echocardiography in the Critically Ill*, De Backer D, *et al.* (eds). Springer-Verlag, Heidelberg.

6. Kitakule M, Mayo P (2010) Use of ultrasound to assess fluid responsiveness in the intensive care unit. *Open Crit Care Med J*, 3:33.

7. Denault AY, Personal communication.

8. Miller A, Mandeville J (2016) Predicting and measuring fluid responsiveness with echocardiography. *Echo Res Pract*, 3(2):G1.

9. Cecconi M , Parsons AK, Rhodes A (2011) What is a fluid challenge? *Curr Op Crit Care*, 17:290.

10. Kim D-H, Shin S, Kim N, Choi T, Choi SH, Choi YS (2018) Carotid ultrasound measurements for assessing fluid responsiveness in spontaneously breathing patients: corrected flow time and respirophasic variation in blood flow peak velocity. *Br J Anaesth*, 121:541.

11. Monge García MI, Gil Cano A, Díaz Monrové JC (2009) Brachial artery peak velocity variation to predict fluid responsiveness in mechanically ventilated patients. *Crit Care*, 13:R142.

12. Godfrey GEP, Dubrey SW, Handy JM (2014) A prospective observational study of stroke volume responsiveness to a passive leg raise manoeuvre in healthy non-starved volunteers as assessed by transthoracic echocardiography. *Anaesthesia*, 69:306.

13. Desai N, Garry D (2018) Assessing dynamic fluid responsive using transthoracic echocardiography in intensive care. *BJA Education*, 18:218.

14. Kenny J-ÉS, Barjaktarevic I, Eibl AM, *et al.* (2020) A carotid Doppler patch accurately tracks stroke volume changes during a preload-modifying maneuver in healthy volunteers. *Crit Care Explorations*, 2:e0072.

15. Monnet X, Teboul JL (2015) Passive leg raising: five rules, not a drop of fluid! *Crit Care*, 19:18.

16. Vignon P, Repessé X, Bégot E, *et al.* (2017) Comparison of echocardiographic indices used to predict fluid responsiveness in ventilated patients. *Am J Respir Crit Care Med*, 195:1022.

17. Millington SJ (2019) Ultrasound assessment of the inferior vena cava for fluid responsiveness: easy, fun, but unlikely to be helpful. *Can J Anesth*, 66:633.

18. Delannoy B, Wallet F, Maucort-Boulch D, *et al.* (2016) Applicability of pulse pressure variation during unstable hemodynamic events in the intensive care unit: a five-day prospective multicenter study. *Crit Care Res Pract,* 2016:7162190.

19. Gavelli F, Teboul JL, Monnet X (2019) The end-expiratory occlusion test: please, let me hold your breath! *Crit Care,* 23:274.

20. Rola P (2016) Volume responsiveness and volume tolerance: a conceptual diagram. www.thinkingcriticalcare.com/2016/02/21/volume-responsiveness-and-volume-tolerance-a-conceptual-diagram-foamed-foamcc-foamus [accessed 16 March 2022].

21. Tang WH, Kitai T (2016) Intrarenal venous flow: a window into the congestive kidney failure phenotype of heart failure? *JACC Heart Fail,* 4:683.

22. Beaubien-Souligny W, Rola P, Haycock K, *et al.* (2020) Quantifying systemic congestion with Point-Of-Care ultrasound: development of the venous excess ultrasound grading system. *Ultrasound J,* 12:16.

23. Miller A, Peck M, Clark T, *et al.* (2021) FUSIC HD. Comprehensive haemodynamic assessment with ultrasound. *J Intensive Care Soc,* doi. org/10.1177/17511437211010032.

24. Pivetta E, Goffi A, Nazerian P, *et al.* (2019) Study group on lung ultrasound from the Molinette and Careggi Hospitals. Lung ultrasound integrated with clinical assessment for the diagnosis of acute decompensated heart failure in the emergency department: a randomized controlled trial. *Eur J Heart Fail,* 21:754.

25. Orde S, Slama M, Hilton A, Yastrebov K, McLean A (2017) Pearls and pitfalls in comprehensive critical care echocardiography. *Crit Care,* 21:279.

26. Lema PC, Kim JH, St James E (2017) Overview of common errors and pitfalls to avoid in the acquisition and interpretation of ultrasound imaging of the abdominal aorta. *J Vasc Diagnostics Intervent,* 5:41.

27. Dietrich CF, Mathis G, Blaivas M, *et al.* (2016) Lung B-line artefacts and their use. *J Thoracic Dis,* 8:1356.

28. Lichtenstein DA (2014) Lung ultrasound in the critically ill. *Ann Intensive Care,* 4:1.

CHAPTER 25

POCUS IN TRAUMA

25

Dipak Mistry

POCUS is now established as an almost universal standard of care in emergency departments and major trauma centres. It is formally recognized and included in courses such as ATLS (Advanced Trauma Life Support) and has been adopted as a curriculum requirement by the Royal College of Emergency Medicine in the UK [1]. Sonography in trauma first originated in Scandinavia in the 1970s as a method of identifying splenic injuries in patients who had suffered road traffic accidents [2]. Over time, the practice was adopted in the USA and the protocol was extended to a more comprehensive focused exam with four main views centred on identifying free fluid in the abdomen and around the heart. Most recently, the protocol has been extended to include focused lung windows to identify a pneumothorax or haemothorax.

25.1 Sensitivity of ultrasonography in the trauma patient

There are several studies showing the sensitivity of focused assessment with sonography for trauma (FAST) scanning which range from 73% to 99% sensitivity and 95 to 100% specificity for detecting haemoperitoneum [3,4]. Studies using diagnostic peritoneal lavage to instil fluid into the abdominal cavity have shown that the volume required to be present in the abdomen ranges from 500ml to around 100ml for experienced operators [5]. Sensitivity for detecting solid organ injury is notably lower at around 40% because there may not be significant associated haemoperitoneum [6].

25.2 Computed tomography versus ultrasonography

POCUS should not be considered as a replacement for contrast-enhanced computed tomography (CT), which remains the gold standard for imaging in trauma, but instead as an adjunct to the primary survey and a guide to resuscitation. The main advantages of POCUS are that it can be performed rapidly at the bedside, typically in under a minute, and that it acts as a rapid triage tool to identify patients who may need immediate transfer to theatres with or without CT, depending on haemodynamic status. It also improves the detection of simple pneumothoraces compared to supine chest radiography alone [7]. A further advantage of POCUS is that it does not use ionizing radiation and so may be applied to children and pregnant women, with some caveats. It is also very portable, with hand-held devices now commonplace, and so can be used in rural or prehospital settings including aeromedicine.

25.3 Limitations of ultrasonography in trauma

POCUS in trauma is limited by the fact that it can only detect the presence of free fluid, be it in the thoracic, abdominal or pericardial space, when it is present in sufficient quantities, and it cannot show where the bleeding has arisen from. The other limiting factor is that it may be initially negative, particularly if the patient is assessed very soon after injury, as may be the case in inner city hospitals, or if the haemorrhage is slow. It also does not image the retroperitoneal space which can conceal large volumes of blood. Finally, one also needs a trained, competent clinician with a robust auditable process of image acquisition and interpretation. Studies have shown that the initial skill competence can be acquired quickly, but without regular practice, skills can fade. See *Table 25.1* for a comparison of CT and point-of-care ultrasound.

Table 25.1. Comparison of CT and ultrasound in the assessment of trauma patients

CT scanning	Ultrasound
Advantages	*Advantages*
Detailed views of anatomy including retroperitoneum and bony structures	Can be performed rapidly using defined protocols (eFAST)
Can be combined with intravenous contrast to localize the source of bleeding	Does not use ionizing radiation
Can be used for pre-operative planning or serial follow-up of conservatively managed injuries	Repeatable if there is a change in clinical condition
May be combined with interventional radiology approaches	May be used where CT is inaccessible, e.g. remote areas or prehospital environment
Limitations	*Limitations*
Requires a relatively stable patient due to the scanning time	Sensitivity is operator-dependent
Uses ionizing radiation and so caution needed in pregnant and paediatric patients	eFAST should only be used in a *rule-in* capacity
	May be negative if performed early or if there is solid organ injury without significant free fluid
	Sensitivity reduced in children due to relatively small volumes of free fluid

25.4 When should it be performed?

In the typical in-hospital trauma patient assessment, extended focused assessment of sonography for trauma (eFAST) is performed either during the 'circulation' assessment or after completion of the primary survey and initiation of resuscitation, depending on total resource and setting. Typically, the full protocol can be achieved in 1–2 minutes in experienced hands. eFAST should be used only to '*rule-in*' injury, i.e. the absence of detectable free-fluid or pneumothorax does not rule out an injury. For those patients in whom serious injury is suspected, even with a negative eFAST scan, a contrast CT should ideally be performed for definitive injury delineation or exclusion.

25.5 eFAST sequence by views

eFAST is normally performed in the supine patient with the abdominal windows first and the thorax last. The order of scanning is designed to assess the most dependent areas first thereby maximizing positive yield. The abdominal views are usually obtained first in the following order: right upper quadrant, left upper quadrant, suprapubic, subxiphoid views, followed by thoracic views (*Figs 25.1* and *25.2*). The sequence may be altered in specific circumstances, such as isolated penetrating chest trauma, e.g. stabbing, whereby the thorax may be scanned first with the patient in the sitting position to rapidly identify a pneumothorax, basal haemothorax or a haemopericardium.

25.5.1 Abdominal views: curvilinear probe 3–5MHz

Right upper quadrant (RUQ) view
Start by placing the probe on the midaxillary line with the probe marker cephalad and aim to initially target the interface between the liver and the kidney. This is known as the hepatorenal space or Morison's pouch. The view may be improved by gently tilting or sliding the probe so that it sits in the intercostal space, thereby removing the acoustic shadow cast by the ribs. This is the most dependent area in a supine patient and blood will show as an anechoic black stripe between the liver and kidney. If possible, fan through the renal profile and aim to image the medial edge of the liver where you may see small volumes of free fluid. Next, slide the probe cephalad and image the base of the lung to look for basal haemothorax.

Left upper quadrant (LUQ) view
Place the probe on the posterior axillary line around the T10 level and scan the interface between the spleen and the kidney. Again, the view may be improved by tilting into the intercostal rib space and dynamic scanning with respiration. Free fluid will appear as an anechoic stripe between the spleen and the kidney and can sometimes collect in the subphrenic space or inferior to the spleen, so try to fan through the space dynamically. The base of the lung should also be inspected for the presence of haemothorax by moving the probe cephalad.

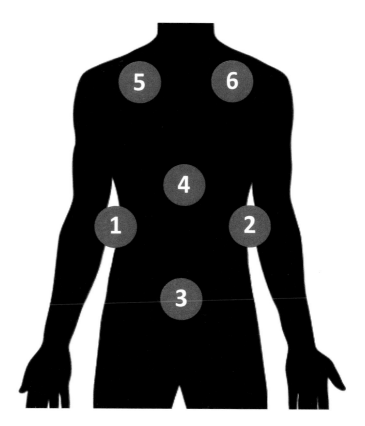

Figure 25.1. eFAST imaging order for the typical trauma patient.

Suprapubic view

The suprapubic region should be scanned in both the transverse and sagittal planes. Fluid will usually collect posterior to the bladder in the rectovesical pouch or rectovaginal pouch. Take care to scan above the dome of the bladder to ensure that free fluid is not missed. Detection is improved with a full bladder acting as an acoustic window; small volumes of free fluid may be missed when the bladder is decompressed with a urinary catheter.

In female patients, volumes up to 50ml may be considered as physiological, but interpretation must be made in clinical context and, if there is a high suspicion of injury, progress to CT after ruling out pregnancy with urine or serum testing [8].

Subcostal view

Place the probe into the subxiphoid area transversely with the tail upwards and then slowly lower the probe until almost parallel to the abdomen. Using the liver as an acoustic window, the entire heart is visualized. Look for global contraction and the presence or absence of an anechoic rim of fluid around the heart (*Fig. 25.3*). Rotating the probe and scanning in a sagittal plane will allow visualization of the inferior vena cava to aid assessment of filling status. Although not a classical part of the eFAST protocol, it can be a useful marker of blood loss. One of the pitfalls of the subxiphoid view is that it can

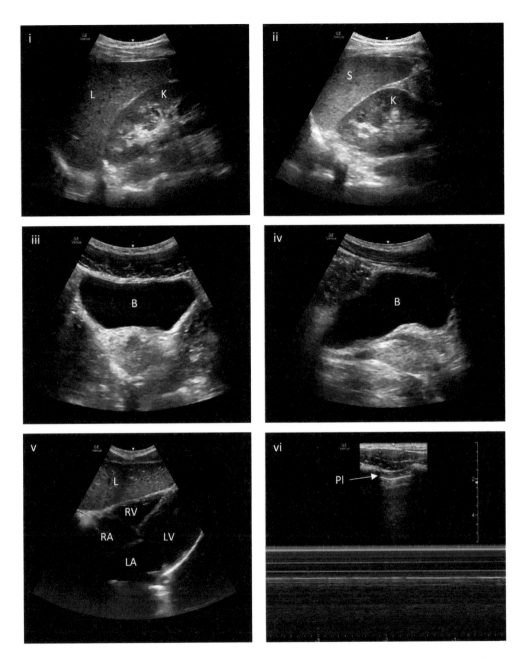

Figure 25.2. Complete set of images for eFAST sequence in a male patient. (i) Right upper quadrant view, (ii) left upper quadrant view, (iii) transverse suprapubic view, (iv) sagittal suprapubic view, (v) subxiphoid view, (vi) lung window with B-mode showing normal lung and the seashore sign. B – bladder; K – kidney; L – liver; LA – left atrium; LV – left ventricle; Pl – pleural line; RA – right atrium; RV – right ventricle; S – spleen.

be obscured by overlying bowel gas or a tense abdomen. In this case, the operator can ask an awake patient to gently take a deep breath in, which will bring the heart closer to the probe, or utilize a single transthoracic view such as the parasternal long-axis view or apical four-chamber view.

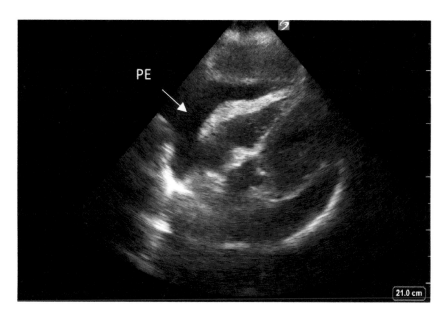

Figure 25.3. Subcostal echocardiographic view demonstrating a large pericardial effusion (PE).

25.5.2 Thoracic views: linear probe >5MHz

Lung windows

Finally, the chest is scanned for a pneumothorax. Using a high frequency linear probe for best resolution, scan initially in the 2nd or 3rd intercostal space in the midclavicular line in the sagittal plane. There are several sonographic markers that confirm the presence of normal lung. First, look for the presence of lung-sliding and B-lines; pneumothorax is suggested by the absence of lung-sliding and B-lines. This can be confirmed further using M-mode scanning focused on an intercostal space. In the presence of normal lung, you will see a pattern resembling a seashore with 'waves' in the top half and 'sand' in the lower half. This represents reverberation artefact from the pleural line which is highly reflective to sound waves. In the presence of a pneumothorax, the seashore is replaced by a continuous horizontal linear pattern known as the barcode or stratosphere sign.

Detection of a pneumothorax can be difficult in the presence of subcutaneous emphysema, which will obscure the sonographic window. Also, be aware that other conditions which cause the lung not to move, such as mainstem bronchus intubation, may mimic a pneumothorax. It is not necessary to comprehensively scan through every rib space, but a sensible screening pattern is to perform three focused windows: apical, mid-chest and basal. For more details on lung ultrasound see *Chapters 11* and *12*.

25.6 Special use cases: trauma in children

eFAST can be used in children and young adults. A sector transducer with a small footprint is advantageous when scanning small children. Most modern ultrasound machines also have pre-sets or automatic image optimizations for paediatric scanning. However, the sensitivity of eFAST in paediatric trauma is lower compared to adults at around 40% [9]. Two important factors must be appreciated when using POCUS in trauma. First, solid organ injury in children is more common than in adults and may not be associated with significant haemoperitoneum. Secondly, free intraperitoneal blood volumes may be much smaller than in an adult and so below detectable limits. However, even with those caveats, eFAST may still provide useful information to *rule-in* injury if positive.

The other main driving factor for the limited use of POCUS in children is the lack of formal adoption within paediatric emergency training schemes. This is changing and POCUS in paediatric trauma is being increasingly adopted by non-radiologists.

25.7 Special use cases: trauma in the pregnant patient

eFAST may be used with caution in pregnant patients. There are few formal studies, but sensitivity has been reported to be as high as 83% and specificity 98% [10]. However, these studies have had small sample sizes and included very experienced practitioners.

A common clinical scenario is a pregnant patient who has suffered blunt force trauma to the abdomen in a car accident. There is no alteration in protocol, but several cautions must be noted. Depending on gestational age, the suprapubic view may be difficult to obtain due to the gravid uterus, hence limiting usefulness [11]. Also, it must be appreciated that eFAST does not formally include assessment of the fetus or *rule-out* placental abruption which is a major cause of fetal loss in blunt force trauma. In patients in whom this is suspected, specialist co-assessment by an obstetrician and admission for 24 hours of cardiotocography monitoring is recommended.

25.8 eFAST in non-trauma patients

The eFAST protocol can be used in non-trauma patients to identify free fluid and is known as focused assessment of free fluid (FAFF) (*Fig. 25.4*).

One example where FAFF is particularly useful is for patients in whom a ruptured ectopic pregnancy is suspected. The abdominal views of eFAST provide a quick and easy method for identification of intra-abdominal free fluid. Visual estimation of the amount of free fluid helps to expedite surgical management for these patients who will often show little physiological abnormality due to their relatively young age. In addition, experienced operators may be able to identify an ectopic pregnancy in the suprapubic views. Similarly, the abdominal views of the protocol can be used to identify the presence of ascites in medical patients.

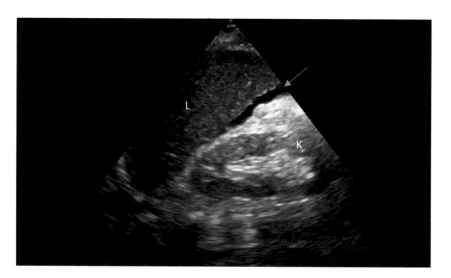

Figure 25.4. Ultrasound image of the right upper quadrant in a patient with a perforated bowel demonstrating fluid (orange arrow) between the liver (L) and kidney (K).

This protocol is also useful for patients who present with undifferentiated breathlessness. Utilizing the subxiphoid window, the heart can easily be scanned for a global view and the presence of a pericardial effusion can be checked. This can be augmented with thoracic views to image the lungs to look for effusions and assessment of lung parenchyma for signs of interstitial consolidation or overload (see *Chapters 11* and *12* for a more detailed explanation).

25.9 Prehospital POCUS and eFAST

POCUS is rapidly expanding as a prehospital tool. Advances with ultrasound machine sizes leading to the development of hand-held devices and multifrequency probes have allowed POCUS to be used in the prehospital environment. Combined with the simplicity of the eFAST protocol, POCUS is now routinely used by many helicopter emergency medical services, retrieval teams and the military as an adjunct to the assessment of the shocked patient. It also has an extended role in helping to make critical decisions such as performing resuscitative thoracotomy in penetrating chest trauma and to guide procedures such as resuscitative endovascular balloon occlusion of the aorta (REBOA) in critically unwell patients.

25.10 Training, competence and future adoption

In current UK practice, the majority of eFAST scans are now performed by emergency physicians, radiologists, anaesthetists, intensivists and to a lesser extent trauma surgeons. There has been no competency consensus between the groups, but studies looking at accuracy between radiologists and non-radiologists show that it is a skill that can be learnt relatively easily with proper training. Basic scanning competence may be achieved after as few as 10 scans, following which most large errors are reduced and may plateau after 25–50 scans. POCUS in trauma will probably continue to gain widespread acceptance as specific curricula are adopted by specialty training bodies, the equipment costs reduce, portable devices become more available and artificial intelligence augmented scans become more accessible.

25.11 Summary

eFAST is a simple, powerful algorithm that can enhance decision making in the trauma patient when combined with clinical history, examination, and an appropriate index of suspicion for injury. Clinicians should remember that the protocol should be used to *rule-in* injury and that it serves as a rapid screening tool prior to more definitive imaging or direct surgical intervention.

25.12 References

1. www.rcem.ac.uk/RCEM/Exams_Training/UK_Trainees/Ultrasound_Training/RCEM/Exams_Training/UK_Trainees/Ultrasound_Training.aspx

2. Kristensen JK, Buemann B, Kühl E (1971) Ultrasonic scanning in the diagnosis of splenic haematomas. *Acta Chir Scand*, 137:653.

3. Moore CL, Copel JA (2011) Point-of-care ultrasonography. *N Engl J Med*, 364:749.

4. McKenney KL, McKenney MG, Cohn SM, *et al.* (2001) Hemoperitoneum score helps determine need for therapeutic laparotomy. *J Trauma*, 50:650.

5. Von Kuenssberg Jehle D, Stiller G, Wagner D (2003) Sensitivity in detecting free intraperitoneal fluid with the pelvic views of the FAST exam. *Am J Emerg Med*, 21:476.

6. McGahan JP, Rose J, Coates TL, Wisner DH, Newberry P (1997) Use of ultrasonography in the patient with acute abdominal trauma. *J Ultrasound Med*, 16:653.

7. Ianniello S, Di Giacomo V, Sessa B, Miele V (2014) First-line sonographic diagnosis of pneumothorax in major trauma: accuracy of e-FAST and comparison with multidetector computed tomography. *Radiol Med (Torino)*, 119:674.

8. Ormsby EL, Geng J, McGahan JP, Richards JR (2005) Pelvic free fluid: clinical importance for reproductive age women with blunt abdominal trauma. *Ultrasound Obstet Gynecol*, 26:271.

9. Patel NY, Riherd JM (2011) Focused assessment with sonography for trauma: methods, accuracy, and indications. *Surg Clin North Am*, 91:195.

10. Goodwin H, Holmes JF, Wisner DH (2001) Abdominal ultrasound examination in pregnant blunt trauma patients. *J Trauma*, 50:689.

11. Brown MA, Sirlin CB, Farahmand N, *et al.* (2005) Screening sonography in pregnant patients with blunt abdominal trauma. *J Ultrasound Med*, 24:175.

CHAPTER 26
POCUS IN CARDIAC ARREST

Luke Flower & Pradeep Madhivathanan

POCUS is a valuable tool in cardiac arrest, with the UK Resuscitation Council's most recent guidelines further acknowledging the vital role it can play [1]. Its core benefit lies in its unrivalled ability to rapidly identify reversible causes and provide a real-time assessment of cardiac function.

In this chapter we will discuss the cardiac arrest diagnoses POCUS can help identify, its potential use in prognostication and share our proposed algorithm for approaching such scenarios.

26.1 Ultrasound for diagnosis in cardiac arrest

The primary use of POCUS in cardiac arrest is in the identification and treatment of reversible causes. In the correct hands it allows for rapid recognition of several life-threatening pathologies [2]. It is important to remember that all ultrasound findings should be interpreted in conjunction with the clinical history and examination.

26.1.1 Cardiac tamponade

Cardiac tamponade occurs when fluid or thrombus accumulates in the pericardial space, resulting in pericardial pressures exceeding those of the cardiac chambers. The resultant impaired ventricular filling and cardiac output leads to haemodynamic compromise and potentially cardiac arrest. Echocardiographic findings in cardiac tamponade reflect these pericardial pressure effects, with both visual and quantitative measurements available (these are discussed in depth in *Chapter 10*).

The volume of pericardial fluid should be assessed in all available windows, allowing for a global estimate of its size and effect. Fluid is usually seen as a black anechoic strip within the pericardial space, with thrombus appearing as a hyperechoic structure (*Fig. 26.1*).

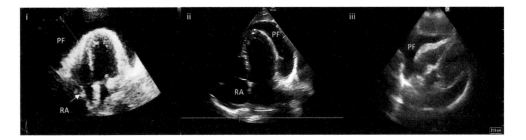

Figure 26.1. (i) Apical four-chamber view of a large pericardial effusion with RA collapse. (ii) Apical four-chamber view of a large pericardial effusion with no RA collapse – suggestive of a chronic effusion. (iii) Subcostal view of a pericardial effusion. PF – pericardial fluid; RA – right atrium.

It is important to acknowledge that the rate of accumulation of an effusion is often more important than its size. A large effusion may develop slowly over time without haemodynamic effect, whilst a small but rapidly accumulating effusion may cause cardiac arrest [3].

The right atrium (RA) is usually the first chamber affected due to its low internal pressures. Collapse is first seen in diastole, with the duration of RA collapse associated with the presence of tamponade. RA collapse for more than one-third of the cardiac cycle is 100% sensitive and specific for cardiac tamponade [4].

As the effusion grows the external pressure it exerts on the cardiac chambers will increase. If this pressure exceeds that of the right ventricule (RV), then it will lead to RV collapse. This is initially seen in early diastole and will then progress over a larger proportion of the respiratory cycle. Once RV collapse begins, there is reduced ventricular filling, stroke volume and cardiac output with subsequent haemodynamic instability.

More advanced methods to assess for the presence of cardiac tamponade include the following.

- Measurement of changes in right and left ventricular diameter during the respiratory cycle (from parasternal long-axis (PLAX) and parasternal short-axis (PSAX) windows), with >5% variation suggestive of compromise.

- The presence of a distended inferior vena cava (IVC) with reduced respiratory variation, however, the caveats mentioned in *Section 24.3* remain relevant.

- Respiratory variation of ventricular inflow during respiration. The use of pulsed wave Doppler over the cardiac valves allows calculation of inflow velocities throughout the respiratory cycle. Velocity variations of >25% through the mitral valve, >40% through the tricuspid valve and >10% over the aortic and pulmonary valves, are suggestive of physiological tamponade [5].

Despite the above, it is important to remember that cardiac tamponade is a clinical diagnosis. Whilst transthoracic echocardiography (TTE) may aid diagnosis, the echocardiographic signs of tamponade can appear in haemodynamically stable patients, thus clinical correlation is essential. Having said this, the presence of pericardial fluid in cardiac arrest should lead to the consideration of pericardiocentesis.

26.1.2 Pulmonary embolism

Echocardiography can be an extremely helpful tool in the assessment of suspected massive pulmonary embolism (PE). However, its strength lies in its role as a *rule-in* rather than a *rule-out* investigation, with a negative predictive value of 40–50% [6]. Importantly, if no signs of RV pressure overload are seen in a haemodynamically compromised patient, then a PE is unlikely to be the cause.

TTE is recommended as a first line investigation for suspected PE by both the European Society of Cardiology (ESC) and The British Thoracic Society. The ESC goes on to state that if computed tomographic pulmonary angiography is not immediately available or feasible, and signs of RV pressure overload are present, then treatment of suspected PE may be justified.

Echocardiographic signs of pulmonary embolus are discussed in more depth in *Section 8.8.4,* but *Table 26.1* and *Figure 26.2* highlight some of the common findings. The majority of these are a result of increased resistance to RV outflow and include an enlarged RV, McConnell's sign (characterized by akinesia of the mid free wall and hypercontractility of the apical wall),

Table 26.1. Echocardiographic signs of pulmonary embolism

Echocardiographic sign	Comments
Enlarged RV – measure in PLAX/A4Ch	Seen in around 25% of PEs; multiple other causes
McConnell's sign (akinetic free wall with hyperdynamic apex)	Poor sensitivity (20%), potentially high specificity (close to 100%)
Flattening of the interventricular septum	High sensitivity (81%), low specificity (41%)
Distended non-collapsing IVC	Multiple caveats (see *Section 24.3*)
Direct clot visualization in the RA, RV or RVOT	Not commonly seen
RV dysfunction (i.e. TAPSE <17mm)	Non-specific, may aid in prognostication; requires more training than basic FTTE
Systolic notching of the pulmonary artery ejection waveform	Requires more training than FTTE
60:60 sign (pulmonary acceleration time <60msec, RVSP <60mmHg)	Low sensitivity (25%) but high specificity (>90%); requires more training than basic FTTE

A4Ch – apical four-chamber; FTTE – focused transthoracic echocardiography; IVC – inferior vena cava; PE – pulmonary embolism; PLAX – parasternal long-axis; RA – right atrium; RV – right ventricle; RVOT – right ventricular outflow tract; RVSP – right ventricular systolic pressure; TAPSE – tricuspid annular plane systolic excursion.
Reproduced from J. *Intensive Care Soc.,* 2021;22:230, with permission from Sage Publishing.

septal flattening, right ventricular dysfunction and visualization of a clot in transit. When assessing for signs of increased resistance to RV outflow it is important to consider other potential causes such as a tension pneumothorax or established pulmonary hypertension.

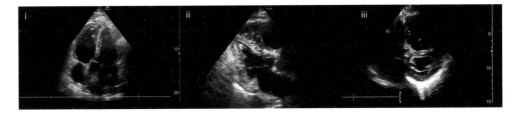

Figure 26.2. Echocardiographic signs of pulmonary embolism. (i) Apical five-chamber view demonstrating McConnell's sign. (ii) Parasternal long-axis view – dilated right ventricle with septal bowing. (ii) Parasternal short-axis view – dilated right ventricle with septal bowing and a 'D'-shaped left ventricle.

The diagnosis of PE in cardiac arrest remains a subject of ongoing discussion. Previous teaching implied the presence of a dilated RV was akin to the diagnosis of a PE, however, multiple studies have demonstrated the RV to be dilated in cardiac arrest of almost any origin [7–9]. It has been suggested that the RV is proportionally more dilated in cases of massive PE, but this cannot be accurately relied upon during cardiac arrest. Vascular POCUS may also be performed to assess for the presence of deep vein thrombosis in association with PE. This should be performed as per the technique described in *Section 18.2*, although this may be technically challenging if cardiopulmonary resuscitation (CPR) is ongoing.

To summarize, echocardiography for assessment of PE must be used in the context of clinical history and examination, with other causes of obstructive shock considered simultaneously.

26.1.3 Ventricular failure

Whilst it may not be possible to assess cardiac function in cardiac arrest, it can be useful in the peri-arrest setting or when assessing pulseless electrical activity (PEA). The methods referred to in *Chapters 7* and *8* can be incorporated to assess for regional wall motion abnormalities or the presence of severe global impairment. Such findings may indicate an ischaemic cause of arrest and highlight the need for discussion with a cardiologist.

26.1.4 Hypovolaemia

In the arrest setting, accurate assessment of a patient's fluid status can be extremely challenging. It may, however, be possible to make a rough assessment, especially in the setting of extreme hypovolaemia and PEA. The IVC may grant us some insight into the patient's intravascular fluid pressures but should be interpreted with caution. The presence of a small and collapsible IVC would be an unusual finding during cardiac arrest and may suggest a fluid deficient state [2].

Another common finding in cardiac arrest, as alluded to in *Section 26.1.2* above, is the dilation of ventricular chambers. The presence of small ventricles, especially in the context of PEA, may be suggestive of extreme hypovolaemia and a fluid challenge should be considered [2]. More detail on assessment of fluid status can be found in *Chapter 24.*

26.1.5 Tension pneumothorax

Tension pneumothorax represents a potentially reversible cause of arrest that can easily be identified and treated with the help of POCUS. The techniques discussed in *Chapters 11* and *12* remain appropriate in the cardiac arrest setting.

During ventilation, the pleura should be visualized bilaterally using windows that do not compromise the quality of compressions. The pleural line should be closely examined to ensure lung sliding is seen and M-mode may be used to confirm the presence of the 'seashore sign' (a sign of lung sliding); an absence of lung sliding, suggestive of pneumothorax, is often referred to as the 'stratosphere' sign (see *Fig. 26.3*) [10-12].

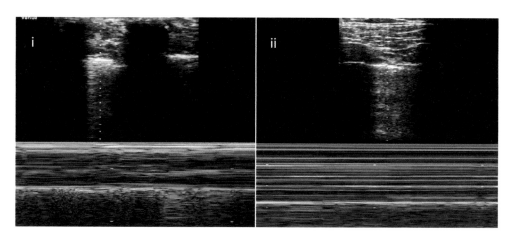

Figure 26.3. Lung ultrasound findings in a pneumothorax. (i) Lung sliding is seen on M-mode with the 'seashore' sign visible. (ii) An absence of lung sliding is demonstrated with the 'stratosphere' or 'barcode' sign seen.

Note that multiple other pathologies, such as endobronchial intubation or the presence of bullae, can also result in reduced lung sliding. Consensus advice is to look for a 'lung point' (the point at which a lung stops sliding) and confirm the absence of a lung pulse to increase confidence in diagnosis [11,13,14].

Another echocardiographic sign of tension pneumothorax is the presence of a vertically oriented heart from the subcostal view, with the absence of parasternal or apical cardiac windows and an A-line profile visible immediately next to the heart [15]. In such cases a tension pneumothorax should be considered, and lung ultrasound performed.

26.2 The POCUS pulse

The POCUS pulse has been proposed as an adjunct to manual pulse palpation. Clinicians are not good at accurately recognizing PEA, incorrectly diagnosing it in up to 75% of cases. This is probably due to the unreliability of manual pulse palpation, with numerous factors (e.g. a raised body mass index) significantly affecting its accuracy [16,17].

Using the skill set mentioned in *Section 18.2*, the ultrasound probe may be placed over the carotid or femoral arteries during pulse checks to assess for the presence of a pulse. This provides equally quick and more reliable results than manual palpation and may aid in prognostication.

26.3 Prognostication in cardiac arrest

A newer role of POCUS in cardiac arrest is in prognostication through identification of the true underlying rhythm. The use of an ultrasound pulse in combination with focused TTE appears to present a different cohort of 'pseudo-PEA' patients, with significantly increased survival rates compared to PEA diagnosed by manual palpation alone. These 'pseudo-PEA' patients with spontaneous cardiac movement (SCM) demonstrate a 7-fold increase in survival to admission (55% vs 8%) [16,17].

A similar pattern occurs in asystole, with the use of focused TTE finding 35% of these patients to have SCM. The presence of SCM more than doubled their survival to hospital (24% vs 11%). Absence of spontaneous cardiac activity is associated with significantly reduced survival to discharge (3.8% vs 0.6%) and reduced chance of return of spontaneous circulation (OR 12.4) [16,17]. Thus, whilst not to be used in isolation, the use of intra-arrest POCUS may help us estimate chances of survival and make decisions around termination of CPR.

26.4 Transoesophageal echocardiography

The use of intra-arrest TOE is growing, although its application remains limited predominantly because of a lack of the requisite skillset and equipment. It can be a useful diagnostic adjunct, especially in patients with challenging cardiac windows, and may help avoid prolonged interruptions to CPR. It can provide a continuous view of the heart and so permits optimization of chest compressions, delivering a real-time view of the cardiac chambers and thus allowing adjustment of hand position to ensure optimal filling and ejection [18,19]. As we see an increase in the utilization of extracorporeal CPR, intra-arrest TOE and TTE will probably also have an increased role to play in assisting cannulation and initiating mechanical support [20,21].

26.5 Putting it all together

In the majority of cardiac arrest settings, the most easily accessible form of echocardiography is transthoracic, with lung and vascular ultrasound adding to the examination. To provide readers with a structure with which to approach the use of POCUS in cardiac arrest, we have created the algorithm shown in *Figure 26.4*. As with all uses of POCUS, findings do not replace thorough history taking and examination, and repeat imaging should be considered following any intervention or change in clinical picture.

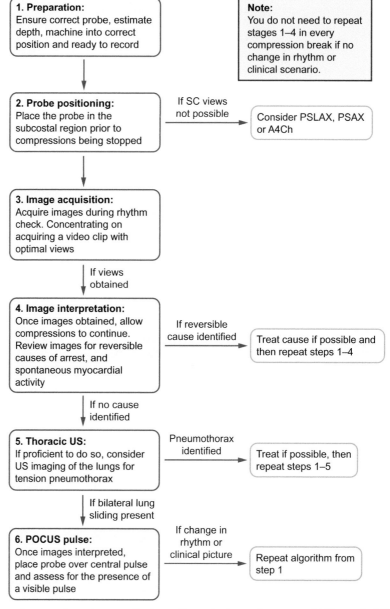

Figure 26.4. Suggested approach to the use of echocardiography in cardiac arrest. A4Ch – apical four-chamber; PLAX – parasternal long-axis; PSAX – parasternal short-axis; SC – sub-costal; US – ultrasound.. Reproduced from *J. Intensive Care Soc.*, 2021;22:230, with permission from Sage Publishing.

26.6 Summary

The importance of POCUS in cardiac arrest is now widely recognized and reflected in its inclusion in several life support algorithms. It provides clinicians with an unrivalled ability to diagnose and treat several causes of cardiac arrest in a rapid, noninvasive and reliable manner. It does, however, remain vital that POCUS findings are interpreted in the context of the clinical picture and serve as an extension of thorough history and examination, not as a replacement.

26.7 References

1. Resuscitation Council UK (2021) Resuscitation Guidelines: www.resus.org.uk/library/2021-resuscitation-guidelines.

2. Zafiropoulos A, Asrress K, Redwood S, Gillon S, Walker D (2014) CRITICAL CARE ECHO ROUNDS: Echo in cardiac arrest. *Echo Res Pract,* 1(2):D15.

3. Sagristà-Sauleda J, Mercé AS, Soler-Soler J (2011) Diagnosis and management of pericardial effusion. *World J Cardiol,* 3:135.

4. Gillam LD, Guyer DE, Gibson TC, King ME, Marshall JE, Weyman AE (1983) Hydrodynamic compression of the right atrium: a new echocardiographic sign of cardiac tamponade. *Circulation,* 68:294.

5. Schneider M, Binder T (2018) Echocardiographic evaluation of the right heart. *Wien Klin Wochenschr,* 130:413.

6. Konstantinides SV, Meyer G, Becattini C, *et al.* (2019) 2019 ESC Guidelines for the diagnosis and management of acute pulmonary embolism developed in collaboration with the European Respiratory Society. *Eur Respir J,* 54:1901647.

7. Dresden S, Mitchell P, Rahimi L, *et al.* (2014) Right ventricular dilatation on bedside echocardiography performed by emergency physicians aids in the diagnosis of pulmonary embolism. *Ann Emerg Med,* 63:16.

8. Casazza F, Bongarzoni A, Capozi A, Agostoni O (2005) Regional right ventricular dysfunction in acute pulmonary embolism and right ventricular infarction. *Eur J Echocardiogr,* 6:11.

9. Aagaard R, Caap P, Hansson NC, Bøtker MT, Granfeldt A, Løfgren B (2017) Detection of pulmonary embolism during cardiac arrest – ultrasonographic findings should be interpreted with caution. *Crit Care Med,* 45:e695.

10. Zhang M, Liu ZH, Yang JX, *et al.* (2006) Rapid detection of pneumothorax by ultrasonography in patients with multiple trauma. *Crit Care,* 10:R112.

11. Ding W, Shen Y, Yang J, He X, Zhang M (2011) Diagnosis of pneumothorax by radiography and ultrasonography: a meta-analysis. *Chest,* 140:859.

12. Chen L, Zhang Z (2015) Bedside ultrasonography for diagnosis of pneumothorax. *Quant Imaging Med Surg,* 5:618.

13. Lichtenstein DA (2014) Lung ultrasound in the critically ill. *Ann Intensive Care,* 4:1.

14. Lichtenstein DA, Mezière GA (2011) The BLUE-points: three standardized points used in the BLUE-protocol for ultrasound assessment of the lung in acute respiratory failure. *Crit Ultrasound J,* 3:109.

15. Olusanya O, Lashin H (2020) An unusual echocardiographic sign in tension pneumothorax. *Intensive Care Med,* 46:1046.

16. Badra K, Coutin A, Simard R, Pinto R, Lee JS, Chenkin J (2019) The POCUS pulse check: a randomized controlled crossover study comparing pulse detection by palpation versus by point-of-care ultrasound. *Resuscitation,* 139:17.

17. Gaspari R, Weekes A, Adhikari S, *et al.* (2016) Emergency department point-of-care ultrasound in out-of-hospital and in-ED cardiac arrest. *Resuscitation,* 109:33.

18. Pell AC, Guly UM, Sutherland GR, Steedman DJ, Bloomfield P, Robertson C (1994) Mechanism of closed chest cardiopulmonary resuscitation investigated by transoesophageal echocardiography. *J Accid Emerg Med,* 11:139.

19. Lin T, Chen Y, Lu C, Wang M (2006) Use of transoesophageal echocardiography during cardiac arrest in patients undergoing elective non-cardiac surgery. *Br J Anaesth,* 96:167.

20. Smith S, Madhivathanan PR (2019) The "double-barrel view": a useful point-of-care ultrasound (POCUS) view in extra- corporeal membrane oxygenation patients. *Perfusion,* 34:82.

21. Ahn HJ, Lee JW, Joo KH, *et al.* (2018) Point-of-care ultrasound-guided percutaneous cannulation of extracorporeal membrane oxygenation: make it simple. *J Emerg Med,* 54:507.

POCUS IN INTENSIVE CARE UNIT ACQUIRED WEAKNESS

Sunil Patel & Zudin Puthucheary

Intensive care unit acquired weakness (ICUAW) is common during and after critical illness. ICUAW is a complex process, and its cause is almost always multifactorial which makes a timely diagnosis difficult. Mechanistically, there is an imbalance between catabolic and anabolic pathways leading to net loss of muscle. To further complicate matters, the Intensive Care Unit (ICU) patient population is often heterogeneous with a wide range of pre-existing comorbidities. Despite this, ICUAW can occur in all patients with varying degrees of severity.

ICUAW prolongs the duration of mechanical ventilation and ICU length of stay as well as being a leading cause of physical disability up to 5 years later [1]. Whilst significant advances have been made in ICU-related technology and novel therapies for specific diseases, ICUAW has unfortunately continued to represent a significant cause of morbidity in ICU survivors.

ICUAW is difficult to diagnose in early critical illness. Patients are often deeply sedated, receiving mechanical ventilation and unable to engage with formal clinical assessments, particularly relating to strength. The current approach is therefore to combine clinical examination, various volitional tests and specialist neurophysiological diagnostics to obtain the diagnosis when it is feasible – this can be weeks after the initial ICU admission. Unfortunately, ICUAW occurs early in critical illness and affects both respiratory and skeletal muscle. There is a genuine need to develop methods and diagnostic tools to facilitate early recognition of ICUAW that may lead to early intervention and possibly prevention.

Ultrasound has advantages over computed tomography and magnetic resonance imaging, which convey a risk of radiation as well as the logistical concerns of moving critically ill patients to the imaging department, making repeated prospective measurements difficult. Furthermore, musculoskeletal ultrasound allows quantitative and qualitative data to be obtained that may identify the onset of significant wasting. Longitudinally, some quantitative measurements may serve as predictors for ventilatory weaning success (see below) [2,3]. The availability of ultrasound in the ICU and opportunity to repeat studies more freely make it an attractive option in the assessment of ICUAW.

27.1 Muscle groups

Assessment of skeletal and respiratory muscle in the ICU patient assumes that the muscle group is relatively superficial (to provide reliable recognition and image resolution) and that changes in its bulk or function can be reliably quantified, repeated and studied. Therefore, posterior muscle groups of the torso, despite their bulk are not easily studied in the ICU patient.

The quadriceps muscles (rectus femoris, vastus lateralis, vastus intermedius and vastus medialis) represent a large, superficial muscle group in the anterior compartment of the thigh (*Fig. 27.1*). In health, they are highly active and important in all weight-bearing postures and locomotion, thus detecting changes in their bulk is widely considered the standard group in the assessment of muscle wasting both in critical illness and other chronic respiratory diseases. In contrast, respiratory muscles are smaller. The diaphragm is the principal respiratory muscle and dysfunction is common in critical illness. During mechanical ventilation, 'lung rest' often leads to ventilatory 'over-assistance' as much as 50% of the time on mechanical ventilation and may lead to ventilator-induced diaphragm dysfunction (VIDD) – defined as the loss of diaphragmatic force-generating capacity associated with mechanical ventilation. Diaphragm ultrasound has been validated in

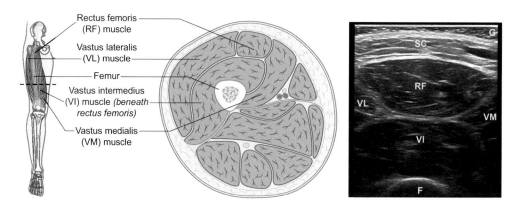

Figure 27.1. Ultrasonography of the quadriceps muscle. The anterior thigh comprises four large muscle groups: rectus femoris (RF), vastus lateralis (VL), vastus intermedius (VI) and vastus medialis (VM). Cross-sectional anatomy is shown in the middle figure. Corresponding ultrasound anatomy is shown in the image on the right. The four groups are easily distinguishable by the echogenic fascia that borders each muscle. The femur (F) lies deep to these muscles and is a useful anatomical reference point and helps to align the ultrasound probe. Minimal compression to allow visualization of a gel (G) layer is important because it prevents distortion of the image through excessive pressure. Subcutaneous fat lies superficially to the RF. SC = subcutaneous tissue.

healthy subjects, is feasible in mechanical ventilation patients and found to be highly reproducible in the context of ICU clinical trials [4–6].

Diaphragm ultrasound is best used to assess spontaneous activity and therefore it is ideally performed during spontaneous modes of ventilation. However, assessment of thickening can still be made during mandatory and partial-assist modes of mechanical ventilation as well as at end-expiration [7]. Some patients may exhibit recruitment of accessory respiratory muscles (both appropriately and inappropriately) such as the sternocleidomastoid, intercostals or trapezius, and others may have paradoxical abdominal breathing. This has led to the study of smaller, non-diaphragm, respiratory muscles in the assessment of ICUAW.

This chapter will discuss the quadriceps (specifically rectus femoris) and diaphragm, and introduce the study of another accessory respiratory muscle, the parasternal intercostal muscle group.

27.2 The basics

27.2.1 Setup and probe selection

Musculoskeletal ultrasound in ICUAW is best performed using a high-frequency linear probe (i.e. at least 9MHz, but ideally greater than 12MHz). Healthy, normal adult muscle appears hypoechoic and is delineated by hyperechoic fascia that borders the muscle (*Fig. 27.1*). Depth and gain should be standardized for each muscle group once an adequate view is obtained, and certainly between images for the same patient. This is to ensure reliable quantitative comparisons over time. If images lack a measurement scale, then one should be added to the image using a commonly available calliper function for offline analysis using appropriate software.

A unique image labelling system should be applied if the images are part of a formal study, for example, side of study, day of study, etc. (see *Section 27.3*). We also suggest keeping a logbook of scans, difficult aspects encountered as well as duration of study. Quantitative anomalies can sometimes be rationalized if the study was particularly challenging. The critically ill patient can pose many technical difficulties over time, and these will impact on image quality (e.g. fluid status, procedural sites in the vicinity of study, skin breakdown, etc.).

27.2.2 Anatomy

A robust knowledge of surface anatomy relating to key muscle groups is essential (*Fig. 27.2*). This ensures reliability and reproducibility between operators and within the patient.

27.2.3 Patient positioning

Patients receiving mechanical ventilation are often nursed 30° head up to prevent ventilator-associated complications. This is the ideal position for respiratory muscle assessment. However, depending on the severity of illness, positions such as prone (ARDS) and fully supine (trauma) may lead to variation in quantitative assessments and in some cases make the study impossible. Furthermore, intercostal drains and surgical access sites often overlie the lateral chest wall and prevent adequate contact of the probe. Drains, catheters, and invasive vascular devices are often secured in the vicinity of the diaphragm site and strict adherence to their care should be taken – however, this may prevent adequate/consistent landmarks and views of the anatomy and prevent imaging altogether. When studying the rectus femoris, the leg should be in a neutral position at the hip and lightly supported by a pillow under the knee to prevent contraction. Overall, maintaining identical positioning for the individual patient is essential and enables reliable longitudinal comparisons.

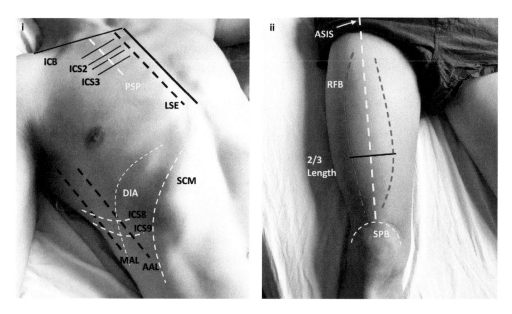

Figure 27.2. *Essential surface anatomy in musculoskeletal ultrasound in ICUAW. (i) Diaphragm and parasternal surface anatomy. (ii) Lower limb anatomy for quadriceps ultrasound.*

AAL – anterior axillary line; ASIS – anterior superior iliac spine; DIA – diaphragm; ICB – inferior clavicular border; ICS2 – 2nd intercostal/parasternal space; ICS3 – 3rd intercostal/parasternal space; ICS8 – 8th intercostal space; ICS9 – 9th intercostal space; LSE – lateral sternal edge; MAL – midaxillary line; PSP – parasternal muscle imaging point; RFB – rectus femoris muscle bulk (outlined with red dotted line); SCM – sub-costal margin; SPB – superior border of patella.

27.3 Developing a protocol and reliability testing

There are currently no official standards or guidelines concerning musculoskeletal ultrasound in ICUAW and critical illness in general, and so technique, approach and publication of results are open to interpretation. In the first instance, expert opinion should be sought, and the literature reviewed for technique and methods. Prior to a clinical study, pilot data or a feasibility trial should be performed to ensure the ultrasound technique is reliable and robust and these results should be published with clear detail of the methodology. An adequate sample size should be used and statistical papers concerning reproducibility studies can be referred to for ease [8]. Images should be taken in triplicate with inter-image variability ideally less than 7.5%. An intra- and inter-class correlation coefficient (ICC) should be calculated to provide statistical reliability between measurements and operators, respectively. Subsequent visual representations through Bland–Altman plots may highlight systematic error and patterns of potential bias. Whilst an ICC of >0.75 confers excellent agreement, in clinical imaging studies an ICC of >0.9 is generally reported. An ICC of 0.9 can be interpreted as 90% of the total variability is between subjects, rather than between operators. To further reduce bias in a feasibility study, anatomical landmark markings can be agreed and marked, or can be independently determined by the operator.

Images should be anonymized and analyzed offline by an independent person that is blinded to all data. Identical ultrasound machines and probes should be used, and depth and gain settings should be reported for all images. Finally, analysis of images should be performed on the same software application.

27.4 Key muscle groups in ICUAW

27.4.1 The diaphragm

The diaphragm is the principal respiratory muscle and in the absence of mandatory mechanical ventilation, remains continuously active. The last decade or so has seen more research in VIDD and the emergence of the concept of 'diaphragm protective ventilation' has been reported [9].

For diaphragm thickening fraction (DTF), a high-frequency linear probe is placed in the 8th or 9th intercostal space between the anterior and midaxillary line on the right or left side (*Fig. 27.2*). This site represents the *zone of apposition*, where the abdominal contents meet the chest wall. At this point, the diaphragm appears as a non-echogenic structure bounded by the echogenic pleura superiorly and the echogenic peritoneum inferiorly (*Fig. 27.3*). The DTF is dynamically assessed using B-mode and thickness measurements calculated at end-expiration using M-mode (*Fig. 27.3*). Maximum inspiration is taken at the peak of the M-mode trace and end-expiration at the narrowest point just before the next inspiratory cycle begins. A slow sweep (scrolling) speed of 10mm/sec is used to obtain three consecutive and visually consistent breaths.

Diaphragm muscle bulk and activity are the two most important aspects. Normal diaphragm thickness at functional residual capacity ranges from 1.8 to 3mm. A thickness of less than 2mm is often used to define atrophy and a 10% change in DTF is associated with a higher chance of failed extubation, prolonged ICU stay and higher incidence of tracheostomy. The technique has been extensively validated in healthy subjects, is feasible in mechanical ventilation patients and was found to be highly reproducible in ICU clinical trials. It is best performed during spontaneous ventilation. However, assessment of thickening can still be made during mandatory and partial-assist modes of mechanical ventilation, and even when neuromuscular blockade has been administered [12]. The two most common measurements of the diaphragm are:

1. **DTF** – calculated as:

$$\frac{\text{(thickness at end-inspiration} - \text{thickness at end-expiration)}}{\text{thickness at end-expiration}}$$

2. **Diaphragmatic excursion (DEX)** – defined as the distance travelled by the diaphragm during spontaneous breathing.

DTF is often used as a quantitative measure of inspiratory effort in non-mechanically ventilated, spontaneously breathing patients and mechanically

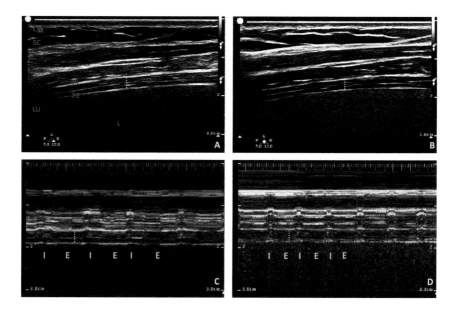

Figure 27.3. Diaphragm thickness. Diaphragm ultrasound in a 54-year-old man receiving mechanical ventilation for severe acute respiratory distress syndrome in a partial-assist mode of ventilation. All breaths recorded are spontaneous in nature. E is end-expiratory thickness, I is end-inspiratory thickness. (A) Taken on day 0 of the admission and (C) is the corresponding M-mode image of (A). In (C), E = 2.6mm and I = 2.8mm (DTF = 7%). In contrast on day 7 (B and D), E = 2.2mm and I = 2.3mm (DTF = 4%). There has been a change in expiratory thickness of 15%. Three complete breaths have been studied. The dotted vertical line in (A) and (B) depicts the trajectory of the M-mode line and resulting M-mode images in (C) and (D), respectively. Dotted vertical line illustrates the end-expiratory thickness point. CW – chest wall; D – diaphragm; E – expiration; I – inspiration; L – liver; LU – lung; PE – peritoneum; PL – pleura; SC – subcutaneous fat.

ventilated patients. The threshold of DTF that may predict successful extubation is variable, but is generally quoted to be greater than 30–35% (however, the normal range varies from 28 to 95%) or a change of no more than 10%. DEX is commonly measured during a spontaneous breathing trial or when disconnected from mechanical ventilation (i.e. during a T-piece trial) to help predict the likelihood of extubation (*Fig. 27.4*). DEX measurement during mandatory modes of mechanical ventilation is less useful because effects of mechanical insufflation and true diaphragm contraction cannot be separated. DTF has been shown to have excellent correlation with specialist diagnostics, including tracheal twitch and trans-diaphragmatic pressures.

DEX is measured using a low frequency (<6MHz) curvilinear or cardiac probe and is positioned below the right costal margin in the 8th or 9th intercostal space in the anterior axillary line or sub-costal in the mid-clavicular line (*Fig. 27.4*). When approaching laterally, the probe should be kept perpendicular to the chest wall and directed medially and cephalad to visualize the diaphragm. Because there is little difference between medial and posterior movements of the diaphragm, to enhance reproducibility the best delineation of the diaphragm can be sought using the cursor in M-mode and kept as perpendicular as possible to the diaphragm (*Fig. 27.4*). Inspiratory diaphragmatic movement is towards the probe and therefore

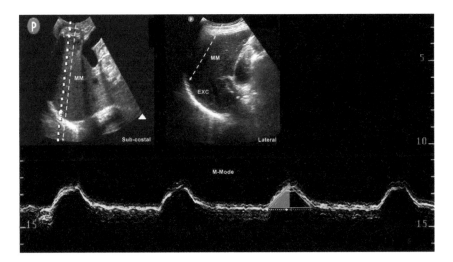

Figure 27.4. Diaphragm excursion in a 47-year-old male who has recovered from severe acute respiratory distress syndrome and is now undergoing a spontaneous breathing trial on FiO_2 0.3, PEEP 5, PS 0 for 5min. In the sub-costal view (upper left), the M-mode line (MM) is directed straight towards the diaphragm. In the lateral approach (upper middle), the MM is not as linear. Despite the difference in trajectory, the resulting M-mode image (lower trace) provides consistent quantitative data. The M-mode trace here shows three complete breaths. The double-headed red arrow represents expiratory time, the double-headed yellow arrow represents inspiratory time. The gradient of the orange triangle = contractility of the diaphragm and the amplitude/height of the triangle is the excursion. In this example the DEX = 1.4cm during the spontaneous breathing trial.

creates an upward deflection in M-mode. A slow sweep speed of 10mm/sec is advised so that multiple consecutive and visually consistent breaths are recorded. M-mode images can then be used to calculate excursion (cm) (wave amplitude), inspiratory time (sec), contraction (cm/sec) (slope) and respiratory cycle time (sec) offline (*Figure 27.4*). It is often difficult to visualize the left hemidiaphragm due to a smaller acoustic window from the spleen and the need to position the probe more posteriorly. It is not necessary to record bilateral diaphragm function because adequate imaging of the right hemidiaphragm provides reliable information about global diaphragmatic function. However, the exception to this is when phrenic nerve injury or evidence of diaphragm palsy is suspected. In this situation, study of the contralateral side is of course warranted. If the lateral approach is unable to obtain adequate views, a sub-costal approach can be attempted and involves placing the probe under the costal margin in the mid-clavicular line, directed upwards and to the posterior portion of the diaphragm (*Fig. 27.4*). Normal DEX values during quiet tidal volume breathing in healthy volunteers are reported as 1.1–2.5cm in men and 1.0–2.2cm in women. In the critical care cohort, cut-off values of DEX during spontaneous breathing trials that may predict extubation failure are quoted as <1.1cm.

27.4.2 Quadriceps

In health, the quadriceps are frequently active and weight-bearing and therefore important in physical activity and locomotion. As a result, they are particularly prone to atrophy during illness (both acute and chronic) compared to other muscle groups. Rectus femoris (RF) muscle bulk has been shown to be lower in patients with chronic respiratory disease (such as COPD) and subsequently associated with poorer lung function, lower physical activity and more severe disease.

Ultrasound studies of ICUAW have largely focused on the quadriceps muscles. RF cross-sectional area (RF_{CSA}) (*Fig. 27.5*) is closely associated with muscle strength (as determined by concurrent volitional and non-volitional tests in both chronic disease and ICUAW). Studies in the ICU have shown that muscle mass declines quickly and a 10% decline in RF_{CSA} within 7 days is associated with a greater number of organ failures, longer mechanical ventilation and ICU length of stay and a higher incidence of post-critical care weakness and physical restriction. RF muscle bulk can be quantitatively measured by the anatomical cross-sectional area, muscle thickness (although this has repeatedly been shown to be less reliable) and/or muscle volume. Information about muscle structure and quality can also be gained through assessment of the pennation angle, fascicle length and echogenicity/echo intensity (see below), but here we focus on anatomical cross-sectional area only. Excellent review articles are available for further reading [10,11].

To image the RF, the patient should be positioned at 30° head up on a suitable bed/couch. The knee should be relaxed to avoid artificial contraction. The high-frequency linear probe is placed on the anterior thigh at a pre-determined point. The point is often taken as two-thirds the distance between the anterior superior iliac spine and the superior aspect of the patella (*Fig. 27.2*), however, three-fifths and half-way is also reported. The chosen point should be marked with a horizontal line and a generous amount of gel placed on top. Minimal compression techniques must be used to prevent distortion of the muscle area whilst balancing effects of the oedema which may distort the image. It is vital that the transducer is placed perpendicular to the point and that no angle is created in either plane, otherwise significant variation in the appearance of the muscle occurs. Visualization of the femur serves as a good reference point.

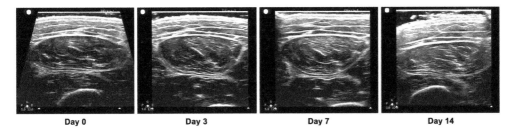

| Day 0 | Day 3 | Day 7 | Day 14 |

Figure 27.5. Rectus femoris ultrasound. High-frequency ultrasound (12MHz) of the rectus femoris from a 54-year-old male admitted with severe refractory respiratory failure requiring veno-venous extracorporeal membrane oxygenation therapy. Gain and depth settings are identical between images. Between day 0 and day 14 there is a 20% decline in RFCSA (517mm^2 to 414mm^2). Preservation of skin and muscle convexity as well as the visible layer of gel between skin and probe provides optimal image acquisition.

27.4.3 Parasternal muscle

Two distinct muscle fibre layers comprise the intercostal muscles (ICM). The outermost layer is the *external intercostal muscles* and these are active during inspiration, interacting with the diaphragm and accessory muscles to support inspiration. The inner muscle layer is the *internal intercostal muscles,* and their fibres run in an opposite direction to the external intercostal muscles. As a result, the lateral ICM has two layers comprising the ICM and a single layer in the ventral aspect. The thickest portion of the sole ventrally positioned internal intercostal muscles are often referred to as the *parasternal intercostals.*

The role of parasternal muscles in the context of ventilatory weaning and recovery is unknown but is gaining interest as an important susceptible muscle in ICUAW. The superficial location and level of activity during acute illness mean they serve as useful muscles to study in critical illness. The sonographic appearances and physiological assessment of this muscle group was well described by Cala *et al.* and the reader is advised to review its appearance and function in more detail there [12].

The measurement of muscle thickness and cross-sectional area as well as echogenicity may support other respiratory muscle tests in the diagnosis of ICUAW. The technique involves a high frequency linear probe placed longitudinally in the intercostal space (usually 2nd or 3rd) approximately 2–3cm laterally to the sternal edge (*Fig. 27.6*). The probe is kept perpendicular to the skin and a layer of gel and minimal pressure is applied. Video capture of multiple, complete respiratory cycles allows for maximal inspiratory and expiratory thickness measurements (either visually or using M-mode) as well as the cross-sectional area to be calculated (*Fig. 27.6*). The relationship between parasternal muscle activity during mechanical ventilation and ICU outcomes is currently not known. To enhance reproducibility, the upper and lower rib lines can be marked on the patient and a line 2–3cm lateral to the sternal edge should bisect these lines. The choice of parasternal muscle to image can vary. If the anatomical site is obscured (i.e. from wounds, dressings, etc.) then it is acceptable to image an intercostal space lower. Multiple parasternal muscles can be measured for comparison, but it is a necessity to compare data of the same muscle, because parasternal muscle contraction varies at different levels.

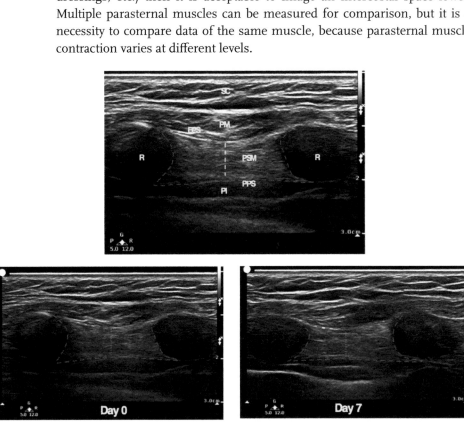

Figure 27.6. Parasternal muscle ultrasound. The high frequency probe is placed longitudinally in the 3rd intercostal space. The subcutaneous tissue (SC) lies superficially and above the pectoralis major (PM) muscle. The parasternal muscle (PSM) is a biconcave structure bound by the external parasternal surface (EPS) superficially, the pleural parasternal surface (PPS) inferiorly, and the ribs (R) bilaterally. The cross-sectional area (dashed red line) is the area bound by these four structures. The parasternal muscle thickness (vertical yellow dashed line) is from the centre of the PSM and from the inner EPS to the inner PPS. The pleura (Pl) is often the deepest structure seen. In this example in a 44-year-old man with severe acute respiratory distress syndrome, the PSM area on day 0 was 1.44cm²; on day 7 this reduced by 15% to 1.22cm². Similarly, the PSM thickness (vertical dotted line) was 5.4mm on day 0 and 4.8mm on day 7 (11% decline).

27.4.4 Echogenicity and basic qualitative assessment

Echogenicity relates to the differential acoustic impedance of tissue with ultrasound. It is a method of assessing muscle quality. Normal muscle has a low echogenicity due to low fibrous and fat content of the tissue. In critical illness, a change in echogenicity has been found to be strongly associated with the presence of quadriceps myofibre necrosis on histology and may offer a completely non-invasive tool to assess myonecrosis in critical illness alongside clinical assessment [13]. Echogenicity is commonly measured using grey scale analysis in most image software packages. Echogenicity values are machine dependent and vary with different depth, gain and frequency settings.

27.5 Protocol development suggestions

Musculoskeletal ultrasound in ICUAW is evolving; however, formal evidence-based guidelines are required. We suggest the following approach if the reader wishes to develop a protocol and utilize it in clinical studies. This advice assumes the reader has basic knowledge of ultrasound and understands functional aspects of the equipment required.

1. A working knowledge of the anatomy is essential, and the reader should invest adequate study time alongside practical sessions before any formal application.

2. Develop the protocol in healthy and patient cohorts before formal study to identify barriers to data collection, logistical aspects and projections of study time per patient.

3. Ensure continuous availability of the same machine and strict application of the protocol across machines.

4. Do not alter settings within the same (and ideally between) patients – this is to enhance intra-patient comparisons. However, gain and depth are highly likely to be different between patients due to body habitus and so this is often unavoidable.

5. Save all images to a secure drive immediately after image acquisition.

6. Analyze images using the same software package using a standard 'protocolized' method.

7. Record B-mode video when possible, for dynamic assessments offline.

8. Review images with an expert in the initial stages to ensure technique and data capture are correct.

9. Perform reliability testing, as detailed above, before and during formal studies to ensure continuation of reliability.

10. Use no more than two operators for a study, both of whom should have demonstrated knowledge and practical application in advance.

11. Disclose the methodology in full in all published work.

27.6 Summary

ICUAW is a common complication of critical illness, associated with significant morbidity and mortality. Early diagnosis is important but challenging. POCUS may provide a method for early identification of ICUAW, assessment of muscle wasting and ICU outcomes.

27.7 References

1. Herridge MS, Tansey CM, Matté A, *et al.* (2011) Functional disability 5 years after acute respiratory distress syndrome. *N Engl J Med*, 364:1293.

2. Goligher EC, Dres M, Fan E, *et al.* (2018) Mechanical ventilation-induced diaphragm atrophy strongly impacts clinical outcomes. *Am J Respir Crit Care Med*, 197:204.

3. Dres M, Goligher EC, Dubé B-P, *et al.* (2018) Diaphragm function and weaning from mechanical ventilation: an ultrasound and phrenic nerve stimulation clinical study. *Annals Intensive Care*, 8:53.

4. Sarwal A, Parry SM, Berry MJ, *et al.* (2015) Interobserver reliability of quantitative muscle sonographic analysis in the critically ill population. *J Ultrasound Med*, 34:1191.

5. Boussuges A, Gole Y, Blanc P (2009) Diaphragmatic motion studied by m-mode ultrasonography: methods, reproducibility, and normal values. *Chest*, 135:391.

6. Goligher EC, Laghi F, Detsky ME, *et al.* (2015) Measuring diaphragm thickness with ultrasound in mechanically ventilated patients: feasibility, reproducibility and validity. *Intensive Care Med*, 41:642.

7. Goligher EC, Fan E, Herridge MS, *et al.* (2015) Evolution of diaphragm thickness during mechanical ventilation: impact of inspiratory effort. *Am J Respir Crit Care Med*, 192:1080.

8. Walter SD, Eliasziw M, Donner A (1998) Sample size and optimal designs for reliability studies. *Stat Med*, 17:101.

9. Schepens T, Dres M, Heunks L, Goligher EC (2019) Diaphragm-protective mechanical ventilation. *Curr Opin Crit Care*, 25:77.

10. Mourtzakis M, Parry S, Connolly B, Puthucheary Z (2017) Skeletal muscle ultrasound in critical care: a tool in need of translation. *Ann Am Thorac Soc*, 14:1495.

11. Parry SM, Burtin C, Denehy L, Puthucheary ZA, Bear D (2019) Ultrasound evaluation of quadriceps muscle dysfunction in respiratory disease. *Cardiopulm Phys Ther J*, 30:15.

12. Cala SJ, Kenyon CM, Lee A, Watkin K, Macklem PT, Rochester DF (1998) Respiratory ultrasonography of human parasternal intercostal muscle in vivo. *Ultrasound Med Biol*, 24:313.

13. Puthucheary ZA, Phadke R, Rawal J, *et al.* (2015) Qualitative ultrasound in acute critical illness muscle wasting. *Crit Care Med*, 43:1603.

CHAPTER 28

ULTRASOUND EDUCATION IN CRITICAL CARE

Jonathan Aron & Sarah Morton

How do we teach or learn POCUS skills within the critical care setting? This is arguably the most important chapter in this book – the other chapters demonstrate the importance of POCUS and describe what we can achieve with an ultrasound probe in a critical care setting, but without guidance and learning this remains aspirational. Ultrasound education is beginning to be integrated into medical schools, although limitations exist because it is recognized to be resource intensive and require maintenance of skills; as such there is a gap which needs to be filled. These are also two of the main barriers we face as critical care clinicians, alongside the continual expectations of maintaining clinical practice whilst learning a new skill [1]. This chapter therefore aims to outline the current curriculum expectations, the accreditation processes available and the future of POCUS education.

28.1 The curriculum

The current (2021 onwards) intensive care curriculum from the Faculty of Intensive Care Medicine expects trainees to be able to:

- use ultrasound techniques for vascular localization

- understand the indications and limitations of ultrasound

- recognize patients who will benefit from ultrasound-guided chest drain placement

- know the basic principles of ultrasound and the Doppler effect [2].

Regarding echocardiography, it is expected that trainees will understand the indications and limitations of transthoracic (TTE) and transoesophageal echocardiography (TOE) in shocked patients. Whilst this does not enforce knowledge relating to POCUS, the expectation is that future curriculum reviews will further emphasize its importance. Increasingly there is an expectation at critical care consultant interviews that candidates will have some POCUS knowledge. This again highlights the need, and the increasing demand, for POCUS education.

The Royal College of Anaesthetists mention POCUS in various parts of the curriculum, including the specific advanced cardiothoracic knowledge and skills sections and within regional anaesthesia [3]. Within the specific advanced cardiothoracic skills section, it states that anaesthetists wanting to complete advanced cardiothoracic anaesthesia training should demonstrate "advanced skills in image acquisition and interpretation for perioperative trans-oesophageal echocardiography and basic transthoracic echocardiography skills". In both emergency medicine and acute medicine, it is expected that clinicians should be able to use and interpret findings of advanced adjuncts to basic examination including focused assessment with sonography for trauma (FAST) scans and echocardiography [4,5]. The emergency medicine curriculum also expects clinicians to be able to perform and interpret limited echocardiograms in the setting of non-shockable cardiac arrest rhythms, looking at detecting wall motion and treatable causes of pulseless electrical activity. For cardiology specifically, there is an echocardiography curriculum delivery tool which details the progression expected throughout speciality training. Interestingly, the guidelines for the provision of intensive care services issued by the Faculty of Intensive Care Medicine and Intensive Care Society in June 2019 state that "transthoracic echocardiography must be available at all times at the patient's bedside" and so the demand for echocardiography is likely to grow [6].

28.2 How do we teach POCUS?

Learning how to perform ultrasound in critical care is time-consuming and consists of four separate areas:

1. sonoanatomy and 'what is normal?'

2. pattern recognition for disease processes

3. practical skills that are required to obtain images

4. integrating POCUS into clinical decision making.

The teaching and learning required for each of these areas differs and what works for one area may not for another. For example, areas 1 and 2 can be taught to a certain extent with online material and e-resources. Area 3 is the most labour intensive, requiring courses and one-to-one tuition. It is also the area that requires the most time, something which is incredibly scarce and valued amongst learners and trainers alike. We must also recognize that each learner will vary; some will quickly obtain the skills needed to reliably obtain images, whereas others will take longer.

28.2.1 Gaining experience

Simulation is useful for obtaining practical skills, and the safest way to learn techniques such as TOE initially; studies suggest that this method of learning improves knowledge quickly and effectively in trainees with no prior experience [7]. Echocardiography simulators exist to facilitate the learning of both the technical obtaining of images and pattern recognition (because software exists to demonstrate pathologies). As supervised time is at a premium, POCUS students are encouraged to spend as much time as possible using electronic resources to build up their knowledge base, so that when clinical interactions are offered students can focus on building up their practical skills. It is, however, important to gain practical experience scanning patients. This should initially be with direct clinical supervision, moving towards indirect [8]. Unwell intensive care patients carry their own diverse challenges and techniques must be learnt to overcome them, including:

- worsening image quality seen with the use of high positive end-expiratory pressure during mechanical ventilation

- nursing turning schedules

- the movement of bedside equipment around the patient

- infection control considerations.

The cases that a trainee encounters must therefore be clinically relevant, and these situations factored into the feedback given by supervisors.

28.2.2 Ethical dilemmas

With practical experience of POCUS to improve learning there are ethical dilemmas to be considered:

- should we scan for the sake of learning alone?

- do we accept patient discomfort to develop a clinician's ultrasound skills?

- is there a suitable quality control and governance system in place to facilitate a trainee's learning?

- is the clinical data stored in a suitable manner according to local protocols?

- if trainees are obtaining images that they themselves cannot yet interpret, but which could potentially have clinical significance, is there a way of getting them reviewed in a timely manner?

Learning to scan within the limits of training is vital; many mistakes have been made by either interpreting suboptimal images or over-interpreting images beyond the scope of the focused nature of the scan (or indeed the scanner's competence). Trainees must be taught that a key element of using POCUS is understanding the limitations of their ability and not over-reaching this, because doing so may have a negative impact on patient care in the short term, and longer term may result in a loss of confidence in the service by end users. Resources are also scarce – do trainees have access to the appropriate equipment to facilitate learning? Are ultrasound machines used and stored in the correct way and is there education around the correct method of cleaning probes? These are all considerations that must be made by trainees, mentors, and the governance system in which they work.

28.2.3 Integrating findings into clinical decision making

Area 4 (integrating POCUS into clinical decision making) is probably the area which receives the least attention but is perhaps the most important aspect. It is rarely formally taught, although perhaps the European Diploma of Echocardiography (EDEC) comes closest. It is important that alongside the technical skills of obtaining images and recognizing diseases, clinicians can integrate this into their clinical care. The ability to integrate the findings of the ultrasound scan with the clinical pictures is also related to the relevant clinical experience of the individual (i.e. their seniority). This is perhaps why the EDEC qualifications ask for trainees in the UK to be post-membership exam and in Europe to have completed their speciality training. Also, it should be recognized that skills such as echocardiography are not simply used for diagnosis but can be used for dynamic assessments and monitoring of the patient, such as fluid status assessment. One approach has been to gradually step-up the learning throughout a course; for example, one advanced intensive care echo course showed improved confidence in image acquisition when delegates initially concentrated on performing a focused scan and then built up to obtaining more advanced views and identifying pathology; they then finished with more complex case-based discussions, incorporating images and clinical context. As technical skills progress, consideration of how to integrate POCUS into clinical practice is crucial to the benefit of our patients.

28.3 Courses, exams and accreditation

As we have described above, learning a new physical skill such as ultrasound normally requires one-to-one tuition. As such, a variety of courses exist to facilitate this, alongside which a variety of exams and qualifications can be targeted (*Table 28.1*). Clear guidance on what is expected of trainees does not yet exist and thus the choice can seem overwhelming, as can the cost and time commitment. Most of the introductory courses focus on the normal sonoanatomy and skills in obtaining images. From this starting point, the clinical decision making will then develop over time and becomes integrated into their training.

28.3.1 UK critical care ultrasound accreditations

One of the most well-known qualifications amongst the intensive care community is focused ultrasound for intensive care (FUSIC). Within the FUSIC accreditation system there are the following modules: heart

Table 28.1. Summary of critical care and transoesophageal echocardiography training pathways

Accreditation	Level of scan	Logbook	Written exam	Practical exam	Other requirements	Website link
FEEL	Basic	50 scans	No	No	1 day course	www.resus.org.uk/
FUSIC – Heart	Basic	50 scans	No	No	1 day course	www.ics.ac.uk/
BSE Level 1	Intermediate	75 scans	No	Yes	None	www.bsecho.org/
BSE ACCE	Advanced	250 scans[1]	Yes	Yes	None	As BSE Level 1
BSE TOE	Advanced	125 scans[2]	Yes	Yes	None	As BSE Level 1
EACVI TOE	Advanced	125 scans[3]	Yes	Yes	None	www.escardio.org/Sub-specialty-communities/European-Association-of-Cardiovascular-Imaging-(EACVI)
EDEC (TOE and TTE)	Advanced	100 TTE and 35 TOE	Yes	Yes	Recognized intensivist, course attendance	www.esicm.org/education/edec-2/
NBE Advanced PTE	Advanced	300 interpreted & 150 performed	Yes	No	1 year cardiothoracic anaesthetic fellowship	www.echoboards.org/
NBE CCE	Advanced	150 scans	Yes	No	1 year CC training dedicated to CCE or 750 hours CC experience	As NBE Advanced PTE
ANZCA	Goal directed (Basic)	40 scans	Yes[4]	No	None	www.anzca.edu.au/education-training
ANZCA	Comprehensive (Advanced)	200 scans	Yes[5]	No	None	As ANZCA Basic
CICM	Basic	30 scans	Yes	No	Attend CICM accredited course	www.cicm.org.au/Trainees/Training-Courses/Focused-Cardiac-Ultrasound
CICM	Advanced	450 scans – additional 50 TOE for combined accreditation	Yes[6]	No	None	As CICM Basic
CICM	Expert	No	No	No	7 years advanced CCE practice, education, training, or research experience	As CICM Basic

Reproduced from *J. Cardiothor. Vasc. Anesth.* 2021;35:235 with permission from Elsevier.
[1] = 125 scans if BSE or EACVI TTE/TOE accredited, [2] = 75 scans if BSE or EACVI TTE/TOE accredited, [3] = 75 scans if EACVI TTE certified, [4] = demonstrated by university post-graduate certificate, [5] = demonstrated by university post-graduate diploma, NS NBE, BSE or EACVI, [6] = demonstrated by completion of nationally or internationally recognized exit examination.
CC – critical care; CCE – critical care echocardiography; TTE – transthoracic echocardiography; TOE – transoesophageal echocardiography.

(previously called focused intensive care echocardiography (FICE)), focused TOE, haemodynamic assessment, lung, abdomen, vascular and neurological, amongst others. It is applicable for all clinicians, whether medical, nursing or allied healthcare professionals. The heart module is likely to require the longest time to complete (minimum of 50 logbook cases), but all modules must have their own logbooks. For each module there is a process to register with the Intensive Care Society, identify a mentor and supervisor, attend an approved course, complete a logbook (for a minimum number of cases) and have an assessment. A number of places offer the approved courses and these can be found by contacting the Intensive Care Society directly or via internet searches. Potential students are encouraged to look for courses that have the most 'hands-on' scanning time practice, to allow them to improve their practical skills in obtaining images in a safe environment, prior to scanning patients.

The British Society of Echocardiography (BSE) offers Level 1 accreditation for bedside echocardiographic assessment of acutely unwell patients, involving a face-to-face course followed by a logbook collecting 75 cases over 12 months and then an assessment. It is similar to the FUSIC heart course, but also incorporates the use of colour Doppler to assess some valvular pathologies and quantitative ventricular assessment. The BSE also offer the advanced critical care echocardiography (ACCE) accreditation. This is an advanced and detailed certification process, including a 250-case logbook (125 if the candidate is already certified in TOE), a written and a practical assessment. The amount of work required to obtain this often requires a dedicated echocardiography fellowship.

28.3.2 European critical care ultrasound accreditations

The EDEC, offered by the European Society of Intensive Care Medicine, is recognized as an in-depth training process over 2 years, incorporating both TTE and TOE, with a written and practical exam to be completed at the end. It is expected that before commencing the EDEC course the trainee should be at 'consultant' level, which within the UK system is likely to represent a senior registrar with suitable intensive care experience. This is to allow the integration of both the technical skills of obtaining the images and the clinical decision making.

Between FUSIC Heart or BSE Level 1 and ACCE or EDEC, there is currently no formal accreditation process. However, clinicians often want to learn more so they can integrate their technical skills into clinical decision making. Courses such as the ACCE course offered by the South London Intensive Care Echo Society are beginning to be developed across the country, with the expectation that those attending have basic echocardiography skills and a desire to learn more about haemodynamic assessment of the critically ill. It is hoped that this may be recognized further over the next few years.

28.3.3 Emergency medicine ultrasound accreditations

For emergency medicine, core (level 1) ultrasound courses cover FAST scans, abdominal aortic aneurysm (AAA) assessment, focused echocardiography in life support (ELS) and ultrasound-guided vascular access [9]. Above this you can go on to level 2 (advanced point-of-care) ultrasound courses, which include assessing for deep vein thrombosis as well as more echo and lung scanning. It is expected that before proceeding to level two ultrasound, the practitioner should have performed at a level one standard for at least 12 months and they will be able to perform 3–5 ultrasound examinations a week, as well as undertaking a logbook of practice as a level two practitioner.

The courses and accreditation described above are some of the better known ones in the UK, but others do exist. An alternative to face-to-face courses are online courses that can offer an initial insight into the physics of ultrasound and the views that can be obtained. Some online courses are free, for example, intensive care echo and basic ultrasound available through e-Learning for Healthcare, but others charge a fee. Whilst the choice of course can seem daunting, it is often worth asking colleagues for their own recommendations and experience.

28.4 Faculty and sustainability

As we have already described, one-to-one tuition is normally required to facilitate POCUS learning. As the number of courses increases, faculty too must be available at a sufficient standard. This is difficult to achieve and there is often a shortfall. Aside from faculty on the courses, mentors are also required for many of the accreditation processes described above and therefore time is a valuable resource. Unlike in other faculty-intensive courses, such as those for advanced life support which ensure future faculty meet the expected standards, within the POCUS setting there is currently no such process. This a barrier to POCUS education which will have to be overcome in the coming years.

With such diverse terminology, such as 'slide', 'rotate', 'tilt' and 'rock', it is important that all faculty start at the same place so that all trainees learn correctly from the beginning. Some courses have started to implement their own schemes, with, for example, the expectation that if you have qualified through one hospital you will come back to teach on courses or mentor future candidates. The South London Intensive Care Echo Society offer to mentor prospective faculty through their first teaching course and ensure individualized feedback is given at the end of the course. It is, however, mainly enthusiastic teachers that continue to drive the POCUS revolution [10].

We must also recognize that there is inequality across the country; POCUS enthusiasts often tend to congregate in the same place. As it is not yet mandatory in the Faculty of Intensive Care Medicine curriculum, there are hospitals where trainees will struggle to find the support required to undertake POCUS qualifications. Ultimately, as it currently stands, demand outweighs the educational opportunities available, something we hope will begin to change over the next few years.

28.5 Skill maintenance

As with any practical procedure, once a clinician feels they are competent (i.e. they have the required skills to perform the task), it is important to maintain those skills. The accreditation processes described previously should facilitate a clinician reaching a point of competence, often with a qualification to show for this. However, we must recognize our own limitations and seek expert assistance when we are not sure. As described above, it is a requirement of many of the accreditation processes that a logbook be maintained after accreditation, in a similar way to all revalidation processes for clinicians. Indeed, for level 2 practitioners of ultrasound for the Royal College of Emergency Medicine, if these logbooks or level of practice are not maintained they can only consider themselves a "level 1 practitioner by virtue of past experience". Providing teaching or mentoring is an additional way in which skill sets can be maintained. Quality control and governance at all stages of the POCUS process is crucial and maintaining POCUS skills falls under this.

28.6 Social media education

Social media platforms allow POCUS education to continue, as well as helping with disease pattern recognition. If you type 'YouTube POCUS' into Google more than 5 million hits are returned. The ability to upload videos and images for training is valuable. However, it can be difficult to ascertain the quality and accuracy of these videos and so care must be taken. Webinars and podcasts are additional online tools that can facilitate education. Many of the Royal Colleges and Societies have their own YouTube channels featuring videos relating to POCUS, and as such offer an assurance of quality; for example, the European Society of Intensive Care Medicine, Royal College of Emergency Medicine, the Intensive Care Society and the Royal Society of Medicine.

On Twitter, #POCUS and #FOAMus are common hashtags used to broadcast the wide range of images being obtained every day in clinical POCUS practice, so that clinicians can learn from each other's experience. There are a variety of (ever-changing) clinicians with extensive followers on Twitter because of the images and learning around POCUS they publish there. For rare conditions that you may never see in clinical practice these images can be invaluable. Although again there is the caveat around the lack of quality control on the information and images being uploaded.

28.7 The future

POCUS continues to grow and evolve. Echocardiography is no longer only the cardiologist's tool nor ultrasound the radiologist's. The continual development of technology will also help the expansion of POCUS, as smaller probes become more affordable and can therefore be used in more situations. It may be that in the future everyone has an ultrasound probe attached to their smartphone.

It is likely that POCUS will be incorporated more and more into medical school teaching, again as the technology becomes more affordable. It may be that students no longer buy a stethoscope when starting medical school but instead an ultrasound probe. Despite this, it is important to recognize that all ultrasound imaging must be interpreted within the clinical context and, however good the images obtained are, they are meaningless if clinicians do not know what to do with them.

For those of us who are practising now the expectation is likely to be that in specialities such as emergency medicine (including pre-hospital care), anaesthesia, acute medicine and intensive care, we must simply learn on the job. The expectations from the Royal Colleges, and the curriculum relating to these expectations, are likely to become clearer. This will take time and dedication but the potential benefit for our patients is immense.

28.8 References

1. Lane N, Lahham S, Joseph L, Bahner DP, Fox JC (2015) Ultrasound in medical education: listening to the echoes of the past to shape a vision for the future. *Eur J Trauma Emerg Surg*, 41:461.

2. The Faculty of Intensive Care Medicine. *ICM Curriculum*: www.ficm.ac.uk/trainingexamstrainingcurriculaandassessment/icm-curriculum [accessed 19 March 2022].

3. Royal College of Anaesthetists (2010) *CCT in Anaesthetics Annex E Advanced Level Training*, Edition 2 Version 1.8: www.rcoa.ac.uk/media/4606 [accessed 22 March 2022].

4. Joint Royal Colleges of Physicians Training Board. *Acute Internal Medicine*: www.jrcptb.org.uk/specialities/acute-medicine [accessed 22 March 2022].

5. Royal College of Emergency Medicine. *Curriculum*: https://rcem.ac.uk/curriculum/ [accessed 22 March 2022].

6. The Faculty of Intensive Care Medicine. *Guidelines for the Provision of Intensive Care Services*: www.ficm.ac.uk/standardssafetyguidelinesstandards/guidelines-for-the-provision-of-intensive-care-services [accessed 22 March 2022].

7. Sharma V, Chamos C, Valencia O, Meineri M, Fletcher SN (2013) The impact of internet and simulation-based training on transoesophageal echocardiography learning in anaesthetic trainees: a prospective randomised study. *Anaesthesia*, 68:621.

8. Blackstock AMS, Powell-Tuck J, Aron J (2018) Development of an ICU advanced echo course. ESICM Lives 2018; Paris, France2018. doi.org/10.1186/s40635-018-0201-6 - number 0481

9. Royal College of Emergency Medicine. *Curriculum Ultrasound*: https://rcem.ac.uk/curriculum-ultrasound/ [accessed 22 March 2022].

10. Morton SFR, Powell-Tuck J, Zilahi G, Aron J (2020) Future FICE Faculty: ensuring the standard of future faculty with a mentorship scheme. *Intensive Care Med Exp*, 8(2): 000008.

Index